# Recent Advances in Microneedle-Mediated Drug Delivery

# Recent Advances in Microneedle-Mediated Drug Delivery

Guest Editors

**Xin Pan**
**Guilan Quan**

MDPI

Basel • Beijing • Wuhan • Barcelona • Belgrade • Novi Sad • Cluj • Manchester

*Guest Editors*
Xin Pan
School of Pharmaceutical Sciences
Sun Yat-sen University
Guangzhou
China

Guilan Quan
College of Pharmacy
Jinan University
Guangzhou
China

*Editorial Office*
MDPI AG
Grosspeteranlage 5
4052 Basel, Switzerland

This is a reprint of the Special Issue, published open access by the journal *Pharmaceutics* (ISSN 1999-4923), freely accessible at: https://www.mdpi.com/journal/pharmaceutics/special_issues/recent_advances_in_mmdd.

For citation purposes, cite each article independently as indicated on the article page online and as indicated below:

Lastname, A.A.; Lastname, B.B. Article Title. *Journal Name* **Year**, *Volume Number*, Page Range.

**ISBN 978-3-7258-6712-7 (Hbk)**
**ISBN 978-3-7258-6713-4 (PDF)**
**https://doi.org/10.3390/books978-3-7258-6713-4**

# Contents

# About the Editors

**Xin Pan**

Xin Pan is a professor and PhD supervisor at the school of Pharmaceutical Sciences, Sun Yat-sen University. Dr. Pan obtained her bachelor's degree in pharmacy from Sun Yat-sen University in June 2006 and earned her doctoral degree in pharmaceutics from Sun Yat-sen University in June 2011. Dr. Pan was recognized for three consecutive years on Stanford University and Elsevier's 2025 Global Top 2% Scientists list, and was featured as a"Young Yangtze River Scholar"by the Ministry of Education and Pearl River Science and Technology Star Talent. As a key contributor, she received awards including the Second Prize of 2018 Guangdong Provincial Science and Technology Award, the First Prize of 2019 China Industry-University-Research Cooperation Innovation Achievement and the Second Prize of the 2020 China Invention & Entrepreneurship Award, etc. She personally obtained the China Biopharmaceutical Industry China Innovation Elite U45 Influential Youth Award and the Young Pharmaceutics Award of the China Pharmaceutical Formulation Conference. Dr. Pan has led more than ten scientific research projects, including the General Program of the National Natural Science Foundation of China, Guangdong Natural Science Foundation—Outstanding Youth Project, Sub-project of the National High-tech R&D Program of China (863 Program), etc. Her academic concurrent positions include Youth Member of the Drug Formulation Professional Committee of the Chinese Pharmaceutical Association, Deputy Director of the 11th Drug Formulation Professional Committee of the Guangdong Pharmaceutical Association, editorial board member of *Pharmaceutics*, youth editorial board member of the following: *Asian Journal of Pharmaceutical Science*, *Chinese Chemical Letters* and *Progress in Pharmaceutical Sciences*, etc.

**Guilan Quan**

Guilan Quan received her Ph.D. degree (2016) at Sun Yat-Sen University majoring in Pharmaceutics. She is currently a Professor and Ph.D. Supervisor of the College of Pharmacy, Jinan University, China. She was selected as a Young Talent in Science and Technology Innovation of Guangdong Province and was among the World's Top 2% Scientists (2024 and 2025). Her research interests focus on novel pharmaceutical technology, especially on dissolving microneedles for transdermal drug delivery. Dr. Quan has been responsible for more than 10 scientific research projects including three within the National Natural Science Foundation of China. She has published more than 60 scientific papers in renowned peer-reviewed journals with an H-index of 39, and holds 12 authorized patents, four of which have been commercialized. Dr. Quan has contributed to the publication of five books as an Editorial Board Member. She was awarded multiple honors including the Chinese Innovation and Entrepreneurship Award, the Chinese Cooperative Innovation Award, and the Guangdong Provincial Science and Technology Prize. Dr. Quan currently serves as Editorial Board Member of *Pharmaceutics*, and Early Career Board Member of the *Asian Journal of Pharmaceutical Sciences*, *Chinese Chemical Letters*, *Research*, and *View*.

*pharmaceutics*

MDPI

*Review*

# Recent Advancements in Microneedle Technology for Multifaceted Biomedical Applications

**Deepak Kulkarni [1,†], Fouad Damiri [2,†], Satish Rojekar [3,4,†], Mehrukh Zehravi [5], Sarker Ramproshad [6], Dipali Dhoke [7,†], Shubham Musale [8], Ashiya A. Mulani [8], Pranav Modak [8], Roshani Paradhi [8], Jyotsna Vitore [9], Md. Habibur Rahman [10,*], Mohammed Berrada [2], Prabhanjan S. Giram [8,11,*] and Simona Cavalu [12,*]**

1 Department of Pharmaceutics, Srinath College of Pharmacy, Bajajnagar, Aurangabad 431136, India; deepakkulkarni68@gmail.com
2 Laboratory of Biomolecules and Organic Synthesis (BIOSYNTHO), Department of Chemistry, Faculty of Sciences Ben M'Sick, University Hassan II of Casablanca, Casablanca 20000, Morocco; fouad.damiri@outlook.fr (F.D.); berrada_moh@hotmail.com (M.B.)
3 Department of Pharmaceutical Sciences and Technology, Institute of Chemical Technology, Mumbai 400019, India; rojekarsatish@gmail.com
4 Departments of Medicine and Pharmacological Sciences, Icahn School of Medicine at Mount Sinai, New York, NY 10029, USA
5 Department of Clinical Pharmacy Girls Section, Prince Sattam Bin Abdul Aziz University, Alkharj 11942, Saudi Arabia; mahrukh.zehravi@hotmail.com
6 Department of Pharmacy, Ranada Prasad Shaha University, Narayanganj 1400, Bangladesh; ramproshad131135@gmail.com
7 Department of Pharmaceutical Sciences, Rashtrasant Tukadoji Maharaj Nagpur University, Nagpur 440033, India; dipalidhoke7@gmail.com
8 Department of Pharmaceutics, Dr. DY Patil Institute of Pharmaceutical Sciences and Research, Pimpri, Pune 411018, India; shubhammusale1010@gmail.com (S.M.); ashiyaayubmulani@gmail.com (A.A.M.); pranavmodak0079@gmail.com (P.M.); roshanisparadhi@gmail.com (R.P.)
9 National Institute of Pharmaceutical Education and Research, Ahmedabad 160062, India; vitorejyotsna@gmail.com
10 Department of Global Medical Science, Wonju College of Medicine, Yonsei University, Wonju 26426, Korea
11 Department of Pharmaceutical Sciences, University at Buffalo, The State University of New York, Buffalo, NY 14260, USA
12 Faculty of Medicine and Pharmacy, University of Oradea, P-ta 1 Decembrie 10, 410087 Oradea, Romania
* Correspondence: pharmacisthabib@gmail.com (M.H.R.); prabhanjanpharma@gmail.com (P.S.G.); simona.cavalu@gmail.com (S.C.)
† These authors contributed equally to this work.

**Abstract:** Microneedle (MNs) technology is a recent advancement in biomedical science across the globe. The current limitations of drug delivery, like poor absorption, low bioavailability, inadequate skin permeation, and poor biodistribution, can be overcome by MN-based drug delivery. Nanotechnology made significant changes in fabrication techniques for microneedles (MNs) and design shifted from conventional to novel, using various types of natural and synthetic materials and their combinations. Nowadays, MNs technology has gained popularity worldwide in biomedical research and drug delivery technology due to its multifaceted and broad-spectrum applications. This review broadly discusses MN's types, fabrication methods, composition, characterization, applications, recent advancements, and global intellectual scenarios.

**Keywords:** MNs; drug delivery; nanoparticles; permeation; skin; transdermal

## 1. Introduction

Oral delivery is the most accepted route of administration for the treatment of disease, diagnosis, treatment, and the most widely studied topic by formulation scientists during the first and second generations of drug delivery. Oral drug delivery has the disadvantages of systemic metabolism, poor absorption, and a lack of tissue selectivity, leading to decreased therapeutic effects [1]. This necessitates the development of other dosage forms such as parenteral, transdermal, intravesical and other novel drug delivery systems. Ancient medicines for therapeutic effect applied on skin surface area, for various types of skin disease, wound healing activity, and cosmetic dermatological applications. However, the skin has an impermeable barrier for efficient and targeted delivery [2]. Scientists developed syringes and needles for local drug delivery applications to overcome this limitation. Although, these developed systems also have some disadvantages, such as poor patient compliance due to the pain in administration and the invasive nature that requires trained medical practitioners. Furthermore, with the advent of polymer science, nanotechnology, and applied engineering, the concept of MNs was introduced in the literature report [3].

MNs are micro projections ranging 25–2500 µm in height available in different shapes with the attachment of a base for support. MNs are used to sample fluid from the body and deliver therapeutic agents to cells [4]. MNs are tiny, unique, novel, and promising devices made using microelectromechanical systems to detect, diagnose, and treat several diseases. Vaccines, nanoparticles, high or low molecular weight drugs of various categories, high molecular weight protein, and antibodies are easily loaded into MNs to deliver it into different layers of skin and deep within the skin to neutrophil Langerhans, dendritic cells for immunological effect. MNs are classified into various classes depending upon their fabrication methods, such as solid, hollow, dissolving coated and hydrogel-forming MNs. The associated advantages and limitations vary with the type of MNs desired for the targeted site of action. MNs fabrication depends on the material used and the intended application [5]. For the design of MNs, various materials have been used, such as silicon, zeolite, glass, metals, polymers and sugars. MNs array density was developed using instant microfabrication techniques (prototyping), including hot embossing, micro-molding, lithography, deep reactive ion etching, thin film deposition, etc. [6,7]. One of the most important applications of MNs in vaccine delivery to the skin is patient compliance, high immunogenic nature of skin, vaccine targeting at desired skin site, and reliable vaccine delivery methods [8]. Numerous drugs, growth hormones, insulin, vaccines, DNA, and oligonucleotides are in the preclinical and clinical stages designed as MNs [5,9].

In this present article, we review various types of MNs, different materials used for fabrication, properties of the MNs, characterization of MNs for biological and mechanical properties, toxicity assessment of MNs with various in vivo and in vitro methods, application of MNs in several diseases, as well as the regulatory aspect, marketed product, and patent of the MNs.

## 2. Types and Fabrication of MNs

Several types of MNs are majorly categorized based on the fabrication method and applications of MNs [10,11]. Each type of MNs has its merit and pitfalls over others for drug delivery applications. MNs are classified based on their fabrication methods [12,13]. Figure 1 and Table 1 show the types of MNs.

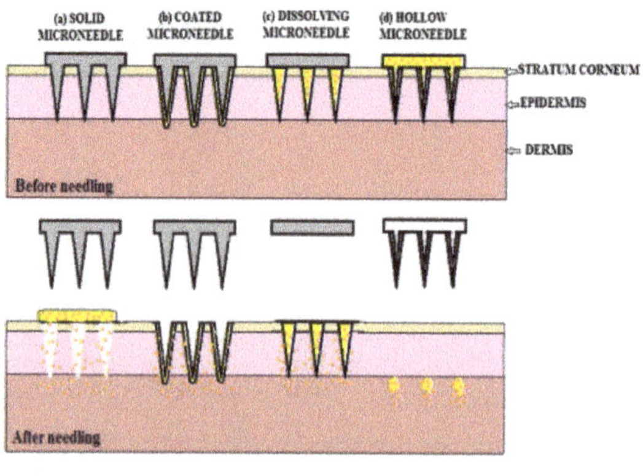


**Figure 1.** Types of MNs [14]. (Adapted from Ref. [14]).

### 2.1. Solid MNs

The drug delivery from solid MNs is based on the "poke-and-patch" approach. The drug delivery mechanism is the disruption of the stratum corneum and the creation of microchannels by the solid MNs. After the formation of microchannels, the drug patch is applied to the skin, through which the drug is efficiently diffused through the microchannels into the skin [12].

The solid MNs were used to transfer the drug through micronized channels formed inside the skin layer and improved drug diffusion [15,16]. In solid MNs, the drug is bound to the channel, and the microchannel is closed to prevent the entry of toxic materials by using termination therapy [17–19]. Solid MNs serve as reservoirs for drugs [20,21]. Non-biodegradable metals can be used to fabricate solid MNs. The fabrication is conducted by forming pointed tips at the end, which helps to make micronized pores on the epidermal surface of the skin [22,23]. Materials used to prepare solid MNs are biodegradable and non-biodegradable materials such as silicon, stainless steel, titanium, nickel with polymers methyl vinyl ether polymethylmethacrylate, maleic anhydride, polycarbonate, maltose, Poly(lactide), Poly(lactide-co-glycolide), etc., [24,25]—various parameters affecting solid MN's performance strip sharpness, insertion force, and density [26,27]. Solid MNs can be fabricated by microfabrication (micro-electromechanical system) and other methods such as using microreactors and micropumps [4,28].

### 2.2. Dissolving MNs

"Poke-and-release" is the drug delivery approach seen with dissolving MNs. In this approach, the drug is encapsulated within MNs. After insertion into the skin, these MNs are retained in the skin and not removed. The encapsulated drug is released when these MNs are degraded within the skin [26]. The dissolving MNs are not removed from the skin after the insertion as the biocompatible composition of natural, semisynthetic and synthetic biodegradable polymers such as poly (propylene), dextrin, chondroitin sulphate, polyvinylpyrrolidone (PVP) albumin, polylactic acid, poly (methyl vinyl ether-maleic anhydride) polyvinylpyrrolidone, polyglycolic acid, polylactic-co-glycolic acid, and poly (vinylpyrrolidone methacrylic acid) [4,29]. The advantage of this technology is the easy fabrication, high drug loading and convenient drug delivery.

Furthermore, these MNs do not leave any biologically harmful waste behind after dissolution, so the drug delivery is safe. The first research work on dissolving MNs and their utility were reported by Miyano et al. in 2015 as a pioneering study within this field [30,31]. The important step for the fabrication of dissolving MNs was the selection of the appropriate polymer, considering its effects on the release kinetics [32].

The literature has reported various examples regarding dissolving MNs for its synergistic drug delivery system and other techniques [32,33]. The application of the dissolving MN load cargo for delivery and improved permeation of MN array patches is clear for the vaccine delivery of influenza, adenovirus vector, etc. [34,35]. Various methods for preparing dissolving MNs include solvent casting, droplet-born air blowing, laser machining, hot embossing, microinjection molding, ultrasonic welding, and lithography [36]. The most frequently used method is the solvent casting method for the fabrication of dissolving MNs. In this method, the ultrasonic wedding fuses the polymer without heating [37]. The dissolving MNs were reported to show poor mechanical performance due to the high hygroscopicity nature [38].

### 2.3. Coated MNs

The drug delivery through the coated MNs is by a "coat-and-poke approach". In this approach, the drug coating is applied to the MNs, and then these MNs are inserted into the skin. The drug coating present on inserted MNs gets dissolved into the skin, and after the dissolution of the drug, the MNs are removed. The advantage of this approach is that it only requires one step and has simple delivery, while a disadvantage is that a much smaller amount of the drug is delivered by this technique [39]. Coated MNs surface completely covered with the drug enables sustained release. Coated MNs were successfully studied for DNA, gene, protein, and peptide delivery [40]. These non-invasive MNs comprise steel for siRNA [41]. Important parameters that need to be optimized in these MNs preparations are the homogenous coating, stability, the method used for MN coating (spraying or dip coating) and release from the MN [15]. Gill and Prausnitz et al. showed a reduction in the surface area and a high viscosity could improve the efficiency of these MNs for drug delivery [42]. In the case of the layer coating of MNs, it has been reported that MNs are immersed in oppositely charged solutions for effective coating. The coating of antifungals on MNs was reported using piezoelectric inkjet printing [43].

**Table 1.** Types of MNs [44]. (Adapted with permission from Ref. [44]. Copyright 2019 Elsevier).

| Sr. No. | Type of MNs | Material Used for Fabrication | Drug Delivery Approach | Benefits | Limitations |
|---|---|---|---|---|---|
| 1. | Solid | Silicon, stainless steel, acrylic | Poke and Patch | High mechanical strength | • Two-step process<br>• Poor patient compliance |
| 2. | Coated | Stainless steel, titanium, polymer | Coat and Poke | • Single step process | • Limited amount of drug can be coated on to the tip and shaft of MN |
| 3. | Dissolving/ Biodegradable | polyvinylpyrrolidone (PVP), carboxymethyl cellulose, sugar, dextran, polyvinyl alcohol (PVA), poly(lactic acid), chitosan, poly(glycolic acid), poly (lactide-co-glycolide) (PLGA) | Poke and Release | • Single step process<br>• Physical removal is not required<br>• Easy fabrication process<br>• Controlled drug delivery<br>• Better patient compliance<br>• Low cost | • Chances of polymer deposition in the skin with dissolving MNs.<br>• In the case of biodegradable MNs, high temperature is needed, which may affect payload |
| 4. | Hollow | Silicon, metal, glass, ceramic and polymers | Poke and Flow | • Large dose administration is possible<br>• Can be used for large molecular weight substances | • Chances of needle blockage<br>• Critical fabrication process<br>• Costly |
| 5. | Hydrogel forming | Chitosan, PVA, PLGA, poly(methyl vinyl ether-co-maleic acid) | Poke and Release | • Intact removal is possible from the skin<br>• Do not leave any polymer residue<br>• Less chances of infection | • Less mechanical strength<br>• Difficult to maintain the shape geometrically |

### 2.4. Hydrogel Forming MNs

Hydrogel forming MNs fabricated with cross-linking polymers. The drug release approach of hydrogel-forming MNs is "poke-and-release". The factors affecting MNs fabrication for solution parameters include a swelling index, molecular weight, and concentration of the foaming agent. This strategy was first established by Donnelly et al. for highly swellable polymers [45]. Iontophoresis, along with MN formation, enhances the efficiency of therapy [46]. The array does not contain a drug, but it imbibes through the skin layer during penetration.

This type of MNs can overcome the pitfalls of the conventional microarray technique by reducing drug loading capacity and modifying release [47]. These hydrogel-based MNs prefer sustained-release formulations [48].

## *2.5. Hollow MNs*

The drug delivery approach used in Hollow MN is the "poke-and-flow". The drug delivery from Hollow MNs is similar to the hypodermic injection. The micropump is generally used to execute them under pressure drug delivery into the skin. The advantage of hollow MN is the fast drug delivery as compared to other approaches as the drug delivery is pressure-driven. Another advantage of this technology is the painless and precisely controlled drug delivery into the skin [49]. The Hollow MNs are micron-sized hollow needles, unlike other MNs in length and diameter [50]. The usual size of the hollow MN is 30 gauge of the hypodermic needle of 300-micrometer length, and the materials mainly used in the fabrication are silicone, glass, ceramic and polymer, etc. [51]. It delivers drugs more promptly through the passive diffusion technique than the other types of MNs [52]. It is investigated that various parameters, including tip dimension, length, pressure, inner diameter, insertion and retraction of depth, affect the drug flow rate through hollow MNs [53]. Various techniques are available, such as MEMS techniques, deep reactive ion etching of silicon, deep X-ray photolithography, wet chemical etching, an integrated lithographic molding technique, and microfabrication to fabricate hollow MNs [54]. In the current era, hollow MNs are engaged in fabrication through the 3D printing method [55]. Figure 2 shows MNs drug delivery approaches.

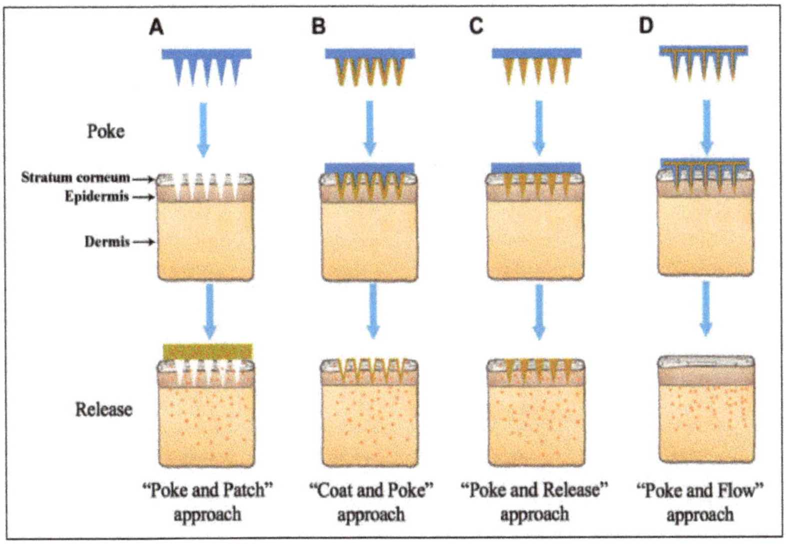


**Figure 2.** Diagrams showing various microneedle drug delivery approaches. (**A**) Solid microneedles, for skin pretreatment to create microchannels, followed by the application of transdermal patch; (**B**) coated microneedles, for deposition of drug formulations into the skin, followed by removal of microneedles; (**C**) dissolving microneedles, incorporated into the substrate of microneedles, remaining in the skin and dissolving over time to release the drugs; and (**D**) hollow microneedles, for inserted into the skin and continuous infusion of the drug through the created microchannels [56]. (Adapted from Ref. [56]).

## 3. Material Used for Fabrication of MNs

Various materials have fabricated MNs like silicon, zeolite, glass, metals, polymers, and sugars. After more continuous research, the fabrication complexity gets reduced and improves their mechanical strength, geometrical shapes, and sharpness of needles. MNs can be divided into two categories based on their fabrication material: biodegradable and non-biodegradable MNs. Table 2 shows the prototype material and its percentage used for MN fabrication.

**Table 2.** Material used for fabrication MNs.

| Material Used for MNs | Material Used in a Publication (in %) |
|---|---|
| Metal | 14 |
| Glass | 5 |
| Ceramic | 3 |
| Silicon | 10 |
| Polymer | 68 |

Silicon was the first fabrication material for MNs; author Henry et al. reported the first silicon MN in 1998. The specific reason behind silicon MNs fabrication is that silicon MNs were precise, 3D structures and widely used for target drug delivery. Still, there is a high risk of breaking the needle during insertion into the skin due to its brittleness [57].

The percentage of MNs was published in various materials. Based on hits for various keywords, percentages were determined. Best Match sorted search results at https://www.ncbi.nlm.nih.gov/pubmed accessed on 30 March 2022. Some of the keywords utilized are MNs of metal glass, ceramic, silicon, and polymer [58].

### 3.1. Metal Material

The initial metal utilized in the fabrication of MN arrays was stainless steel. Metal MNs are designed by physically pushing the smallest size of stainless steel hypodermic needles through a predetermined thickness supporting material or laser cutting metal sheets into MN forms and twisting them out of the plane [58]. This type of MNs is non-biodegradable and is more suitable than silicon as it avoids brittleness. Stainless steel, palladium, titanium, and nickel are common metals used to fabricate MNs [57]. Various methods used to fabricate metal MNs are laser micromachining [59], laser ablation [60] and photochemical etching. The stainless-steel MN was prepared by author Gill et al., who drafted MNs on Auto CAD for the required shape, and the orientation of array and then laser beam ablated onto the stainless-steel sheet to cut the MN, which are manually bent at 90° from the sheet [61]. The other method, lithographic masking, was used to fabricate titanium MNs by Choi et al. They prepared a row of five in one plane MN followed by a wet etching process [62]. The comparative study was performed for the in vitro transdermal permeation of atenolol in the porcine ear skin by the silicon, stainless-steel MN array or gold—titanium MN roller; the presence of atenolol analyzed the result at the receptor site by LC-MS, and the stainless-steel MN array has a greater transcutaneous flux than the other materials [63]. The advantages of metal material are toughness and its mechanical properties within the transdermal drug delivery system.

### 3.2. Polymers

Polymers are the most promising material for MNs fabrication compared to metals and inorganic materials. The polymeric material has been used to make solid, coated and hollow MNs [64]. The polymers are less expensive, biocompatible, and have viscoelasticity to improve resistance against shear-induced breakage. The compatibility and biodegradation ability of the polymers make them one of the prominent materials of choice in the fabrication of MNs. Polymers are mostly used to prepare dissolving and hydrogel-forming MNs, whereas the poke-and-release approach is used for drug delivery. Very few polymers used as a fabricating material are seen with solid coated and hollow MNs. The dip coating, inkjet printing, and spray drying are generally used to coat drugs and polymers on MNs. In the case of dissolving needles, high drug encapsulation can be achieved due to polymer degradation-based drug release. The use of biodegradable polymers can provide sustained release due to dissolution over a period [65].

The variety of polymers used for the fabrication of MNs are polylactide-co-glycolide acid (PLGA) [66], poly-L-lactic acid (PLA) [67], polycaprolactone (PCL) [68], poly-glycolic acid (PGA) [69], hyaluronic acids (HA) [70], polyvinyl pyrrolidone (PVP) [71], polyvinyl alcohol (PVA) [72], fibroin [73], sodium alginate [74], chitosan [75], carboxymethyl cellulose (CMC) [76] and more [64].

### 3.2.1. Biodegradable

The polymeric biodegradable MNs are made up of natural and synthetic polymers to improve drug delivery at the targeted site with a prolonged or sustainable release. The synthetic materials are mainly Polyglycolic acid (PGA), polylactic acid (PLA), polycarbonate and their copolymers (poly(lactic-co-glycolic acid) (PLGA), polycaprolactone (PCL), polystyrene (PS)), and silk, chitin, chitosan are natural biodegradable polymers used for the fabrication of MNs, which dissolves or degrades into the body by a metabolic process without producing any poisonous side effects [77]. Some other examples of natural biodegradable polysaccharides are amylopectin, dextrin, hydroxypropyl cellulose, carboxymethyl cellulose, alginate, chondroitin, and hyaluronic acid, which have been used as biodegradable MNs [58].

The fabrication of MNs using biodegradable polymers by a molding method is a novel approach that provides inexpensive and robust mass production. The polyglycolic acid (PGA), Poly-L-lactic acid (PLA) and their co-polymers polylactide-co-glycolide acid (PLGA), polycaprolactone (PCL) are used for the manufacture of biodegradable MNs as this polymer has biocompatibility, is mechanically robust, cost-effective, and resorbable. Eventually, biodegradable MNs break when poked into the skin, which has additional safety concerns as it degrades and is transported into the skin. Biodegradable polymers have minimal severe side effects. The drug can be encapsulated into MNs and then inserted into the dermal layer; as the polymer degrades or dissolves simultaneously, the drug gets released into the skin. This method does not produce any biological hazard like sharp tips waste. This polymer material can process at a low melting temperature, so the micro-molding technique is mostly used as, with these certain advantages, the polymer becomes a promising material for the fabrication of MNs. The downside with polymers is that most polymers are soft and induce catastrophic buckling during injection or blood sampling. The author Chu and Prausnitz et al. prepared the biodegradable polymer MN of an arrowhead sharp tip with the base of a metal shaft. This intellectual design fabrication requires complex processing and extra cost. Some carbohydrates are an excellent natural material resource for the fabrication of MNs as they are very effective, cheap and safe. Carbohydrates have significant biocompatibility and less toxicity and produce products with great strength. Carbohydrates are a good source of a biodegradable polymer as they show biocompatibility, are less costly and have good mechanical strength for insertion into the skin. This includes various sugars, maltose, sucrose, trehalose, mannitol, and galactose used for MN fabrication [30,78].

### 3.2.2. Non-Biodegradable

The non-biodegradable polymers are usually synthesized using living organisms in one way or another. They have been found in the xenobiotic class, which are originally synthetic, i.e., these compounds are chemicals and do not fall into a natural polymer. Not all xenobiotics are non-biodegradable; there are many examples of biodegradable xenobiotics. We cannot say that all-natural polymers are biodegradable; lignin is the amplest natural polymer material, but it degrades by selective micro-organisms at a very slow rate. The polythioester is a biopolymer obtained by recombinant E. coli bacterial strain fermentation and can produce large quantities [79]. There are also subsequent methods available like in vitro enzymatic synthesis, i.e., immobilization of lipase enzyme of Candida Antarctica in the attendance of Epsilon-caprolactone and 11-mercaptoundecanoic acid [80]. The polythioesters are non-biodegradable as these polymers cannot produce from simple organic carbon compounds (lipids, carbohydrates) and inorganic sources (sulphur, sulphates) but from precursor substrates. In 1951 the chemical synthesis pathway of polythioester was mentioned; recent studies revealed that due to the shortage of precursor substrates and their occurrence in very few natural habitats, other than the carbon sources, the yield of polythioesters is low and not scalable for commercializing purposes. The degradation of polythioesters occurred by extracellular enzymes, that is, the enzymes located at the cell surface. The degradation of polythioesters is restricted by the molecular weight and insolubility of polymer into the water, which reduces the entry of polymer into a cell or the periplasm (cell surface); this mechanism does not cause enzymatic degradation. Polyolefin is the example of a non-degradable polymer (polyethylene) as they are found in higher molecular weights, whereas the molecular weight lowers (Hexadecane) as they are degraded by many micro-organisms [81]. Polyphenols and polyisoprenoids are water-insoluble, poor biodegradable polymers that degrade at a low rate. Lignin is a cellulose material found abundantly, and sporopollenin degrades by only white-rot fungi or other particular fungi. Polyisoprenoids include natural rubbers (cis-1,4-isoprene) obtained from the Hevea brasiliensis rubber tree and can only be degraded by Gram-positive bacteria [82,83].

#### 3.2.3. Natural Polymers

Polymers have lower tensile strength than metal and silicon materials, but have a tough nature. Many naturally occurring polymers are used to prepare MNs, including polysaccharides, proteins, and synthetic and semisynthetic polymers. These polymers are mainly used to fabricate solid, dissolvable MNs and coat the other material [58].

Carbohydrates are an excellent natural material resource for MNs fabrication as they are very effective, cheap, and safe. Carbohydrates have significant biocompatibility and less toxicity and produce products with great strength [84]. By using the master plate method, carbohydrates can be molded into suitable MNs, low in cost and biodegradable. They can be mixed with active ingredients to produce active ingredients–carbohydrates mixtures and then molded; upon insertion, the drug–carbohydrate mixture gets dissolved into the skin [85]. Many sugars can be used to fabricate MNs like maltose, sucrose, mannitol, trehalose and galactose. Maltose is mainly used to prepare MN array as it is the FDA-approved excipient in the parenteral preparation. The author, Gouhua et al., studies the in vitro study on the transdermal delivery of monoclonal antibodies using maltose MN on the human IgG protein model. The cryosection MN was pierced into the skin after the methylene blue was taken out by the maltose MN. As the MN increases in length and arrays, the delivery of human IgG increases. The other materials like starch and gelatine can also be used as they dissolve into the skin within five minutes after insertion. They can insert into porcine skin up to a depth of 200 μm, similar to the depth of rat skin. The rat model was used to investigate hypoglycemic activity by MNs and shows the equivalent hypoglycemic activity with subcutaneous injection [30,86]. The material used to fabricate protein-based MNs is collagen and its derivatives, gelatine, zein and silk, which are assumed to deliver better high molecular weight protein-based drugs and vaccines into high-capacity drug loading MNs with improved stability. These proteins are becoming a good choice for fabrication as they are mostly inexpensive and easily fabricated using micro-molding [58].

### *3.3. Natural Polysaccharides for MNs*

Polysaccharides are primarily used in transdermal drug delivery due to their biocompatibility, biodegradability, cost, easy availability, ease of fabrication and sustainable delivery. They are obtained from natural sources such as plants, animals, microorganisms, etc. These include hyaluronic acid, dextran, Chitosan, and other biopolymers [87–89]:

(1) Hyaluronic acid MNs;
(2) Chondroitin sulphate MNs;
(3) Cellulose-based MNs;
(4) Chitin and chitosan MNs;
(5) Starch-based MNs.

#### 3.3.1. Hyaluronic Acid MNs

HA is a natural and major extracellular component of matrix and cartilage and possesses mucoadhesive properties [90]. It is widely present throughout the human body, including the dermis, synovial fluid, dental pulp, and vitreous humor in the form of non-sulfated glycosaminoglycan. It bears a negative charge and is present in water-soluble salt form. It is reported in several lengths ranging from 200, 300 and 800 μm. HA MNs are highly dissolvable in water; that serves many benefits in terms of fabrication, including high drug loading and improved economic benefits.

Jinjin Zhu et al. studied 5-Aminolevulinic acid-loaded HA MNs for the effective pharmacodynamics therapy for the penetration of superficial tumors that showed long-term stability and deep penetration [91]. Hyaluronic acid is used as part of a combination therapy of gene and phototherapy for immunochemotherapy. The combination of p53 DNA and IR820 is readily incorporated into the HA MN patch for effective delivery [92]. Ying Hao et al. fabricated HA-based MNs to treat epidermal cancer and melanoma. MNs showed controlled release of the incorporated drug [93]. Hongyao et al. fabricated HA-based MNs to treat psoriasis and improve solubility and mechanical properties. The FDA-approved product is Microhyala, which dissolves in intestinal fluid, with degradation observed by lysosomal enzymes. Saha et al. showed the application of the HA MN array in the cosmetics and medical field [70]. A few methods used to fabricate MNs are micromolding, photopolymerization, and drawing lithography [94].

#### 3.3.2. Chondroitin Sulphate MNs

It is a natural polysaccharide compound used in the form of sodium chondroitin sulfate. It possesses certain potential features such as superior hydrophilicity and biodegradability, and hence it is used in the fabrication of dissolving MNs. It is present as the necessary component in the extracellular matrix and cartilage in the body. Fukushima et al. have developed desmopressin and rhGH-loaded sodium chondroitin sulfate and dextran MNs, which showed dose-dependent concentration [95]. In addition to this, Poirier et al. fabricated an MN array by using CS and hydroxyethyl starch. The Prepared MN array loaded hepatitis B surface antigen and QS-21 saponin as an adjuvant. A stability study suggested that at 37°, antigenicity was retained after a six month time duration, and 10% loss was observed at 50 °C [96].

#### 3.3.3. Cellulose-Based MNs

Cellulose is a natural biomaterial obtained from various sources such as wood, cotton, bacteria, and algae. It contains a beta (1,4) linkage of glucose monomers. Cellulose was reported for biomedical application. Cellulose nitrate is a film former in cosmetics [97]. The application of cellulose-based MNs has been patented in the treatment of cancer therapy [98] (US20160136407A1).

In addition, some scientists at the University of Pittsburgh and Carnegie Mellon University studied carboxymethyl cellulose (CMC) MNs for incorporating various chemotherapeutic agents and immune-stimulating agents for skin cancer [99]. These MNs have been patented for gene delivery and anti-cancer drug delivery [100]. Yong-Hun Park et al. demonstrated cellulose-based MNs fabrication by using laser writing and replica molding for transdermal drug delivery. The fabricated MNs observed a three-fold enhancement in permeability, and thus, it was considered an efficient fabrication process for even cosmetic products. Dissolvable hyaluronic acid (HA) and bacterial nanocellulose (BC) MNs have been used for dermo-cosmetic application. It was observed that an HA and BC blend provides sufficient mechanical strength to the MNs, and BC promotes the controlled release of drug molecules. The safety profile of this MN has been proven by in vivo studies [101].

3.3.4. Chitin and Chitosan MNs

Chitosan is a polysaccharide prepared by deacetylation from chitin. Its linear structure of β-(1,4) linkage contains D-glucosamine and N-acetyl-D-glucosamine units. It is water-insoluble and has a molecular weight of this polymer in the range of 300 and 1000 kDa. The lower molecular weight corresponds to poor mechanical strength, and this bottleneck can be overcome by blending it with PLGA [102]. However, Chitosan shows antibacterial and wound healing properties naturally [103]. Micro-molding and electrospraying techniques were combined to fabricate these MNs to deliver doxorubicin and AuMSS nanorods. It was observed that Dox@MicroN patches showed good photothermal capacity upon increased temperature by 12 °C under near-infrared irradiation. However, these MNs have penetrated through a tumor-mimicking agarose gel and promote a layer-dependent drug release [104]. However, with the addition of the thiol group, the mechanical property has been improved, and hence thiolated MNs possess sharpness and good mechanical strength [105]. Mei-Chin Chen et al. studied bovine serum albumin-loaded chitosan-based MN for transdermal application. The prepared MN showed 95% in vitro drug release within eight days and a penetration depth of 300 μm [106].

3.3.5. Starch-Based MN

Starch is a versatile biomaterial and has been explored in various applications in the biomedical field. It provides brittleness and is applicable for various topical purposes. There are numerous reports on starch-based MNs, such as that by Yujie Zhang et al., who fabricated dissolving glucose-responsive insulin-releasing MN patches for diabetes. Starch improved the mechanical strength of MNs [107]. The starch and gelatin combination used for the fabrication of MN-loaded losartan was studied as proof of concept for transdermal applications [108].

## 4. Techniques of Preparation of MNs (MNs)

Investigators have used various methods over the past few years to manufacture a wide variety of MNs. The applications of the MN are considered first while designing an MN, which includes the type of drug, its dose, desirable pharmacokinetics/pharmacodynamics, and the targets and properties of the material used for MN [109]. Achieving the uniformity and reproducibility of the needle geometry at micron-scale resolution is the main goal in the fabrication of MN to facilitate easy penetration of the needles in the skin. However, mostly as a result of the conical three-dimensional (3D) geometry and higher aspect ratio of the MNs structures, the fabrication of MNs is very challenging. The most optimized MN design and materials are considered for the fabrication of the MN. Depending on the design (various sizes and shapes), different types (solid, hollow, coated, dissolving, sharp, or flat) and different materials (silicon, metal, polymer, glass, ceramic), the manufacturing method for MNs varies [110].

MNs are fabricated in various ways for different applications [6]. The two basic and primary designs of MNs are in-plane, out-of-plane, and an amalgamation of both MNs. The in-plane MNs are the simple and precisely controlled fabrication method with different lengths in the fabrication process. In the case of out-of-plane designs, the MNs are perpendicular to the fabrication surfaces [111]. Sivamani et al. are at ease generating arrays that are in-plane [112–114]. Figure 3 SEM images of MNs for out-of-plane and combined in-plane.

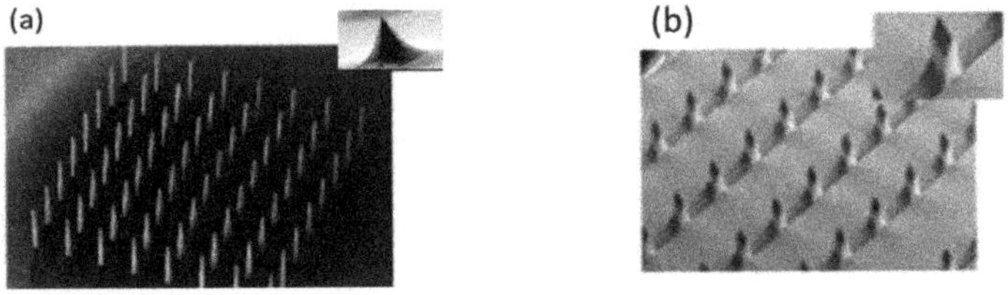


**Figure 3.** Scanning electron microscope (SEM) images of (**a**) out-of-plane MNs Source [115] (Adapted from Ref. [115]). (**b**) combined in-plane and out-of-plane MNs [116]. (Adapted with permission from Ref. [116]. Copyright 2008 Elsevier).

### 4.1. Microfabrication Basics

Microfabrication technology (micro-machining or micro-electromechanical) systems (MEMS) is the most encouraging method used for MNs fabrication and precise application [117]. MEMS technique exploits various tools and methods to produce smaller 3D structures with the dimensions (sub-centimeter to sub-micrometer). MN production through the MEMS technique is vastly specific and consists of multifaceted multi-step processes [118]. MEMS techniques have been potentially utilized in the biomedical fields, i.e., DNA sequencing devices, drug delivery, chemical analysis systems and biosensors [113]. A series of consecutive processes are required before the actual device is generated in the MEMS process. The three primary techniques in the MEMS technology include: (i) thin film of material deposition on a substrate; (ii) application of the patterned mask on the top of a film by photolithographic imaging; and (iii) selective etching of the films for masking [119,120].

### 4.2. Thin Film Deposition

Thin-film deposition leads to the addition of the material in the thin-film layer over the substrates. These thin layers could act as spacers with a few nm thicknesses to 700 μm [121]. Thin-film deposition occurs in two types, subject to whether the process is mainly chemical vapor deposition or physical vapor deposition (PVD) [122]. In the PVD process, the raw materials, i.e., solid, liquid or vapor, are freed and transferred directly from source to material to be coated and the substrate through the gas phase, e.g., thermal evaporation, ion plating and sputtering. In thermal evaporation, the source (e.g., aluminum) is heated by a radiofrequency or electron beam and the silicon wafer is located inside a vacuum chamber. A source boils on heating, and vapors are condensed on the substrate surface to form a film. In the sputtering technique, high-energy particle bombardment atoms or molecules are expelled from the target material. The expelled atoms or molecules could condense on the substrate, such as a thin film [123]. In ion plating, the material used for coating is ionized and vaporized with the assistance of an electric arc and then forced toward the target at high speed [124]. A thin film is formed in the CVD process by a thermally induced chemically driven reaction among the inert-carrier gases in a chamber and hot substrate. This flexible method works at atmospheric pressure at moderately lower temperatures [125,126]. The two most common CVD technologies in MEMS are the LPCVD (Low-pressure CVD) and PECVD (Plasma-enhanced CVD). The LPCVD could allow uniform deposition of many thin-film materials on substrates without damaging effects on film homogeneity at higher temperatures, >600 °C. Conversely, PECVD functions at low temperatures (200 to 400 °C) due to thermal cycle concerns or material limitations, but the films grow faster [127]. In conclusion, a specific deposition process depends on several factors, e.g., source, substrate structure, apparatus, working temperature, deposition rate, and production time. Afterward, the thin layer deposition is decorated using photolithographic techniques and then etched away to create the final structure [119,120].

### 4.3. Photolithography

Most of the developments in microelectronics and micromachining fabrication start with lithography. The different types of lithography include ion beam lithography, photolithography, X-ray lithography and electron beam lithography. The maximum widely utilized type of lithography is photolithography [128]. Photolithography is used to decoratively create dissolving, hydrogel, solid, and hollow MNs. This method is also used to manufacture silicon MNs and polymer MNs by making an inverse mold based on MNs structure [14]. This technique transfers copies of a master design on the substrate surface of some material, e.g., a silicon wafer. For this purpose, a thin layer of oxide is developed onto the surface of the silicon wafer by heating it at 9000–11,500 °C in the occurrence of steam or humidified oxygen steam. This is followed by the deposition of a thin layer of a photoresist organic polymer, sensitive to ultraviolet radiation on the silicon wafer's oxide surface (Figure 4a). A spin coating process carries out this deposition (spun, 1500 and 8000 rpm) to produce a photoresist of a well-defined thickness (Figure 4a) [129]. The solvent in the resist layer is taken out through heating at 750 and 100.80 °C for 10 min after the spin coating step. Along with solvent evaporation, this process indorses devotion of the photoresist layer to the silicon wafer. When the solvent is taken out, a glass plate (transparent) coated chromium pattern (opaque) and a photomask are positioned to contact the photoresist-coated surface [130]. The silicon wafer is exposed to UV radiation (150 and 500 nm), shifting the photomask's design to the photoresist-coated wafers (Figure 4c). The radiation treatment stimulates a chemical reaction in exposed sections of the photoresist, which are of two types; negative and positive (Figure 5). The solubility of the exposed photoresist is altered after this reaction. Afterward, in the course of the development processes, this resistant region could be dissolved by a rinsing solution that removes either the exposed areas or the unexposed areas of the photoresist, either by wet (solvent) or dry (plasma or plasma or dry vapor phase) techniques [131]. Thus, it leaves a design of photoresist-coated and straightforward oxides on the wafer surface (Figure 4d). Subsequently, unwanted photoresist left after the advancement process is detached by the de-scumming-induced oxygen-plasma treatment called de-scumming [110]. The final oxide design (positive or negative) is then a photomask pattern used as a mask in subsequent processing steps (Figure 4f) [132]. In the MEMS method, the oxide is utilized as successive masking to form either a new layer on which further layers are to be built, or further etching to form deep 3D holes, subsequent in a complete 3D structure or device [120].

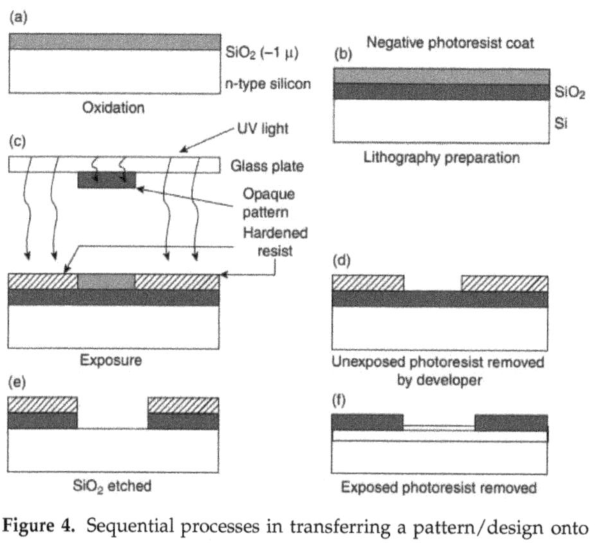


**Figure 4.** Sequential processes in transferring a pattern/design onto the substrate surface [114]. (Adapted with permission from Ref. [114]. Copyright 2013 Elsevier).

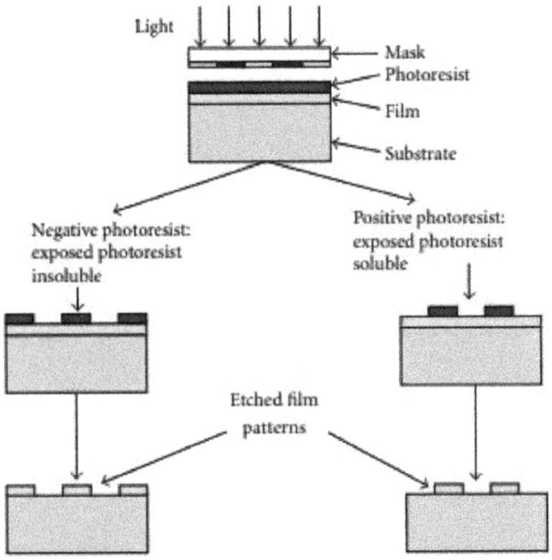


**Figure 5.** Positive and negative photoresist [133]. (Adapted from from Ref. [133]).

### 4.4. Etching

Etching is an important process to fabricate the final and optimized functional type of MEMS structure onto the substrate after lithography. This technique creates a design on a substrate surface by incising the thin films (unprotected parts) previously deposited/placed on a substrate and/or removing layers of the substrate itself by using strong acid or a physical process. It is mainly carried out after the photolithography process, through which a uniform layer of photoresist is deposited over the substrate and patterned for fabricating the etching pattern [4]. Any photoresist layer or a film resistant to the etching process can be used as the masking material, e.g., silicon dioxide, silicon nitride, and metal films. Etching is also used to determine the tapered shape of MNs tip, the size of MNs base and gap among the MNs before the etching process and the length and shape of the MN after the etching process [134]. Multiple applications use etching, including silicon micromachining [135], fabrication through nanoscale etching [136], IC fabrication [137], biosensors [138], accelerometers [139], phosphoric acid etching of the human enamel for enhancing resin adhesion for dental applications [140], PDMS [141] and the development of microfluidic devices via the etching of Parylene [142,143]. The critical parameters of an etching process are structuring with high resolution, cutting direction of the etchant and higher aspect ratios. In general, the etching processes are dry etching and wet etching, subject to the physical state of the etchant [4].

#### 4.4.1. Wet Etching

Wet etching is a patterning method. The material (typically a silicon wafer) or metal is removed/etched by submerging in a liquid bath containing a chemical solution or etchant [144]. In this process, the film designed/patterned by etching is covered by another layer of pattern that is resistant to an etchant (Figure 6A,B). The layer to be patterned is the metal film, and the masking layer is often a designed/patterned photoresist film [145]. The etchants used for wet etching are classified into isotropic and anisotropic (Figure 7).

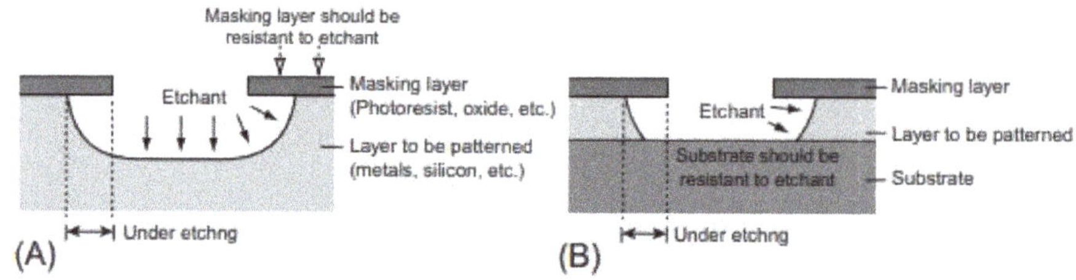


**Figure 6.** Wet etching (side view). (**A**) indicates a case where a substrate or a thick material is being etched, and (**B**) shows a case where a thin film deposited on a substrate is patterned [134]. (Adapted with permission from Ref. [134]. Copyright 2014 Elsevier).

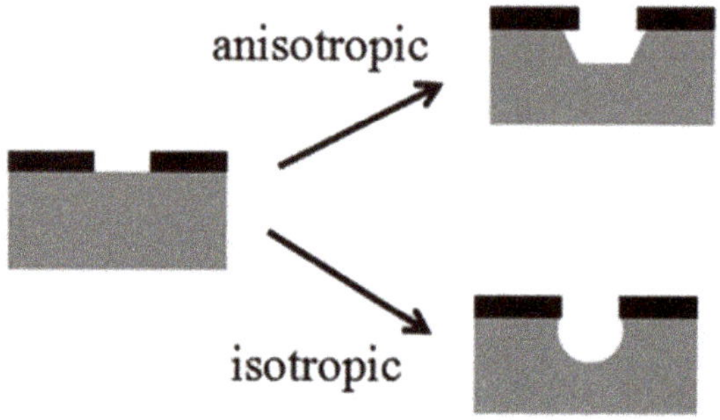


**Figure 7.** Etching profiles generated with [146] isotropic and anisotropic etching. (Adapted from Ref. [146]).

The isotropic etchants engrave the material, such as oxide, aluminum, nitride, polysilicon gold and silicon, at the same rate in all directions. Hence, they take off material horizontally under the etch mask at the same rate as they etch through it. For instance, a thin oxide film on a silicon wafer is etched with isotropic etchants (hydrofluoric acid) that etch the oxide quicker than the underlying silicon, as shown in Figure 8. In amalgamating with water or methanol, isotropic etchants such as hydrofluoric acid, phosphoric acid, and nitric acid could be used [147].

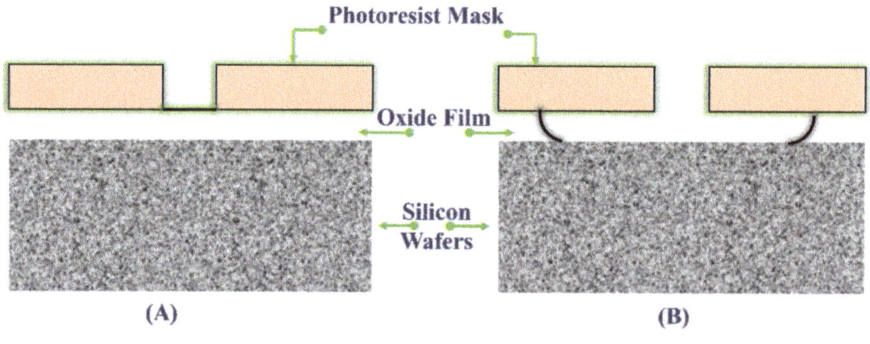


**Figure 8.** (**A**) Oxide film onto the silicon wafer with established photoresist mask, (**B**) after prolonged wet etching; the etch has developed under the mask (not to scale) [120]. (Reprinted from Ref. [120]).

Rounded side wall microchannels are produced by isotropic wet chemical etching. The application of titanium as a receding mask through the wet etching process leads to adjusting the shape and angle of the sidewall of the microchannels (Figure 9). The etch rate and etch duration control the channel's depth, while mask opening to twice the channel depth estimates the width of the channel. A thick layer of negative photoresists (i.e., SU-8) may be a simple, low cost and suitable masking material in case of some shallow etches.

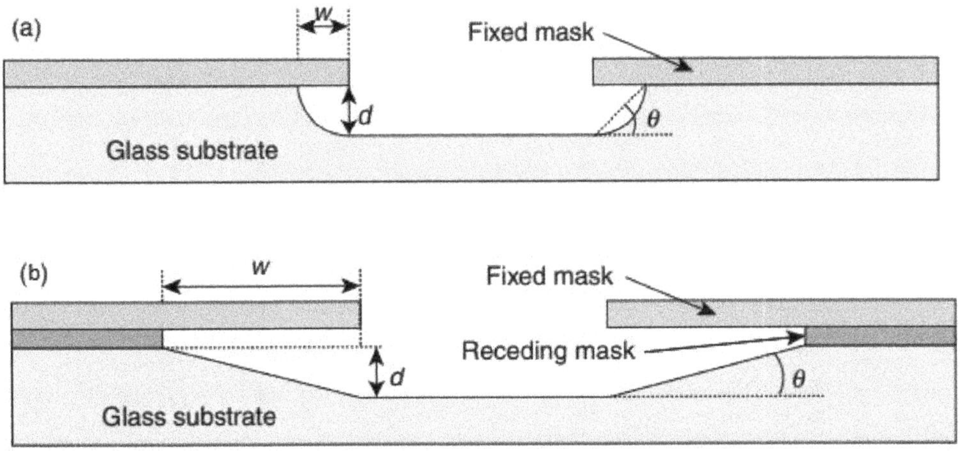


**Figure 9.** Schematic illustration of etching of glass by (**a**) Si passive etch mask, and (**b**) Schematic representation of etching of glass with a bilayer mask made of a fixed mask and a receding mask [148]. (Adapted with permission from Ref. [148]. Copyright 2013 Elsevier).

During the wet etching isotropic process, if the etching time is prolonged or when the etchant is the strong base solution, the photoresist could not offer enough protection and easily get damaged. For example, the photoresist layers are effortlessly etched in a wet etching of silicon where potassium hydroxide (KOH) or tetramethylammonium hydroxide (TMAH) is utilized. Hence, they have not functioned as the masking layer. In such a case, a multistep etching process is employed where the silicon dioxide is designed through a photoresist as the masking layer and HF as the etchant. As a result, silicon dioxide is the vastly resistant mask to KOH or TMAH, and the silicon layer is then etched [149].

HF is employed as the main etchant for all types of silicate glass. The chemical reaction for etching is shown below:

$$SiO_2 + 6HF \rightarrow H_2SiF_6 + 2H_2O$$

It is usually used to etch the oxides, and in strong concentrations, it speedily strips oxides [150]. Buffering with ammonium fluoride is known as buffered HF (BHF), or buffered oxide etch (BOE), which is used to pattern oxides. As a result of the buffering of HF, its etch rate is more precise and controlled, and it could not peel photoresist as it is more concentrated than HF [151]. In mixtures with other compounds, phosphoric acid is utilized to etch either nitride or aluminum substrate, where oxide is used as the mask [152]. Gold is typically etched with an iodine-based solution [153]. Noble metals are etched by aqua regia, a mixture of hydrochloric and nitric acids (3:1) [154].

Anisotropic etchants attack the material at diverse rates in different directions, so they are faster in a favored direction at producing more controlled shapes [121,155]. The most common anisotropic etchants are potassium hydroxide (KOH), tetramethylammonium hydroxide (TMAH), ethylenediamine (EDP) and hydrazine [156]. The crystal orientation of the substrate or wafer decides the structures formed in the substrate.

Depending upon the exposure of the crystal faces of a few crystalline materials, they remain etched at diverse rates. Silicon is a single-crystal material having different crystal planes that allows very high anisotropic etching at different rates. KOH or TMAH is regularly used as an anisotropic etchant. Using KOH, the anisotropic etching of silicon wafers results in the most common crystal orientation (100). The etch rate of a 30% KOH solution in <100> directions is 0.8 μm/min, which is >150 times higher than the <111> directions [157], while the (100)/(111) etch ratio of TMAH is approximately [158] 10–50. Oxide and nitride both etch gradually in KOH. Silicon dioxide could be employed as an etch mask for short periods to form narrow grooves and pits; however, KOH etches silicon dioxide a few nm/min, which is considerable for some applications. For longer periods and deeper etching (>100 μm), silicon nitrides are an enhanced etch mask as it etches more gradually in the KOH. TMAH has good etching discernment between silicon dioxide and silicon [159]. On the requirement of a deep etching with a thickness of a silicon wafer (500 μm), a thermally developed oxide layer could be used as a mask.

The amount of boron in silicon affects its rate of etching. An increased amount of boron in silicon reduces the etching rate in KOH by a greater extent and further stops the etching of the boron-rich silicon, called as concentration-dependent etching method [160]. The diffusion method is used to introduce the boron impurities in silicon. A silicon oxide mask is introduced on the surface of the silicon wafer. It is designed such that the surface of the silicon wafer is exposed for the introduction of boron (Figure 10A). The silicon wafer is now positioned in a furnace in connection with a boron-diffusion source; nevertheless, it is required to retain the time in the furnace as small as possible. The boron atoms transfer to the silicon wafer for 15 to 20 h. After the boron diffusion is finished, the oxide mask is stripped off (Figure 10B). A second mask is deposited and designed over the silicon wafer before immersing it in a KOH etch bath (Figure 10C). The KOH etches around the boron-doped silicon and the silicon, which is not sheltered by the mask (Figure 10D).

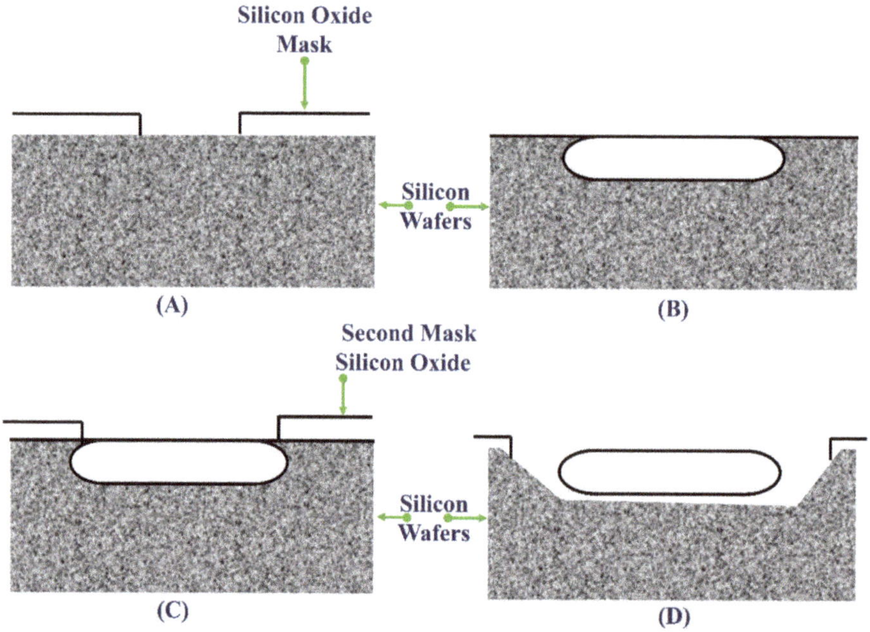


**Figure 10.** Concentration-dependent etching methodology: (**A**) mask for the boron diffusion, (**B**) oxide mask stripped succeeding diffusion, (**C**) mask for the KOH etching, (**D**) boron-doped structure expelled by the KOH etching [120]. (Reprinted from Ref. [120]).

A typical anisotropic etching process with a (100) silicon wafer is shown in Figure 11 A. Anisotropic etching on a silicon wafer continues in the <100> direction and is directed by the (111) surface on all four sides. The (100) surface will shrink as the four (111) surfaces meet at the apex of the inverse pyramid structure during the etching process. Etching in <111> direction is remarkably slower and is detected as an undercut. The shape of the etched cavity could be roughly assessed by considering the angle between a (100) surface and a (111) surface, which is 54.7° (Figure 11B). The etching of a (110) wafer is further complex than that of a (100) wafer (Figure 11C). Several studies have been carried out to examine overall cases of anisotropic silicon etching [161–163]. Good predictions for shapes of etched wafers can be found using numerical analysis [164–166].

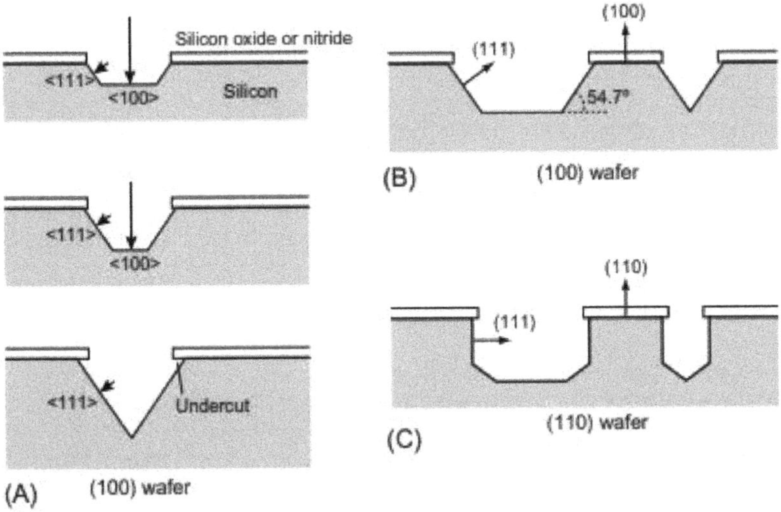


**Figure 11.** The anisotropic silicon wet etching (side view). (**A**) Etching in the <100> direction is much faster than in the <111>direction. (**B**) An angle of 54.7° is observed between (100) and (111) surfaces. (**C**) Vertical walls are created with (110) wafers [134]. (Reprinted with permission from Ref. [134]. Copyright 2014 Elsevier).

Wet etching is used to produce silicon MN, metallic MN and hollow MN arrays of a sharp tip [155]. However, the crystal planes in silicon limit anisotropic wet etching [167]. The etching rate in wet etching is considerably faster than in dry etching.

#### 4.4.2. Dry Etching

Dry etching, or plasma etching, is the etching process in which an accelerating motion of an ion species to the substrate combined with a masking process is used to physically or chemically etch the target materials. This form of etching is carried out at little pressure using inert or reactive gases. The most commonly used dry etchants are hydrogen fluoride [168], fluorocarbons [169], xenon difluoride [170], oxygen [171] and boron trichloride [172]. Dry etching is considered a huge scale integration (VLSI) process as it could be more exactly controlled by regulating parameters like gas pressure, temperature and electric field distribution. Dry etching is a method classified into two types: reactive ion etching (RIE), which involves chemical processes and ion-beam milling, which involves purely physical processes [25]. Depending on the pressure in the plasma chamber and the electric field that provides direction to the ionic species in the plasma, this process can be either isotropic or anisotropic [173]. Dry etching methods were used for patterning metals such as Aluminum [174], Copper [175] and Titanium [176], organic materials [177], Polymers such as PDMS [178], Parylene [179], PMMA [180], Polycarbonate [181], Polyimide, [182] and SU-8 [183], silicon and silicon dioxide [184], silicon nitride [185] and, Glass [186].

#### 4.4.3. Reactive Ion Etching (RIE)

In RIE, a plasma generates high-energy ions in a chamber that reacts chemically with the substrate to be etched. RIE is a form of isotropic etching, primarily embodied as barrel etching; conversely, it is often utilized as an anisotropic etch. In this form, the reactive ions are accelerated toward the substrate to be etched [132]. The electric field accelerates ions, and etching is enhanced in the direction of the travel of the high-energy ions. The degree of etching in an RIE system depends strongly on reactive gases, gas flow, pressures, temperatures, RF power and DC bias [187]. The above parameters have been thoroughly studied to fabricate such deeper structures. Using the RIE system, various materials such as silicon, oxide, and nitride can be etched to form pits (up to several microns) of arbitrary shape, deep trenches, and holes with vertical walls [188]. Despite the anisotropic wet etching, RIE is made inadequate by the crystal planes in the silicon. The table shows different etchant gases used for the plasma etching of various films. Various chemicals are used in plasma etching which ultimately results in etchant gas like Chlorine, Oxygen, Fluorine etc. [189].

The etching rate in RIE is low; hence, to achieve a high width-to-height ratio, a deep RIE (DRIE) process was introduced. A deep RIE (DRIE), often called the Bosch process, was introduced to generate high aspect ratios, height-to-width ratios, and structures in amalgamation with chemical vapor deposition (film forming process). Fabrication parameters can be optimized using the BOSCH process to achieve a high aspect ratio; high etch rate, straight sidewalls and small sidewall scalloping. The possibility of getting non-vertical, tapered sidewalls is limited [190].

In order to generate high aspect ratio troughs or beams with vertical walls in a substrate, two different phases that work repetitively at a reasonable frequency are employed [191]: (1) Etching: employing an isotropic plasma-enhanced etching method, the substrate is etched; (2) Deposition: In the second phase, the entire substrate is deposited with an inert protection layer (e.g., $C_4H_8$) to preserve the etching of the side walls when the plasma etching phase is repeated for the next cycle of fabrication. The Bosch process typically creates undulating sidewalls due to the above two steps. The Bosch method is appropriate for the manufacture of off-plane MNs. This method is also used to yield hollow MNs with a lumen of several hundred μm widths to height ratio of 30:1 [192]. Although wet etching can decrease fabrication costs more than dry etching, distinct and sharp MN tips are fabricated by uniting isotropic dry and anisotropic wet etching [49].

Research by Henry et al., in 1998, fabricated solid silicon out-of-plane MNs arrays employing the DRIE process. The chromium dots formed the masks on the silicon wafers. The patterned silicon wafers were etched using a reactive ion etcher using $SF_6$ and $O_2$ gas as an etchant at a pressure of 150 mTorr and power of 150 W for a run time of about 250 min. These parameters resulted in deep vertical and lateral etching forming MNs from the regions protected by the chromium masks [193]. Howells et al., 2022 fabricated solid silicon MN and hollow silicon in-plane MN arrays with a 54.7° sidewall etch angle from a simple single wet etch process. MNs were fabricated using double-side polished, boron-doped, 300 μm thick (100) orientation silicon wafers with a thermal silicon dioxide layer on both front and back sides. Photolithography processes were used to pattern devices onto silicon dioxide. Using ICP, the device pattern was etched into the silicon dioxide hard mask. The wafer was flipped, and again, the device was patterned and etched. The whole wafer was submerged in 44% KOH solution for etching for 5 h and then removed. V-shaped grooves were achieved as the KOH concurrently etched together the front and back sides of the wafer, which further intersected to form a sharp pyramidal six-sided MN tip. Via bonding of two grooved MNs together, a hollow MN was designed using ICP. The MNs arrays established efficiently pierce in the skin, lacking significant indentation, thus enabling actual delivery of drugs using solid MNs or direct injection using hollow MNs. Effective insulin and hyaluronic acid delivery into the skin was achieved using these MN arrays [194]. Figure 12 shows the Planar plasma etch configuration method.

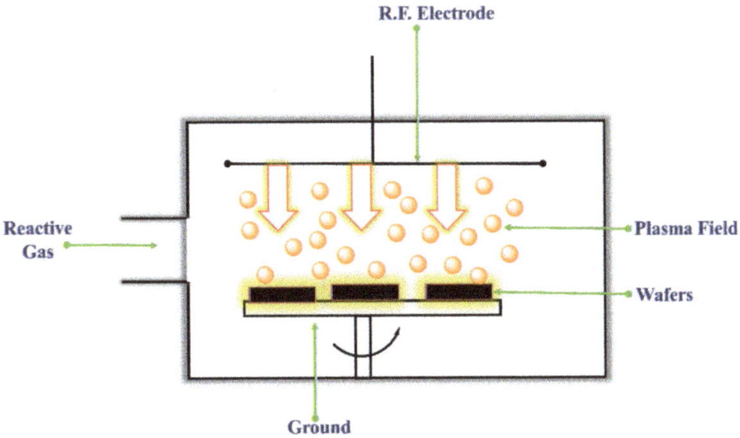


**Figure 12.** Planar plasma etches configuration method. The wafers are held on a grounded chuck close to the RF electrodes. Reactive gas introduced in the chamber is ionized, and the ions help in material removal [189]. (Reprinted from Ref. [189]).

### *4.5. Ion-Beam Milling (IBM)*

The Ion-Beam Milling method, in which inert ions are accelerated from a source to physically eliminate the material etched from the wafer. They are of two types; showered-ion-beam milling (SIBM), and concentrated ion-beam milling (FIBM) [195]. In SIBM, energetic ions are poured over the whole substrate. In FIBM, ions are concentrated on a spot directed to a particular workpiece part [196]. Although SIBM is slower and more controlled, it can be used as RIE. In ion-beam milling, inert gas ions, usually Ar, are used as they exhibit higher sputtering yields due to heavy ions and avoid chemical reactions, e.g., Ar, $O_2$, $N_2$, Xe [197]. The process is not selective or specific, but it is highly directional. Figure 13 shows a Representation of the ion beam etching process methods.

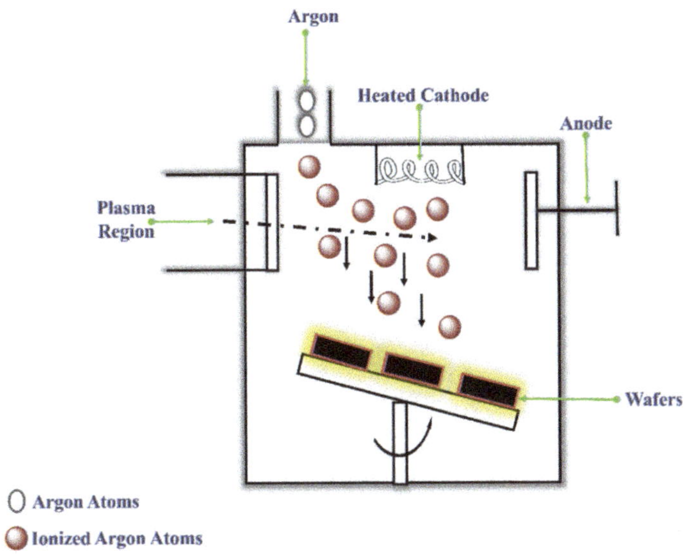


**Figure 13.** Representation of the ion beam etching process methods. Ar gas introduced in the vacuum chamber was ionized by bombarding with electrons. These ions are then directed onto the wafer, where they eliminate material by physical bombardment [189]. (Reprinted from Ref. [189]).

## 5. Characterization of MNs

The characteristic feature of MN advancement is its diversified application. The basic characteristic includes dimensions, i.e., size, shape and geometry. The material (metal, ceramic, silicone) used in designing MNs also has a significant role in the characterization of MNs [198].

These characteristics include: (1) Deep penetration of intact MN into the skin tissue. (2) Optimized dimensions, as the short needle would not be completely pierced into the skin tissue, and with a long needle size, there might be a risk of breaking (due to lack of strength and rigidness) before insertion into the skin [199,200].

### *5.1. Morphology and Geometry*

Morphological characteristics like shape, length, base diameter, and a tip diameter of MN are observed.

#### Scanning Electron Microscopy (SEM)

The study of geometry and dimensions was conducted on two types of MN, i.e., maltose MN and DermaRollerTM (metallic), on a Scanning electron microscope (Hitachi S-4100) for MN imaging. These MNs samples were directly imaged without coating with DermaRollerTM, and detachment of the head embedded with MN from a needle holder was executed, and samples were placed in SEM with 15 eV accelerated voltage. The measurement of the dimensions was recorded by software—Vantage 1.3 (Noran Systems, Middleton, WI, USA). The observed results were as follows; maltose MN consisted of pyramidal shape, 497.41 ± 31.10 μm length, 197.60 ± 17.53 μm base diameter and ~8 μm tip diameter, whereas DermaRollerTM MN had conical shape, 699.38 ± 70.72 μm length, 127.88 ± 15.96 μm base diameter, ~15 μm tip diameter [201].

Amer RI et al. characterized polymeric MNs of Sodium alginate by conducting an SEM analysis. The geometry of the MN was confirmed from the master mold where the visualization of MN length is 600–650 μm, the base width of 300–350 μm with 100–125 μm interspacing. Deformation was observed slightly, i.e., needles were more wide and flat; this was associated with sampling preparation with a low level of electron beam and magnification, which resulted in the interaction of both the sample and electron beam, causing sample degradation by melting.

Uniform sharp tips inter-spacing dimensions of MN were observed and confirmed by a photograph of a light microscope (MN cross-section sample) [202].

### *5.2. Mechanical Integrity*

#### Thermogravimetric Analysis

A TGA was performed for sorbitol, polyvinyl alcohol, and MN patch to ensure the thermal stability of components of MNs where a 3% loss in mass, caused by the evaporation of adsorbed water, was observed for a powdered sample of polyvinyl alcohol (PVA) with temperatures ranging from 25 °C to 200 °C. More than 60% mass loss in PVA was recorded at 300–370 °C, indicating thermal degradation of PVA, and an additional 30% loss in mass at 370–470 °C occurred due to the decomposition mechanism. Sorbitol under thermal exposure reported mass loss <1% at 230 °C and represents thermal stability. A further 50% reduction in mass was observed with a temperature rise of 230–350 °C, representing thermal degradation. The MN patch showed the approximate 85% mass loss is similar to PVA as it consists of PVA in large amounts. About 6% mass reduction at 65–240 °C occurred due to water removal and melting. At 300–370 °C, organic combustion caused mas sample reduction of ~48%. At 380–480 °C the sample showed second phase degradation. This study concluded the efficient thermal stability of sorbitol, polyvinyl alcohol, and MN patch [203].

### 5.3. Swelling Property

The swelling property signifies the mechanical integrity of the MN. The swelling study is carried out as follows; where a blank and dry patch was taken from a known mass (Wd), and was immersed in a petri dish containing phosphate buffer saline solution with pH 6.8. The immersion continued until the swelling caused disruption to the structure and thus the structural integrity collapsed due to water uptake (approx. 30 min). The patch was taken out of the petri dish, and using filter paper, surface water removal was conducted [204]. The swollen patch was weighed ($W_s$), and the determination of the percentage of swelling was calculated using the following formula:

$$W\% = \frac{(W_S - W_d)}{W_d} \times (100)$$

The super swelling MN arrays fabricated using an aqueous mixture containing 20% *w*/*w* Gantrez S-97, 7.5% *w*/*w* PEG 10,000 and 3% *w*/*w* $Na_2CO_3$ were subjected to swelling studies PBS pH 7.4 buffer. First, the weight of the MN was measured in a dry state at a zero time point and then immersed in PBS pH 7.4. The MN films were removed at specific time intervals, surface fluid was wiped, and the MN film's swollen mass was measured. The results showed the highest swelling and fast achievement of the equilibrium state by the super swelling MN compared to the control formulation (15% Gantrez AN-139, 7.5% PEG). At equilibrium, the super swelling percentage of the super swelling MN compared to the control MN was 1708% and 1071%, respectively. Thus, the above study proves the mechanical integrity of the hydrogel MN array when administered transdermally [45]. Swelling of the polymer network hydrogel is presented in Figure 14.

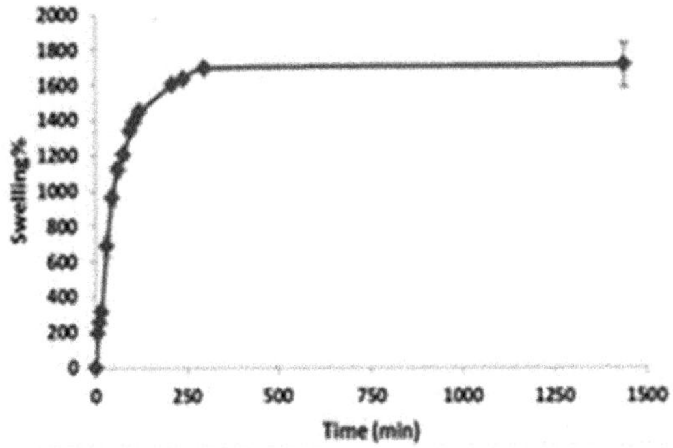


**Figure 14.** Swelling curve for crosslinked hydrogel films prepared from aqueous blends containing 20% *w*/*w* PMVE/MA, 7.5% *w*/*w* PEG and 3% $Na_2CO_3$ based on the increasing mass of the swelling array expressed as a percentage of the mass of a dry array (Means ± SD, n = 3). Adapted from ref [45].

### 5.4. Drug Release and Drug Distribution

MN design aims to ensure drug delivery into the epidermis and dermis of the skin by piercing the stratum corneum. The skin staining technique uses methylene blue stain to confirm these MN holes by piercing the MN. Preparation of methylene blue solution of 10 mg/mL by adding methylene blue powder(M9140, Sigma-Aldrich, St. Louis, MI, USA) and distilled water. For biological stains, methylene blue dye is used. It acts as it binds with the protein in the tissue; due to its hydrophilic nature, it is not absorbed by the stratum corneum hydrophobic nature [205,206].

When coated, PLA MN and dissolvable MN were removed from a skin sample, the deposition of methylene blue on the skin sample was conducted for 10 min on the skin surface, and leftover methylene blue solution was wiped out with ethanol (24,194, Sigma-Aldrich), leaving dye stains in the punctured region of the stratum corneum and highlighting them [67].

MN drug delivery aided the rapid dissolution of the drug into the body. Drug distribution enhances the efficiency of drug release. The interaction of polymer and drug molecules was carried out by multiscale simulation influencing MN drug distribution. The study was carried out with sulforhodamine B (SRB) as a model drug, along with Hyaluronic acid (HA) and polyvinyl alcohol (PVA) for fabricating MNs. Dissolvable MNs were produced to study controlled drug distribution in those MN patches. These observations were studied using an optical microscope under an objective lens by viewing the side and top angle of the MN array. The analysis of SRB in both MN patches was studied and observations made were as follows; limited drug distribution in PVA, as drug molecules, are seen concentrated at the tip, and mild concentration was seen in the middle portion, with no drug molecules at the base of the needle. Conversely, Hyaluronic acid showed poor drug diffusion control ability. Here, SRB distributes largely into the needle body and bottom plate; it has a poor concentration at the needle tip; owing to the high water solubility of HA with a high compatibility drug molecule, Hyaluronic acid faced a significant challenge in achieving controlled control drug distribution [207].

## 6. Mechanical Properties of MNs

Mechanical strength is an important aspect for MNs to perform their function. Mechanical property is often determined by compression strength [208]. The compression strength of MNs assesses the mechanical property of MNs. The measurement of the robust nature of MNs is their integrity for skin penetration. Here, metal-coated MN is assessed by Yang SJ., et al. for compression strength. The MNs skin penetration was performed using porcine skin. The texture analyzer was used with a trigger force of 100 N and 12 mm working distance (from the probe to the skin) for the MNs skin patch (MNP) testing. The probe holding this patch descended at 100 mm/min speed until it reached 10 mm from the target, slowing down towards 10 mm/min speed with 2 mm from the surface. As it approached the skin surface, the needle points penetrated 700 μm. When full penetration of the MNs patch with porcine skin took place, the detachment of the MNs patch from porcine skin and the images were reviewed.

The calculation of compressive strength was made when the MNs patch was penetrated to a length of 50% into porcine skin. There was a slight MNs patch stress change by a 43% compression rate. An optical microscope represented MNs patch deformation. Flat PVP- hydrogel has a compression strength of 268 kPa, while PVP-MNP has 284 kPa of compression strength; PVP-MNP's higher compression strength is due to the larger force applied per unit of arrangement. The compressive strength of Ag coated PVP MNs 278 kPa, and Au coated PVP MNs 276 kPa are slightly less than PVP-MNP due to polymeric chain degradation with polymeric chain heat created during the process of degradation. These Ag and Au coated PVP MNs have higher strength than flat PVP hydrogel. The MNPs have perfectly penetrated the porcine skin, seldom broke or deformed. Furthermore, complete skin penetration occurred at the surface without breaking at contact. The slight reduction in length < 1% when penetrated to 700 μm was observed before (~701–703 μm) and after (~692–695 μm) MNs length skin penetration. The shape was retained well (slight deformation). Results represented effectiveness in drug delivery as PVP-based MNPs are prepared by radiation and have MNs of sufficient strength and flexibility required for insertion through the stratum corneum and to reach the dermis [200].

## 7. In Vitro and In Vivo Evaluations of MNs

### *7.1. In Vitro Studies*

In vitro studies for an assessment of the MNs include penetration and permeability studies. The skin distribution technique evaluates the uniformity and depth of penetration by MNs. The patch is placed on the hairless skin of a Rat or Pig and immediately removed. The skin site is dyed with a cotton swab soaked with India ink. This skin is then stored at −20 °C on dry ice for three days up to processing. The skin is cut in a section of uniform size (6 mm, with a cryotome instrument). The number of stained pathways in each section is counted. The percentage of MNs to have penetrated the skin can be plotted as a function of depth, and the depth at which 50% of the MNs penetrated can be extrapolated [209]. Permeability studies of MNs can help to predict how MNs can help improve drug delivery. In vitro methods for a permeation study are usually carried out by diffusion cell apparatus and rat skin. Kocchar et al. [210] conducted an in vitro permeation study of Bovine Serum Albumin (BSA) MNs on abdominal rat skin with the help of a water-jacketed horizontal diffusion cell. Overnight hydrated skin in 0.005% phosphate-buffered saline was placed as stretched on 10 layers of Kim wipes to absorb and provide mechanical support like tissue [211]. MNs, having different concentrations, were applied to a taken rat skin as a sample, and MNs without any BSA was used as a blank. BSA solution in propylene glycol (PG) was used as a standard to compare the release of BSA by passive diffusion and MNs. The MNs were fixed on the skin with the help of scotch tape. This skin was placed in the middle of the two compartments. About 4.5 mL of receptor solution was placed in the receptor compartment and stirred continuously at 250 rpm. Then, 1 mL of receptor solution was withdrawn at each sampling point. The removed release samples were centrifuged at 10,000 rpm for 5 min. UV A215-A225 method164 calculated the permeation of BSA through the skin. Another study checked Doxorubicin MNs' permeation on the mouse skin spread on a glass slide. The MNs were removed, and a confocal scanning microscope observed the skin to check the penetration of drugs into the skin [212]. In the case of dip-coated MNs, the content of coated material (Lidocaine) was determined by HPLC. The coating of MNs was desorbed into a diluent, and the resulting solution was injected into HPLC, and freebase Lidocaine was used as the standard for the quantification [213]. The study carried out by Kumar et al. [214] used MNs for piercing the skin and permeation of nanoparticles through the skin. The dorsal skin on BALB/c mice was made free of fatty layers. MNs roller was then perpendicularly rolled in four lines for five times, twenty times each. The applying pressure was constantly monitored and kept between 350–400 g. This treated skin was clamped between the donor and receiver compartment of the Franz-diffusion cell. The donor compartment was filled with the pCMV-β-coated nanoparticles in water. The receiver compartment was filled with 5 mL of PBS (pH 7.4). The temperature of the setup was maintained at 37 °C with a continuous circulation of water. At several time intervals, 150 μL of solution from the receiver compartment was removed and replaced by the same volume of PBS. The diffused plasmid into the receiver compartment was evaluated using a microplate reader and compared. Permeation through intact skin was also carried out simultaneously.

### 7.2. In Vivo Studies

The visualization of MNs patches and drug uptake is carried out by an in vivo imaging system (IVIS). It observes the subject animal at a predetermined time interval [215]. Insulin delivery in the induced diabetic Sprague Dawley rats with the help of MNs was conducted [216]. A pneumatically driven insertion device was used for inserting the MNs into the lower back skin of the rat. The MNs were removed with the help of forceps. Around the pierced skin of the rat, a chamber was fixed, which was later filled with Humulin-R insulin (100 u/mL). It was kept for 4 h, and blood glucose measurements were made every 30 min using a human insulin-specific radioimmunoassay. The same protocol was carried out for negative control without MNs insertion in the skin. The positive control, subcutaneous administration of Humulin-R insulin 50 μL diluted with PBS was conducted. The visualization of MNs patch and drug uptake was carried by an in vivo imaging system (IVIS). It observed the subject animal at a predetermined time interval [212]. Figure 14 showed MNs for the delivery of insulin. Here, they found that the insulin that was applied to rats' skin without a microneedle roller was not found to be significantly different ($p > 0.05$) than the time controlled group, approving in-efficiency of passive insulin absorption through the transdermal route. The subcutaneous administration of insulin rapidly decreased the blood glucose level at 1 h, to around 18%. For the 500 micron group, the glucose level was 18% at 3 h, significantly different from the negative control rats ($p < 0.05$). In comparison to the positive control after 3 h, the changes in blood glucose levels persuaded through the microneedle roller are higher ($p < 0.05$), but there was no significant difference 3 h (initial 3 h). This specifies that microneedle rollers might increase the skin permeability in long-term delivery, which is suitable for the delivery of repeated amounts of pharmacologically active insulin.

## 8. Applications of MNs

The MNs were first introduced for drug delivery applications, and the major objective was the enhanced permeation in the skin using solid and hollow MNs compared to conventional hypodermic needles. The MNs were filled with drug solutions or formulations, or they were coated for improved intradermal drug delivery. Nowadays, MNs are the leading novel technology for several fields of drug delivery, such as intradermal, ocular and intracellular drug delivery. However, the transdermal route is still the leading application area for MNs, especially vaccine-based delivery.

### *8.1. Intradermal Drug Delivery through MNs Formulations*

Drug delivery to the skin is challenging as it may be a local application or systemic delivery as a result of the stratum corneum's highly tough and barrier properties. However, the human stratum corneum thickness is (10–15 μm), and it still prohibits the drugs at therapeutic levels [217]. The Food and Drug Administration approves more than 20 drugs for transdermal patches applications with a molecular weight of less than 400 Da and a higher logP [218]. Due to the challenging barrier of the skin, and despite its few micron sizes, novel MNs formulations were developed to pass the stratum corneum and load the drug into the dermal skin without generating any pain or bleeding in the human host [219]. MNs increased the number of drugs administered through the dermis, considering low molecular weight, biomolecules, vaccines or proteins and other materials [220].

### *8.2. Small Molecules (Low Molecular Weight Drugs)*

The small molecule or low molecular weight drugs have higher skin diffusion coefficients than the larger molecule or biomolecule, which could easily penetrate the skin. This is so that the small molecule is quickly delivered into the skin using MNs.

Rojekar et al. have formulated dissolving MNs containing the etravirine and etravirine nanosuspension for long-acting drug delivery and improved HIV infection therapy. They have demonstrated the robust nature of MNs, with significant drug deposition of 12.84 ± 1.33% ex vivo, in neonatal porcine skin for 6 h. The in vivo pharmacokinetic studies demonstrated improved parameters; Cmax exhibited by DMNs containing ETR powder and ETR NS was 158 ± 10 ng/mL and 177 ± 30 ng/mL, respectively. It was also revealed that the improved t1/2, Tmax, and mean residence time (MRT) compared to intravenous ETR solutions indicated the long-acting nature of etravirine delivery using DMNs [220].

Lin Zhu et al. have developed estriol-loaded EMNs to effectively treat radiation-induced injury. For the development of EMNs, biocompatible polymer polyvinyl pyrrolidone K90 was used. The drug is dissolved in methanol and mixed with polymer gel to cast into a mold to obtain the conical-shaped EMNs. The developed EMNs are robust and easily penetrate 200 μm into mouse skin. Most interestingly, these EMNs dissolve very quickly in 5 min, which could help immediately permeate the drug into the skin. The mouse model of the ionizing radiation-induced injury was developed by the source of 6.5 Gy radiation of 60 Co γ ray. Furthermore, EMNs enhanced the peripheral blood leukocytes count in irradiated mice, which protected the bone marrow hematopoietic system and 80% increased the survival rate of the irradiated mice [221].

Alyaa et al. have investigated and developed dissolving MNs using biocompatible and biodegradable polymers, poly(vinylpyrrolidone) (PVP) and hyaluronic acid (HA) to intradermally deliver the Amphotericin-B (AMP-B) to treat the fungal infection. It was found that both polymers used in development reduced the AMP-B cytotoxicity, compared to the drug-free solution. Moreover, it was found that AMP-B-loaded dissolving

MNs showed significant antifungal activity compared to plain drugs. Furthermore, MNs maintain the activity of drugs [222].

Ismaiel A. Tekko et al., have for the first time, developed the MNs array patches (MAP) with the higher Cabotegravir or micronized sodium salt loading of ($\approx$3 mg/0.5 cm$^2$). The MAP was robust with the skin penetration potential. The tips were dissolved in 30 min, giving immediate deposition of the drug in the skin. Moreover, the in vivo dermatokinetic study in Sprague Dawley rats of both forms of drug-loaded MAP deposited into the skin, forming the depot. Both drug forms are released slowly, maintaining the therapeutic concentrations in the blood for one month for a single application [223].

Alejandro J. Paredes et al. have developed tenofovir alafenamide (TAF) loaded dissolving and implantable MAPs to systematically deliver or release the drug. The developed MNs are mechanically strong enough and could pierce the excised neonatal full-thickness porcine skin and deposit the drug as a depot form. The release study performed using dialysis methods demonstrated the relatively fast drug release in both the formulations. The in vivo studies in rats showed rapid metabolization of the TAF into tenofovir, along with quick elimination of the metabolite from the blood plasma [224].

Maelíosa Crudden et al. have developed Rilpivirine nanosuspension-loaded, dissolving MN array patches (MAPs) for the long-acting delivery in HIV for improved therapy and patient compliance. MAPs were mechanically strong enough to pierce the skin and load the drug as depot formulation for a prolonged effect. In vivo pharmacokinetic studies demonstrated that the mean plasma concentration in rats is 431 ng/mL at seven days, which is about ten-fold larger than the trough concentration found after a single dose administered in the previous clinical studies [225].

Mingshan Li et al. developed a novel strategy for co-formulating the dexamethasone and pro-drug dexamethasone sodium phosphate in the DMNs. That could have led to the immediate effect to achieve long-term drug delivery. The 3D printing technique was used the first time to fabricate the baseplate of the MN. The 3D printed base plate is robust, providing excellent support to the drug encapsulated or loaded tips. These novel trilayer-based MNs have shown the effective drug delivery of dexamethasone, which could be the novel promising drug option for oral and injectable drug delivery [226].

### 8.3. Large Molecules (Biotherapeutics)

Protein and peptides are very unstable and degraded after oral administration. Transdermal drug delivery could avoid this issue; however, delivering all kinds of molecules is difficult due to challenging skin barriers [227]. Using MNs, protein and peptide delivery could be an excellent alternative to the traditional transdermal patches. MNs have excellent mechanical properties as they penetrate the dermis and resolve the problem of penetration and permeation associated with conventional drug delivery. It also has good thermostable properties, which could help in protein and peptide drug delivery [228].

Desmopressin is a synthetic form of vasopressin, the potent peptide hormone used to replace the low vasopressin levels in the therapy. This is used to treat diabetes insipidus, which causes bedwetting in children and hemophilia A. The MNs formulation is a novel approach to deliver the desmopressin, which showed an effective and safe delivery compared to the other conventional routes [14].

Liu et al. have formulated GAP-26, a gap-junction blocker containing polyethylene glycol diacrylate MNs to deliver peptides by swelling effect. The developed MNs formulation has improved the permeation of peptides, which leads to improved inhibition of the keloid fibroblasts and the collagen I expression [14,229]. Cyclosporin A is a high molecular weight, a hydrophobic molecule with a cyclic peptide used to treat several skin and dermal diseases. Cyclosporine A loaded dissolving MNs was developed with 600 μm in length, and 250 μm wide was prepared by a molding process. This fabricated MNs formulation delivered 10% *w*/*w* of Cyclosporin A in the porcine skin for 60 min. Approximately 65% of MNs were dissolved with a 34 $\pm$ 6.5 μg drug delivery [14,230].

Insulin is the hormone for modulating blood glucose levels with a 51-amino-acid peptide. However, the exceptionally high pain triggered by frequent subcutaneous injections could adversely affect the patient's compliance [228,231]. Despite this, transdermal delivery of insulin is an eye-catching delivery method. With SC injections, MN-loaded insulin delivery would benefit diabetic patients through self-administration and low pain. The solid MNs fabricated by diverse materials, such as polymer, silicon and metal, have effectively decreased the blood glucose level by improving the insulin permeability by skin pre-treatment [232].

Zhou et al. demonstrated the applicability of the stainless steel MNs with different needle lengths, which were used to evaluate the delivery efficacy of insulin in diabetic rats. The results demonstrated that the skin permeability increased significantly with a rapidly decreasing glucose level within 1 h of application. It is also seen that solid MNs associated with the iontophoresis could effectively improve the intradermal delivery of the insulin [233]. McAllister et al. demonstrated that hollow MNs can deliver the microliter solution to the skin; however, larger pressure could trigger a faster decrease in blood glucose levels. The hollow MNs-based intradermal insulin delivery resulted in faster insulin onset, driven by the passive diffusion, electricity or pressure [232]. Li et al. have optimized and developed MNs to study the effect of insulin delivery on blood levels in mice. It was found that blood glucose level was decreased to 29% of the initial level at 5 h, which could confirm the improved insulin permeability using MN-based drug delivery [14,109].

Ye and co-workers have studied MNs association with pancreatic β-cell capsules, which could sense the glucose level in the blood and secrete insulin as per the requirements. It was found that the patch was not effective enough. MNs matrix-loaded synthetic glucose signal amplifiers were developed. These MNs include α- amylase, glucoamylase, and glucose oxidase; this indicates insulin secretion from the β-cells capsules [14,234]. The clinical study of the parathyroid hormone (I-34) coated MNs demonstrated two times shorter $t_{1/2}$ and three times shorter Tmax than the conventional injectable therapy [235]. These studies demonstrated the MN's potential capability in hormonal drug delivery, suggesting MNs formulations' effectivity and efficiency. These could also be altered for sustained effect by using appropriate polymers. Furthermore, iontophoresis united with MNs could also be discovered to deliver numerous hormones [14,236]. Figures 15 and 16 showed MNs for delivery of insulin.

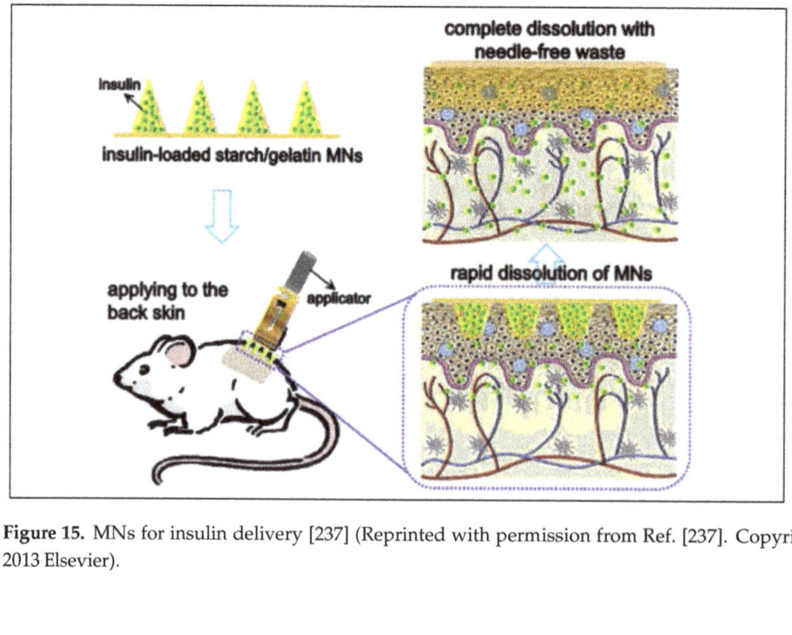


**Figure 15.** MNs for insulin delivery [237] (Reprinted with permission from Ref. [237]. Copyright 2013 Elsevier).

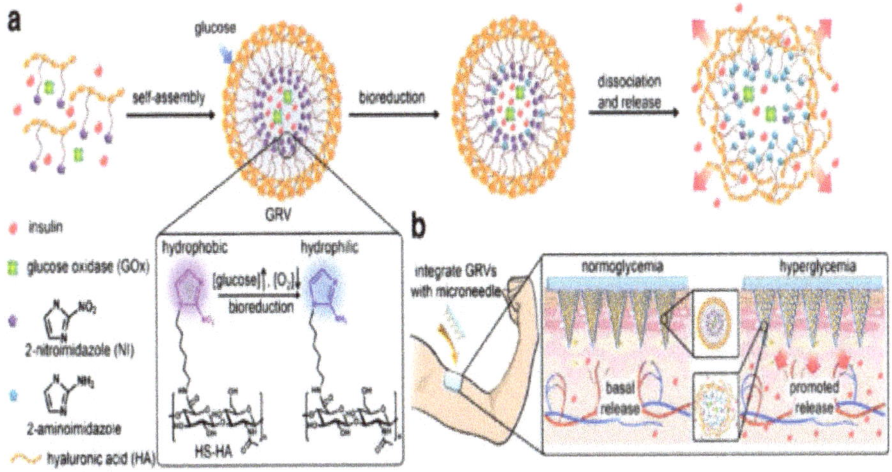


**Figure 16.** MNs for delivery of insulin (**a**) Formation and mechanism of GRVs composed of HS-HA. (**b**) Schematic of the GRV-containing MN-array patch (smart insulin patch) for in vivo insulin delivery triggered by a hyperglycemic state to release more insulin [238]. (Adapted from Ref. [238]).

### *8.4. Other Biomolecules*

The DNA and RNA are short oligonucleotides, basically smaller units than proteins. Delivery of the oligonucleotide is difficult due to their properties, so numerous techniques were employed to deliver these agents. The delivery of the 20-merphosphorothioated oligodeoxynucleotide was conducted using the MNs formulations approach. The solid MNs, made from stainless steel, were used to deliver these oligonucleotides via the poke with the patch approach. It was found that more drugs were delivered using this approach compared to intact skin [14,239].

### *8.5. Vaccine*

A vaccine is a complex biological preparation or formulation. It successfully offers active acquired immunity to a specific disease. Vaccines consist of the killed or weakened form of disease triggering microorganisms, toxins or one of its surface proteins [109]. Vaccines could stimulate the body's immune system and protect the host system against future infections or diseases [240]. The MN-based intradermal vaccine drug delivery was an excellent and effective option. The MNs have delivered the DNA-based vaccine and have obtained immune responses that were much better than regular injections [241]. An attempt to develop an MNs patch to administer the influenza vaccine was made [242]. A lower dose is required when the drug is administered using hollow MNs compared to when using an intramuscular injection. Anthrax and rabies vaccine delivery using hollow MNs have been studied [3]. Ogai et al. have developed hollow MNs by using biodegradable PLGA to improve the delivery and efficiency of the vaccine by intradermal route. It was demonstrated that the drug or vaccine delivery in the upper dermis could provide improved immunity. Furthermore, it was found that the antibody titers were significantly higher than conventional delivery [230,243]. Figure 17 showed Dissolving MNs loaded with vaccines and hydrophobic adjuvants for improved cancer therapy.

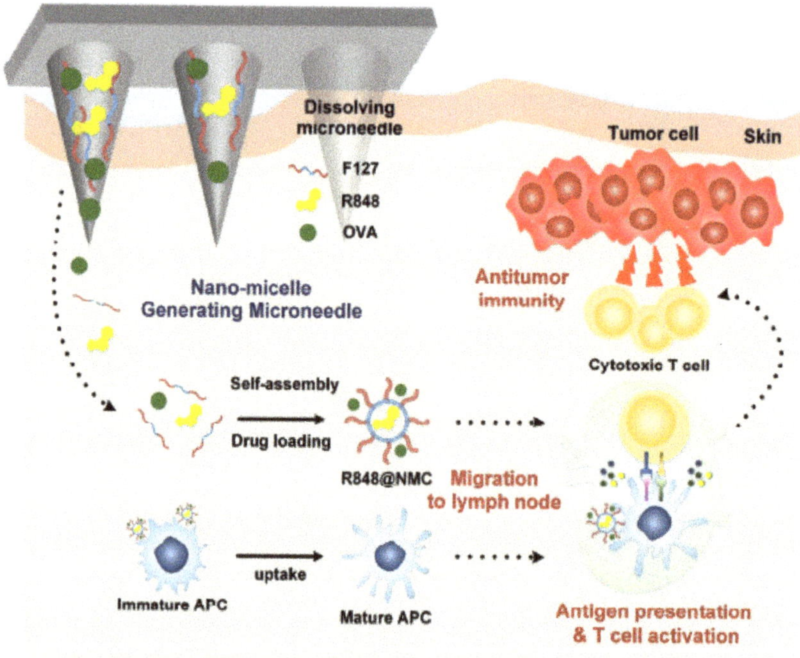


**Figure 17.** Dissolving MNs loaded with vaccines and hydrophobic adjuvants for improved cancer therapy [244]. (Adapted with permission from Ref. [244]. Copyright 2018 American Chemical Society).

### 8.6. Diagnosis

The painless withdrawal of the biological fluids from the body is the major advantage of MNs over conventional blood collection techniques. Various biomarkers present in interstitial fluid beneath the skin can be useful for diagnosing various diseases like diabetes, cancer, arthritis, etc., and helpful, timely medical intervention. Multiple research studies demonstrated the usefulness of MNs for disease diagnosis [245]. Chang et al. revealed the application of MNs in the extraction of interstitial fluid to analyze metabolites. The MNs patch consisting of methacrylate hyaluronic acid efficiently extracted skin interstitial fluid. The extracted fluid can be further used for diagnostic purposes [246]. Jin and coworkers reported the usefulness of MNs in Tuberculosis (TB) skin tests (Mantoux test). The MNs efficiently deliver the purified protein derivative (PPD) in TB skin tests. The precise and controlled delivery in deep skin is advantageous for using MNs [247]. El-Laboudi et al. stated the effective use of MNs array in monitoring glucose, which could be useful in diagnosing diabetes and associated disorders [248]. Pires et al. described the use of MNs in pediatrics. Vital vaccination like tetanus, diphtheria, and pertussis is carried out within a year from the child's birth. The use of MNs can help overcome the discomfort and phobia associated with conventional needles and results in efficient child vaccination.

Along with vaccination, the MNs can be used to diagnose various skin diseases in pediatrics like psoriasis and other inflammatory conditions [249]. One of the prime applications of MNs is in diagnosing various carcinogenic conditions. Multiple anticancer vaccines and drugs are delivered through MNs using nanocarriers. The delivery of these cancer diagnostic agents through MNs shows improved biodistribution and efficient diagnosis [250].

### 8.7. Biosensing

MNs provide significant efficiency in the biosensing of various biomarkers and metabolites. Collection of biofluid is more convenient with MNs than with conventional hypodermic needles. Recent advancements in MNs are resulting in improved biosensing [251]. Strambini et al. demonstrated MN-based biosensors to detect glycemia in interstitial fluid [252]. Electrochemical biosensors are emerging advancements in MNs technology used for biosensing. Innovation geometrical configurations of MNs provide an advantage in biosensing [253]. After their research, Zho et al. reported that the MNs fabricated from silk, polyols, and glucose oxidase could be used for glucose biosensing by electrochemical biosensing technology [254]. Bollela and coworkers reported the development of second-generation MN-based biosensors to detect lactate. The gold MNs were functionalized with nano carbons, through which the electron transfer of lactate oxidase took place, resulting in efficient sensing of lactate [255]. Polymer-based MNs are also frequently used for biosensing. Multiple researchers across the globe have reported the usefulness of polymeric needle-based MNs in biosensing of various endogenous substances [256]. Calio et al. demonstrated the use of MNs fabricated from poly (ethylene glycol) diacrylate in biosensing applications. The prepared polymeric MNs were used to fabricate the electrodes used for biosensing of glucose and lactic acid [257]. Various carbon-based MNs are also used in biosensing. Jin et al. demonstrated the usefulness of hybrid MNs consisting of reduced graphene oxide and platinum nanoparticles for the biosensing of hydrogen peroxide. The in vivo study on pig skin and living mice proved the biosensing efficiency of prepared hybrid MNs [258]. Figure 18 shows commercially available MNs devices.

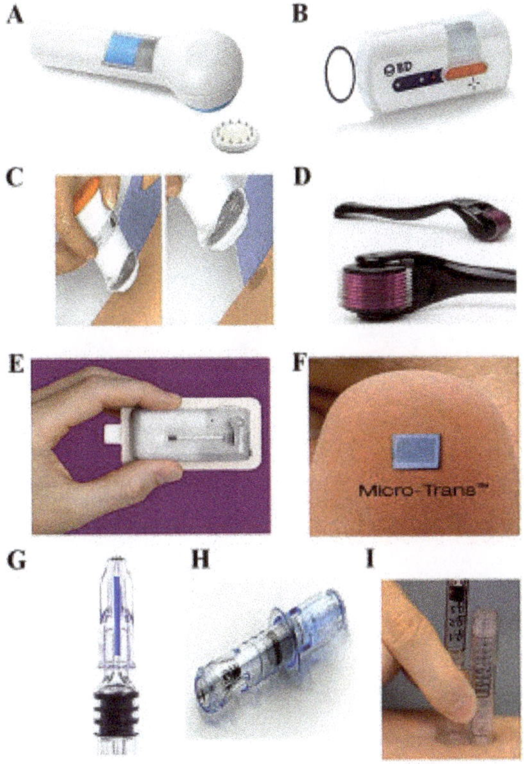


**Figure 18.** Commercially available MNs devices **(A)** Microstructured Transdermal Syst **(B)** BD Microinfuser® **(C)** MicrofluxrTM **(D)** MTS RollerTM **(E)** Vaaleritas h-patchTM **(F)** MicrotransTM **(G)** MicronJet® **(H)** Intanza® **(I)** DebioJectTM [259]. (Reprinted with permission from Ref. [259]. Copyright 2019 Elsevier).

### 8.8. Cancer Therapy

MNs technology creates a new horizon in cancer therapy through efficient drug delivery of anticancer vaccines and drugs. Various chemotherapeutic agents, genes and proteins can be efficiently delivered through MN-based devices [260]. Hao et al. established the usefulness of MNs technology in the treatment of epidermoid cancer therapy. The researchers developed the near-infrared responsive PEGylated gold nanorod and Doxorubicin-containing dissolvable Hyaluronic Acid MNs for the localized efficient therapy of epidermoid cancer, and it showed efficient antitumor activity [261]. Gadag and coworkers also demonstrated the usefulness of MNs in breast cancer therapy. Resveratrol is one of the efficient anticancer agents used to treat breast cancer but is limited by low bioavailability. To overcome this limitation, researchers developed the nanostructured lipid carriers of Resveratrol and delivered them through MNs arrays. The drug delivery through MNs improved permeation and bioavailability at the tumor site [262]. Hao et al. demonstrated the application of MNs in skin cancer therapy. The researchers fabricated the near-infrared responsive 5-indocyanine green and fluorouracil containing monomethoxy-poly (ethylene glycol)-polycaprolactone nanoparticles delivered through dissolvable MNs efficient therapy of human epidermoid cancer and melanoma [93]. Moreira et al. demonstrated the efficient delivery of doxorubicin and AuMSS nanorods through polyvinyl alcohol/chitosan layer-by-layer MNs, resulting in efficient cancer chemo-photothermal therapy [104]. Lan and coworkers also provided MN's significant applications in delivery proteins in cancer immunotherapy. They fabricated an MNs patch containing Ph responsive tumor-targeted lipid nanoparticles loaded with PD-1 and cisplatin, resulting from precise drug delivery and efficient immunotherapy [99]. Figure 19 showed Biodegradable Hyaluronic acid MNs (HAMN) containing antibodies for the treatment of skin cancers.

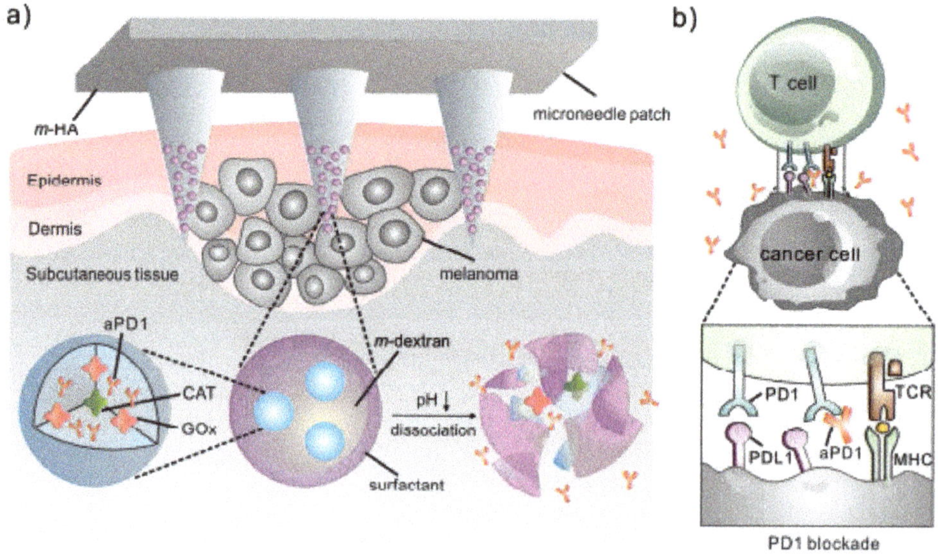


**Figure 19.** Biodegradable Hyaluronic acid MNs (HAMN) containing antibodies for the treatment of skin cancers. (**a**) Schematic of the aPD1 delivered by an MN patch loaded with physiologically self-dissociated NPs. (**b**) The blockade of PD-1 by aPD1 to activate the immune system to destroy skin cancer cells. [263]. (Reprinted with permission from Ref. [263]. Copyright 2016 American Chemical Society).

### 8.9. Ocular Drug Delivery

Bypassing the ocular barrier with minimum invasion is the advantage of MNs over intravitreal injection. Several studies demonstrated the application of MNs in ocular drug delivery. Patel et al. demonstrated the successful delivery of micro and nanoparticle suspension in the suprachoroidal space of pig, rabbit and human eye (ex vivo) using hollow MNs. Optimizing dimension and process parameters concluded that efficient drug delivery could be achieved with a needle length of 800–1000 μm and pressure of 250–300 kPa [264]. Through their research, Jiang et al. also endorsed the application of MNs technology in ocular drug delivery. Using the coated solid MNs, the intrascleral and intracorneal delivery of drugs, protein, and DNA was assessed. The successful delivery of drugs in the ocular system with minimum invasion was observed [265].

## 9. Toxicity Study Methods

The toxicity of MNs is checked by examining the materials used in their fabrication, such as silicon and stainless steel, and polymers, i.e., poly-methyl methacrylate, poly-lactic acid, etc., cause the toxicity of MNs. Sometimes the presence of materials such as photoinitiators can result in the toxic effects of MNs [227].

### 9.1. In Vitro Method

In vitro methods for toxicity assessment of MNs are carried out using cell line assays. Commonly used cell lines are human adult low calcium high temperature (HaCaT) keratinocytes and human embryonic kidney (HEK293) [210]. Piu et al. have carried out the cytotoxicity assay by cell viability for cellulose acetate MNs. NIH-3T3 fibroblasts cells were used for the study. The porous patches made up of polymers cellulose acetate, polysulfone, and polyethersulfone were sterilized with alcohol and soaked with PBS in triplicate to remove the alcohol. Uv irradiation was conducted for 2 h. The fibroblast cells were seeded into 48-well plates, with a cell density of $1 \times 10^4$ per well. The incubation media used was 90% of DMEM and 10% of fetal bovine serum. The sterilized MN patches were put into the wells, and this was kept for incubation for 24 h. Untreated cells were used as control. For analysis, 100 μL of culture media from each well was transferred to a 96-well plate, and the absorbance was checked with a microplate reader at 450 nm [266]. In another study on PEGDA MNs, Human vein endothelial cells (HUVECs) are used. The HUVECs are cultured in 96-well plates with a seeding density of $1 \times 10^4$ for 12 h. The MNs patch of 0.5 $cm^2$ was soaked in 1 mL DMEM media for 24 h and this was used as a soaking solution. Next, 200 μL of soaking solution was poured to each well and incubated for 24 h. Supernatant was replaced by 200 MTT μL agent. Then, 200 μL of DMSO was added to each plate and gently shaken for 15 min. The absorbance was checked at 570 and 630 nm and relative cell viability was calculated [267].

### 9.2. In Vivo Method

Biocompatibility of MNs by in vivo methods is usually assessed by acute dermal toxicity study. An MNs patch is placed on to the shaved skin of rats and observed visually to see whether the inflammation has occurred or not [268]. The material used in the fabrication of MNs is also checked for biocompatibility study with the help of a cell lines study. The cell lines used are the human dermal fibroblasts, HaCaT, and HEK293.

## 10. Regulatory Aspects

For genuine MNs goods, there are currently no agreed regulatory requirements. Precise quality requirements in the framework of Good Manufacturing Practice need to be developed for MNs to be made on an industrial scale. Currently, standardized testing and equipment utilized to validate MNs mechanical characteristics and insertion capacity are missing, making it hard to compare MNs and necessitating the adoption of standardized tests and equipment to evaluate product quality and adequate least requirements. There is the need to perfect the implementation of a pharmaceutical quality system with good manufacturing practice and quality risk management for well-designed MNs to commercialization. A stringent rule and regulation should be applied to meet all drug product requirements before being released for human use. The complex regulatory specifications and time requirements will impact the cost of the end finished product [269,270]. The Food and Drug Administration (FDA or Agency) published a draught guideline titled "Regulatory considerations for micro-needling devices: draught guidance for industry and FDA staff" on 15 September 2017. In the current circumstances, this guideline has not been finalized or applied. However, the guidance is very informative and provides sufficient knowledge, but more test data is needed to investigate the clinical applications of MNs. As a result, data on safety is important. Short-term and long-term safety data should be collected more precisely and effectively to enable the use of MNs devices in today's environment [44]. Table 3 shows the marketed product for MNs for different applications.

**Table 3.** Marketed product for MNs.

| Product Name | Company | Approved for Condition | Description | Reference |
|---|---|---|---|---|
| Fluzone | Sanofi Pasteur Inc. | Influenza Virus Vaccine (USFDA) | Micro-injection system for intradermal delivery of vaccine | [271] |
| Intanza | Sanofi Pasteur Europe | Split virion, Inactivated Influenza vaccine (EMA) (Discontinued due to commercial issues) | Micro-injection system of a prefilled syringe, having a 1.5 mm needle length. The needle shielding system is provided, which covers the needle after use. | [272] |
| C-8 (Cosmetic type) | The Dermaroller Series by Anastassakis K | Cosmetic use. | It has a 0.13 mm needle length. It enhances the penetration of topical agents | [273] |
| C-8HE (Hair-bearing surface) | | Cosmetic Use | It has a 0.2 mm. needle length. The length is below the pain threshold, so painless delivery | [273] |
| CIT-8 (Collagen Induction Therapy) | | Medical type | It is used for collagen induction and skin remodeling therapy. It has a 0.5 mm needle length. | [273] |
| MF-8 | | Creating deeper microchannels on the epidermis | Needle length of 1.5 mm, its deep penetration is targeted for destroying bundles of scar collagen | [273] |
| MS-4 | | Facial acne scars | The needles have 1.5 mm in length and 4 circular arrays. Its use is preferred where better precision and penetration in deep location is required. | [273] |

## 11. Patents

MNs are a new approach to administered medications via the stratum corneum [144]. MNs are well-known for their efficiency, and they have been widely employed in the delivery of insulin, biological macromolecules, and vaccinations. Nevertheless, their minimal invasiveness, stability concerns, and non-compliance are a source of concern, necessitating highly competent medical practitioners to administer them [274]. MNs have shown their potential in this context since they can administer medications with ease, painlessly, and safely without specialized storage conditions. Here, some patents are briefed, which summarize its scope. Table 4 shows recent patents on MNs for different applications.

**Table 4.** Recent patents on MNs.

| Patent No. | Title of Patent | Aim | Description |
|---|---|---|---|
| US 10,898,703 B2 | MNs template and MNs prepared using the same. | Preparation of MNs template; Preparation of MNs, using a prepared template and MNs preparation method. | An MNs template includes a substrate on which a minimum of one MNs shape is projected to which at least one diamond layer is formed on the MNs surface. |
| US 2021/0008360 A1 | Adhesion membrane and MNs patch | To provide a new patch with excellent flexibility to skin, which carries an MNs array patch. | MNs provide excellent skin punctures and also stay on the skin; Provides variation in puncture property depending on the elasticity of the skin. |
| US 2021/0030975 A1 | Application for applying an MNs device to the skin | An applicator, method for application of MNs device to the skin | Applying the MNs device on the skin delivers active ingredients for treatment using applicators and methods. |
| US 10,946,180 B2 | Applicators for MNs | Description of micro projection array for MNs application | Applicator and method for applying MNs for treatment. |
| US 10,973,757 B2 | Biodegradable MNs device | To provide one or more biodegradable MNs capable of drug administration to the skin. | The invented device is embodied in MNs form for skin applications. At least one biodegradable MNs is projected from the cap with the lower surface abutted. MN projection is formed by a polymeric blend of preserved stem cell factors. |
| US2021/0046299A1 | Composite MNs array including nanostructures thereon | A composite MNs array overlays the film (consists of a plurality of nano-sized structures fabricated thereon) with MNs. | MNs array and MNs assembly and film consist of a plurality of nano-sized structures fabricated for drug delivery applications. |
| US 2021/0106520 A1 | Conductive polymer MNs arrays for electronically controlled drug release | A method that delivers a therapeutic agent, provided with an MNs array, also includes a plurality of MNs, including conductive coating disposal. | Conductive coating derived controlled therapeutic agent release by using MNs array implant in and across the dura mater to CNS of the subject. |
| US 10,987, 503 B2 | Dissolvable MNs for skin treatment | A skin treatment includes MNs application on the skin and penetration to the stratum corneum. | Polymeric MNs and their methods as a skin treatment device |
| US 10,994,111 B2 | Drug holding MNs array and manufacturing method thereof | To provide a drug-holding MNs array, where the drug is applied and held on the area of the tip of the MNs, for holding the dose capacity and prevention of drug spillage during insertion. | Technique for drug holding into MNs by step formation on MNs for quantitative dose administration |
| US 2021/0106259 A1 | The electrically functional polymer MN array | A sensor (biosensor) device comprises a polysubstrate substance structured to form MNs. | A device with electrodes, related devices, apparatus and fabrication methods, and devices use |
| US8708966B2 | MNs devices and methods of manufacture and use thereof | A method for delivering the active agent across a biological barrier | Devices with MNs are available for transporting compounds across tissue barriers and serving as microflameholders |

## 12. Conclusions

This review article extensively describes the type of microneedle, fabrication material, detailed casting methods and techniques, and its applications. Microneedles have been fabricated using different materials, like silicon, metals, polymers, and ceramics, by several fabrication methods, i.e., lithography, wet and dry etching, laser cutting and micro molding. The practical use of microneedles has been acknowledged and gained widespread attention. Optimization of sharpness, length, insertion force and velocity, and other parameters have allowed reliable microneedle insertion into the skin. Nowadays, MNs are the leading novel technology for several fields of drug delivery, such as intradermal, ocular and intracellular drug delivery. However, the transdermal route is still the leading application area for MNs, especially vaccine-based delivery. MNs technology creates a new horizon in cancer therapy through efficient drug delivery of anticancer vaccines and drugs. Various chemotherapeutic agents, genes and proteins can be efficiently delivered through MN-based devices. Patients and clinical workers are highly inclined to prefer microneedle-based delivery over hypodermic injections according to surveys. Human subjects report little or no pain associated with most microneedle designs. After microneedle treatment, the skin often shows mild, transient erythema, but there is currently no evidence of increased infection risk at the treatment site. Big pharmaceutical giants are currently working on the developments and commercialization of microneedle-based drug delivery systems; this technology is rated in the top 10 recent technologies. Patients, healthcare providers and companies have established interest in the technology. Microneedles are poised to make an expanded impact on clinical medicine over the coming years.

## 13. Future Scope

Microneedles are being studied worldwide as a drug delivery system for various ailments, including treatment of all diseases and vaccination. The development of sophisticated delivery systems like MNs could boost the efficiency of drug administration and lower the total dose concentration to minimize side effects. Some characteristics, such as the needle dissolution rate, can affect bioavailability. As a result, changing the needle geometry and size could assist us in achieving a more profound transdermal drug release. Novel MNs production technologies have resulted from much research in this field. MNs devices improve patient compliance by avoiding site-specific infections caused by conventional needles. However, the discovery of innovative micro-fabrication processes and stability medicines for MNs devices remains a challenge. Some of the primary reasons driving the market expansion include the increased prevalence of chronic hyperpigmentation and skin infections worldwide. Another factor driving the market over the forecast period is the low cost of microneedle devices compared to plastic surgery. MNs are also anticipated to be a revolutionary tool in the Cosmetic Industry. Furthermore, changing lifestyles are predicted to increase skin infections, and the availability of at-home micro-needling devices is expected to drive market expansion. Lack of experience, lack of public consciousness, and treatment side effects are some of the limitations on market growth.

**Author Contributions:** Conceptualization, D.K., F.D., S.R. (Satish Rojekar), D.D., S.M., A.A.M., P.M., R.P., J.V., M.B., M.Z. and P.S.G., M.H.R.; methodology, S.R. (Sarker Ramproshad), F.D., S.C. and P.S.G.; software, D.D., S.M., A.A.M., P.M., R.P. and J.V.; validation, S.R. (Satish Rojekar) F.D. and P.S.G.; formal analysis, S.R. (Satish Rojekar), D.D., S.M., A.A.M., P.M., R.P. and J.V.; investigation, S.R. (Sarker Ramproshad), F.D. and P.S.G.; resources, S.R. (Satish Rojekar), F.D. and P.S.G.; data curation, S.R. (Sarker Ramproshad) F.D. and P.S.G.; writing—original draft preparation, D.K., F.D., S.R. (Sarker Ramproshad), D.D., S.M., A.A.M., P.M., R.P., J.V., M.B. and P.S.G.; writing—review and editing, D.K., F.D., S.R. (Satish Rojekar), D.D., S.M., A.A.M., P.M., R.P., J.V., M.B. and P.S.G.; supervision, M.B. and S.C. All authors have read and agreed to the published version of the manuscript.

**Funding:** The publication fee for this manuscript was supported by the University of Oradea, Romania.

**Institutional Review Board Statement:** Not applicable.

**Informed Consent Statement:** Not applicable.

**Data Availability Statement:** This research did not report any data.

**Acknowledgments:** Prabhanjan S. Giram would like to acknowledge Dr. DY Patil Institute of Pharmaceutical Sciences and Research, Pimpri, Pune 411018 Sciences and Research, Pimpri, Pune-411018 for the facility providing for literature search and review writing.

**Conflicts of Interest:** The authors declare no conflict of interest.

## References

1. Goldberg, M.; Gomez-Orellana, I. Challenges for the Oral Delivery of Macromolecules. *Nat. Rev. Drug Discov.* **2003**, *2*, 289–295. [CrossRef] [PubMed]
2. Scheuplein, R.J.; Blank, I.H. Permeability of the Skin. *Physiol. Rev.* **1971**, *51*, 702–747. [CrossRef] [PubMed]
3. Nazary Abrbekoh, F.; Salimi, L.; Saghati, S.; Amini, H.; Fathi Karkan, S.; Moharamzadeh, K.; Sokullu, E.; Rahbarghazi, R. Application of microneedle patches for drug delivery; doorstep to novel therapies. *J. Tissue Eng.* **2022**, *13*, 20417314221085390. [CrossRef] [PubMed]
4. Donnelly, R.F.; Singh, T.R.R.; Woolfson, A.D. Microneedle-Based Drug Delivery Systems: Microfabrication, Drug Delivery, and Safety. *Drug Deliv.* **2010**, *17*, 187–207. [CrossRef]
5. Donnelly, R.; Douroumis, D. Microneedles for Drug and Vaccine Delivery and Patient Monitoring. *Drug Deliv. Transl. Res.* **2015**, *5*, 311–312. [CrossRef]
6. Aldawood, F.K.; Andar, A.; Desai, S. A Comprehensive Review of Microneedles: Types, Materials, Processes, Characterizations and Applications. *Polymers* **2021**, *13*, 2815. [CrossRef]
7. Jakka, D.; Matadh, A.V.; Shivakumar, H.N.; Maibach, H.; Murthy, S.N. Polymer Coated Polymeric (PCP) microneedles for sampling of drugs and biomarkers from tissues. *Eur. J. Pharm. Sci.* **2022**, 106203, *in press*. [CrossRef]
8. Kim, Y.C.; Prausnitz, M.R. Enabling Skin Vaccination Using New Delivery Technologies. *Drug Deliv. Transl. Res.* **2011**, *1*, 7–12. [CrossRef]
9. Kabir, M.T.; Ferdous Mitu, J.; Akter, R.; Akhtar, M.F.; Saleem, A.; Al-Harrasi, A.; Bhatia, S.; Rahman, M.S.; Damiri, F.; Berrada, M.; et al. Therapeutic Potential of Dopamine Agonists in the Treatment of Type 2 Diabetes Mellitus. *Environ. Sci. Pollut. Res.* **2022**. [CrossRef]
10. Vora, L.K.; Moffatt, K.; Tekko, I.A.; Paredes, A.J.; Volpe-Zanutto, F.; Mishra, D.; Peng, K.; Raj Singh Thakur, R.; Donnelly, R.F. Microneedle Array Systems for Long-Acting Drug Delivery. *Eur. J. Pharm. Biopharm.* **2021**, *159*, 44–76. [CrossRef]
11. Zhang, W.; Zuo, H.; Cheng, Z.; Shi, Y.; Guo, Z.; Meng, N.; Thomas, A.; Liao, Y. Macroscale Conjugated Microporous Polymers: Controlling Versatile Functionalities over Several Dimensions. *Adv. Mater. (Deerfield Beach Fla.)* **2022**, *34*, e2104952. [CrossRef]
12. Microneedle Technologies for (Trans) Dermal Drug and Vaccine Delivery. Available online: https://www.sciencedirect.com/science/article/abs/pii/S0168365912000740 (accessed on 30 March 2022).
13. Nguyen, T.T.; Nguyen, T.T.D.; Tran, N.M.A.; Nguyen, H.T.; Vo, G.V. Microneedles Enable the Development of Skin-Targeted Vaccines against Coronaviruses and Influenza Viruses. *Pharm. Dev. Technol.* **2022**, *27*, 83–94. [CrossRef]
14. Microneedles: A Smart Approach and Increasing Potential for Transdermal Drug Delivery System. Available online: https://www.sciencedirect.com/science/article/pii/S0753332218348091 (accessed on 8 March 2022).
15. Li, J.; Xiang, H.; Zhang, Q.; Miao, X. Polysaccharide-Based Transdermal Drug Delivery. *Pharmaceuticals* **2022**, *15*, 602. [CrossRef]
16. Benson, H.A.; Grice, J.E.; Mohammed, Y.; Namjoshi, S.; Roberts, M.S. Topical and Transdermal Drug Delivery: From Simple Potions to Smart Technologies. *Curr. Drug Deliv.* **2019**, *16*, 444–460. [CrossRef]
17. Sachdeva, V.; Banga, A.K. Microneedles and Their Applications. *Recent Pat. Drug Deliv. Formul.* **2011**, *5*, 95–132. [CrossRef]
18. Zhang, P.; Zhang, Y.; Liu, C.G. Polymeric Nanoparticles Based on Carboxymethyl Chitosan in Combination with Painless Microneedle Therapy Systems for Enhancing Transdermal Insulin Delivery. *RSC Adv.* **2020**, *10*, 24319–24329. [CrossRef]
19. Yeo, L.Y.; Chang, H.C.; Chan, P.P.Y.; Friend, J.R. Microfluidic Devices for Bioapplications. *Small* **2011**, *7*, 12–48. [CrossRef]
20. Ita, K. Transdermal Delivery of Drugs with Microneedles—Potential and Challenges. *Pharmaceutics* **2015**, *7*, 90–105. [CrossRef]
21. Khandan, O.; Kahook, M.; Rao, M. Fenestrated Microneedles for Ocular Drug Delivery. *Sens. Actuators B Chem.* **2016**, *223*, 15–23. [CrossRef]
22. Aditya, A. *Optimization of Collagen Microneedle Using Taguchi Method*; The University of Texas at El Paso: El Paso, TX, USA, 2017.
23. Pendse, P.A. *Skin Response to Immunogenic and non Immunogenic Material as Applied to Vaccine Delivery and Reconstructive Surgery*; Mercer University: Macon, GA, USA, 2006.
24. Gao, N.; Zhu, J.L.; Su, A.L.; Kou, L.L.; Liu, Z. Five-in-one: A novel, cost-effective yet simple use of micro needle holder. *Int. J. Ophthalmol.* **2022**, *15*, 657–660. [CrossRef]
25. Donnelly, R.F.; Singh, T.R.R.; Larrañeta, E.; McCrudden, M.T. *Microneedles for Drug and Vaccine Delivery and Patient Monitoring*; John Wiley & Sons: Hoboken, NJ, USA, 2018.
26. Microneedle, Bio-Microneedle and Bio-Inspired Microneedle: A Review. Available online: https://www.sciencedirect.com/science/article/abs/pii/S0168365917300627 (accessed on 30 March 2022).
27. Monitoring the Penetration Process of Single Microneedles with Varying Tip Diameters. Available online: https://www.sciencedirect.com/science/article/pii/S1751616114002999 (accessed on 30 March 2022).

28. Shravanth, S.H.; Osmani, R.A.M.; Anupama, V.P.; Rahamathulla, M.; Gangadharappa, H.V. Microneedles-Based Drug Delivery for the Treatment of Psoriasis. *J. Drug Deliv. Sci. Technol.* **2021**, *64*, 102668. [CrossRef]
29. Díaz-Gómez, L.; Concheiro, A.; Alvarez-Lorenzo, C. Polymers in Drug Delivery: Fundamentals. In *Advanced Polymers in Medicine*; Puoci, F., Ed.; Springer International Publishing: Cham, Switzerland, 2015; pp. 319–339. ISBN 978-3-319-12478-0.
30. Nagarkar, R.; Singh, M.; Nguyen, H.X.; Jonnalagadda, S. A Review of Recent Advances in Microneedle Technology for Transdermal Drug Delivery. *J. Drug Deliv. Sci. Technol.* **2020**, *59*, 101923. [CrossRef]
31. Miyano, T.; Tobinaga, Y.; Kanno, T.; Matsuzaki, Y.; Takeda, H.; Wakui, M.; Hanada, K. Sugar Micro Needles as Transdermic Drug Delivery System. *Biomed. Microdevices* **2005**, *7*, 185–188. [CrossRef]
32. Lagreca, E.; Onesto, V.; Di Natale, C.; La Manna, S.; Netti, P.A.; Vecchione, R. Recent Advances in the Formulation of PLGA Microparticles for Controlled Drug Delivery. *Prog. Biomater.* **2020**, *9*, 153–174. [CrossRef]
33. Dissolving Polymeric Microneedle Arrays for Electrically Assisted Transdermal Drug Delivery. Available online: https://www.sciencedirect.com/science/article/abs/pii/S0168365912000089 (accessed on 7 March 2022).
34. Rodgers, A.M.; Cordeiro, A.S.; Donnelly, R.F. Technology Update: Dissolvable Microneedle Patches for Vaccine Delivery. *Med. Devices (Auckl)* **2019**, *12*, 379–398. [CrossRef]
35. Leone, M.; Mönkäre, J.; Bouwstra, J.A.; Kersten, G. Dissolving Microneedle Patches for Dermal Vaccination. *Pharm. Res.* **2017**, *34*, 2223–2240. [CrossRef]
36. Damiri, F.; Kommineni, N.; Ebhodaghe, S.O.; Bulusu, R.; Jyothi, V.G.S.; Sayed, A.A.; Awaji, A.A.; Germoush, M.O.; Al-Malky, H.S.; Nasrullah, M.Z. Microneedle-Based Natural Polysaccharide for Drug Delivery Systems (DDS): Progress and Challenges. *Pharmaceuticals* **2022**, *15*, 190. [CrossRef]
37. Cavalu, S.; Ratiu, C.; Ponta, O.; Simon, V.; Rugina, D.; Miclaus, V.; Akin, I.; Goller, G. Improving osseointegration of alumina/zirconia ceramic implants by fluoride surface treatment. *Dig. J. Nanomater. Biostruct.* **2014**, *9*, 797–808.
38. Swathi, H.P.; Anusha Matadh, V.; Paul Guin, J.; Narasimha Murthy, S.; Kanni, P.; Varshney, L.; Suresh, S.; Shivakumar, H.N. Effect of Gamma Sterilization on the Properties of Microneedle Array Transdermal Patch System. *Drug Dev. Ind. Pharm.* **2020**, *46*, 606–620. [CrossRef]
39. Giri Nandagopal, M.S.; Antony, R.; Rangabhashiyam, S.; Sreekumar, N.; Selvaraju, N. Overview of Microneedle System: A Third Generation Transdermal Drug Delivery Approach. *Microsyst. Technol.* **2014**, *20*, 1249–1272. [CrossRef]
40. Cormier, M.; Johnson, B.; Ameri, M.; Nyam, K.; Libiran, L.; Zhang, D.D.; Daddona, P. Transdermal Delivery of Desmopressin Using a Coated Microneedle Array Patch System. *J. Control. Release* **2004**, *97*, 503–511. [CrossRef]
41. Chong, R.H.E.; Gonzalez-Gonzalez, E.; Lara, M.F.; Speaker, T.J.; Contag, C.H.; Kaspar, R.L.; Coulman, S.A.; Hargest, R.; Birchall, J.C. Gene Silencing Following SiRNA Delivery to Skin via Coated Steel Microneedles: In Vitro and in Vivo Proof-of-Concept. *J. Control. Release* **2013**, *166*, 211–219. [CrossRef] [PubMed]
42. Prausnitz, M.R. Microneedles for Transdermal Drug Delivery. *Adv. Drug Deliv. Rev.* **2004**, *56*, 581–587. [CrossRef] [PubMed]
43. Boehm, R.D.; Daniels, J.; Stafslien, S.; Nasir, A.; Lefebvre, J.; Narayan, R.J. Polyglycolic Acid Microneedles Modified with Inkjet-Deposited Antifungal Coatings. *Biointerphases* **2015**, *10*, 011004. [CrossRef]
44. Sharma, S.; Hatware, K.; Bhadane, P.; Sindhikar, S.; Mishra, D.K. Recent Advances in Microneedle Composites for Biomedical Applications: Advanced Drug Delivery Technologies. *Mater. Sci. Eng. C* **2019**, *103*, 109717. [CrossRef]
45. Donnelly, R.F.; McCrudden, M.T.C.; Alkilani, A.Z.; Larrañeta, E.; McAlister, E.; Courtenay, A.J.; Kearney, M.C.; Raj Singh, T.R.; McCarthy, H.O.; Kett, V.L.; et al. Hydrogel-Forming Microneedles Prepared from "Super Swelling" Polymers Combined with Lyophilised Wafers for Transdermal Drug Deliqvery. *PLoS ONE* **2014**, *9*, e111547. [CrossRef]
46. Griss, P.; Stemme, G. Side-Opened out-of-Plane Microneedles for Microfluidic Transdermal Liquid Transfer. *J. Microelectromechanical Syst.* **2003**, *12*, 296–301. [CrossRef]
47. Nawar, A.E. Modified Microneedle for Suprachoroidal Injection of Triamcinolone Acetonide Combined with Intravitreal Injection of Ranibizumab in Branch Retinal Vein Occlusion Patients. *Clin. Ophthalmol.* **2022**, *16*, 1139–1151. [CrossRef]
48. Raghu, T.; Singh, R.; Mccarron, P.A.; Woolfson, A.D.; Donnelly, R.F. Investigation of Swelling and Network Parameters of Poly (Ethylene Glycol)-Crosslinked Poly (Methyl Vinyl Ether-Co-Maleic Acid) Hydrogels. *Eur. Polym. J.* **2009**, *45*, 1239–1249. [CrossRef]
49. Karelin, A.M.; Orekhov, Y.D.; Luchinin, V.V.; Gareev, K.G.; Khmelnitskiy, I.K.; Testov, D.O. Development of a Modular Reconfigurable Mold for Prototyping of Hollow Microneedles. In Proceedings of the 2022 Conference of Russian Young Researchers in Electrical and Electronic Engineering (ElConRus), St. Petersburg, Russia, 25–28 January 2022; pp. 1531–1533.
50. Mishra, R.; Maiti, T.K.; Bhattacharyya, T.K. Development of SU-8 Hollow Microneedles on a Silicon Substrate with Microfluidic Interconnects for Transdermal Drug Delivery. *J. Micromech. Microeng.* **2018**, *28*, 105017. [CrossRef]
51. Makvandi, P.; Kirkby, M.; Hutton, A.R.J.; Shabani, M.; Yiu, C.K.Y.; Baghbantaraghdari, Z.; Jamaledin, R.; Carlotti, M.; Mazzolai, B.; Mattoli, V.; et al. Engineering Microneedle Patches for Improved Penetration: Analysis, Skin Models and Factors Affecting Needle Insertion. *Nano-Micro Lett.* **2021**, *13*, 93. [CrossRef]
52. Kumar, V.; Pallapa, M.; Rezai, P.; Selvaganapathy, P.R. Polymers. *Ref. Modul. Mater. Sci. Mater. Eng.* **2016**. [CrossRef]
53. Jiang, J.; Moore, J.S.; Edelhauser, H.F.; Prausnitz, M.R. Intrascleral Drug Delivery to the Eye Using Hollow Microneedles. *Pharm. Res.* **2009**, *26*, 395–403. [CrossRef]
54. Anand, P.; Tripathi, N. A Procedural Excursion of Micro Needles for Drug Delivery Systems. *Micro Nanosyst.* **2020**, *12*, 232–239. [CrossRef]

55. 3D-Printed Microneedles in Biomedical Applications. Available online: https://www.sciencedirect.com/science/article/pii/S2589004220312098 (accessed on 31 March 2022).
56. He, X.; Sun, J.; Zhuang, J.; Xu, H.; Liu, Y.; Wu, D. Microneedle System for Transdermal Drug and Vaccine Delivery: Devices, Safety, and Prospects. *Dose-Response* **2019**, *17*, 1559325819878585. Available online: https://journals.sagepub.com/doi/10.1177/1559325819878585 (accessed on 31 March 2022). [CrossRef]
57. Iliescu, F.; Dumitrescu-Ionescu, D.; Petrescu, M.; Iliescu, C. A Review on Transdermal Drug Delivery Using Microneedles: Current Research and Perspective. *Ann. Acad. Rom. Sci. Ser. Sci. Technol. Inf.* **2014**, *7*, 734.
58. Bhatnagar, S.; Gadeela, P.R.; Thathireddy, P.; Venuganti, V.V.K. Microneedle-Based Drug Delivery: Materials of Construction. *J. Chem. Sci.* **2019**, *131*, 90. [CrossRef]
59. Gill, H.S.; Prausnitz, M.R. Coated Microneedles for Transdermal Delivery. *J. Control. Release* **2007**, *117*, 227–237. [CrossRef]
60. Kim, Y.C.; Park, J.H.; Prausnitz, M.R. Microneedles for Drug and Vaccine Delivery. *Adv. Drug Deliv. Rev.* **2012**, *64*, 1547–1568. [CrossRef]
61. Kim, Y.C.; Quan, F.S.; Compans, R.W.; Kang, S.M.; Prausnitz, M.R. Formulation and Coating of Microneedles with Inactivated Influenza Virus to Improve Vaccine Stability and Immunogenicity. *J. Control. Release* **2010**, *142*, 187–195. [CrossRef]
62. Choi, H.J.; Bondy, B.J.; Yoo, D.G.; Compans, R.W.; Kang, S.M.; Prausnitz, M.R. Stability of Whole Inactivated Influenza Virus Vaccine during Coating onto Metal Microneedles. *J. Control. Release* **2013**, *166*, 159–171. [CrossRef]
63. Ita, K. Transdermal Delivery of Drugs with Microneedles: Strategies and Outcomes. *J. Drug Deliv. Sci. Technol.* **2015**, *29*, 16–23. [CrossRef]
64. Amarnani, R.; Shende, P. Microneedles in diagnostic, treatment and theranostics: An advancement in minimally-invasive delivery system. *Biomed Microdevices.* **2021**, *24*, 4. [CrossRef]
65. Ahmed Saeed AL-Japairai, K.; Mahmood, S.; Hamed Almurisi, S.; Reddy Venugopal, J.; Rebhi Hilles, A.; Azmana, M.; Raman, S. Current Trends in Polymer Microneedle for Transdermal Drug Delivery. *Int. J. Pharm.* **2020**, *587*, 119673. [CrossRef]
66. Pawley, D.C.; Goncalves, S.; Bas, E.; Dikici, E.; Deo, S.K.; Daunert, S.; Telischi, F. Dexamethasone (DXM)-Coated Poly(Lactic-Co-Glycolic Acid) (PLGA) Microneedles as an Improved Drug Delivery System for Intracochlear Biodegradable Devices. *Adv. Ther.* **2021**, *4*, 2100155. [CrossRef]
67. Wu, L.; Shrestha, P.; Iapichino, M.; Cai, Y.; Kim, B.; Stoeber, B. Characterization Method for Calculating Diffusion Coefficient of Drug from Polylactic Acid (PLA) Microneedles into the Skin. *J. Drug Deliv. Sci. Technol.* **2021**, *61*, 102192. [CrossRef]
68. Li, X.; Xu, Q.; Wang, J.; Zhang, P.; Wang, Y.; Ji, J. A Gene-Coated Microneedle Patch Based on Industrialized Ultrasonic Spraying Technology with a Polycation Vector to Improve Antitumor Efficacy. *J. Mater. Chem. B* **2021**, *9*, 5528–5536. [CrossRef] [PubMed]
69. Epigallocatechin Gallate/L-Ascorbic Acid–Loaded Poly-γ-Glutamate Microneedles with Antioxidant, Anti-Inflammatory, and Immunomodulatory Effects for the Treatment of Atopic Dermatitis. Available online: https://www.sciencedirect.com/science/article/abs/pii/S1742706121003421 (accessed on 7 April 2022).
70. Saha, I.; Rai, V.K. Hyaluronic Acid Based Microneedle Array: Recent Applications in Drug Delivery and Cosmetology. *Carbohydr. Polym.* **2021**, *267*, 118168. [CrossRef] [PubMed]
71. Zare, M.R.; Khorram, M.; Barzegar, S.; Sarkari, B.; Asgari, Q.; Ahadian, S.; Zomorodian, K. Dissolvable Carboxymethyl Cellulose/Polyvinylpyrrolidone Microneedle Arrays for Transdermal Delivery of Amphotericin B to Treat Cutaneous Leishmaniasis. *Int. J. Biol. Macromol.* **2021**, *182*, 1310–1321. [CrossRef] [PubMed]
72. Zhang, X.P.; Wang, B.B.; Li, W.X.; Fei, W.M.; Cui, Y.; Guo, X.D. In Vivo Safety Assessment, Biodistribution and Toxicology of Polyvinyl Alcohol Microneedles with 160-Day Uninterruptedly Applications in Mice. *Eur. J. Pharm. Biopharm.* **2021**, *160*, 1–8. [CrossRef] [PubMed]
73. Lu, X.; Sun, Y.; Han, M.; Chen, D.; Wang, A.; Sun, K. Silk Fibroin Double-Layer Microneedles for the Encapsulation and Controlled Release of Triptorelin. *Int. J. Pharm.* **2022**, *613*, 121433. [CrossRef]
74. Zhou, Z.; Xing, M.; Zhang, S.; Yang, G.; Gao, Y. Process Optimization of Ca2+ Cross-Linked Alginate-Based Swellable Microneedles for Enhanced Transdermal Permeability: More Applicable to Acidic Drugs. *Int. J. Pharm.* **2022**, *618*, 121669. [CrossRef]
75. Yu, X.; Wang, C.; Wang, Y.; Li, L.; Gao, X.; Zhu, T.; An, P.; Meng, Z.; Wang, W.; Wu, T.; et al. Microneedle Array Patch Made of Kangfuxin/Chitosan/Fucoidan Complex Enables Full-Thickness Wound Healing. *Front. Chem.* **2022**, *10*, 838920. [CrossRef]
76. Nguyen, T.T.; Nguyen, T.T.D.; Tran, N.M.A.; Vo, G.V. Advances of Microneedles in Hormone Delivery. *Biomed. Pharmacother.* **2022**, *145*, 112393. [CrossRef]
77. Azmana, M.; Mahmood, S.; Hilles, A.R.; Mandal, U.K.; Saeed Al-Japairai, K.A.; Raman, S. Transdermal Drug Delivery System through Polymeric Microneedle: A Recent Update. *J. Drug Deliv. Sci. Technol.* **2020**, *60*, 101877. [CrossRef]
78. Martin, C.J.; Allender, C.J.; Brain, K.R.; Morrissey, A.; Birchall, J.C. Low Temperature Fabrication of Biodegradable Sugar Glass Microneedles for Transdermal Drug Delivery Applications. *J. Control. Release* **2012**, *158*, 93–101. [CrossRef]
79. Thakor, N.; Lütke-Eversloh, T.; Steinbüchel, A. Application of the BPEC Pathway for Large-Scale Biotechnological Production of Poly(3-Mercaptopropionate) by Recombinant Escherichia Coli, Including a Novel in Situ Isolation Method. *Appl. Environ. Microbiol.* **2005**, *71*, 835–841. [CrossRef]
80. Iwata, S.; Toshima, K.; Matsumura, S. Enzyme-Catalyzed Preparation of Aliphatic Polyesters Containing Thioester Linkages. *Macromol. Rapid Commun.* **2003**, *24*, 467–471. [CrossRef]
81. Hakkarainen, M.; Albertsson, A.C. Environmental Degradation of Polyethylene. *Adv. Polym. Sci.* **2004**, *169*, 177–199. [CrossRef]

82. Rose, K.; Steinbüchel, A. Biodegradation of Natural Rubber and Related Compounds: Recent Insights into a Hardly Understood Catabolic Capability of Microorganisms. *Appl. Environ. Microbiol.* **2005**, *71*, 2803–2812. [CrossRef]
83. Steinbüchel, A. Non-Biodegradable Biopolymers from Renewable Resources: Perspectives and Impacts. *Curr. Opin. Biotechnol.* **2005**, *16*, 607–613. [CrossRef]
84. Cavalu, S.; Bisboaca, S.; Mates, I.M.; Pasca, P.M.; Laslo, V.; Costea, T.; Fritea, L.; Vicas, S. Novel Formulation Based on Chitosan-Arabic Gum Nanoparticles Entrapping Propolis Extract. Production, physico-chemical and structural characterization. *Rev. Chim.* **2018**, *69*, 3756–3760. [CrossRef]
85. Antonescu, A.I.; Miere, F.; Fritea, L.; Ganea, M.; Zdrinca, M.; Dobjanschi, L.; Antonescu, A.; Vicas, S.I.; Bodog, F.; Sindhu, R.K.; et al. Perspectives on the Combined Effects of Ocimum Basilicum and Trifolium Pratense Extracts in Terms of Phytochemical Profile and Pharmacological Effects. *Plants* **2021**, *10*, 1390. [CrossRef]
86. Ray, S.; Wirth, D.M.; Ortega-Rivera, O.A.; Steinmetz, N.F.; Pokorski, J.K. Dissolving Microneedle Delivery of a Prophylactic HPV Vaccine. *Biomacromolecules* **2022**, *23*, 903–912. [CrossRef]
87. Qi, X.; Tong, X.; Pan, W.; Zeng, Q.; You, S.; Shen, J. Recent Advances in Polysaccharide-Based Adsorbents for Wastewater Treatment. *J. Clean. Prod.* **2021**, *315*, 128221. [CrossRef]
88. Tong, X.; Pan, W.; Su, T.; Zhang, M.; Dong, W.; Qi, X. Recent Advances in Natural Polymer-Based Drug Delivery Systems. *React. Funct. Polym.* **2020**, *148*, 104501. [CrossRef]
89. Qi, X.; Pan, W.; Tong, X.; Gao, T.; Xiang, Y.; You, S.; Mao, R.; Chi, J.; Hu, R.; Zhang, W.; et al. E-Polylysine-Stabilized Agarose/Polydopamine Hydrogel Dressings with Robust Photothermal Property for Wound Healing. *Carbohydr. Polym.* **2021**, *264*, 118046. [CrossRef]
90. Kutbi, H.I.; Asfour, H.Z.; Kammoun, A.K.; Sirwi, A.; Cavalu, S.; Gad, H.A. Optimization of Hyaluronate-Based Liposomes to Augment the Oral Delivery and the Bioavailability of Berberine. *Materials* **2021**, *14*, 5759. [CrossRef]
91. Zhu, J.; Dong, L.; Du, H.; Mao, J.; Xie, Y.; Wang, H.; Lan, J.; Lou, Y.; Fu, Y.; Wen, J.; et al. 5-Aminolevulinic Acid-Loaded Hyaluronic Acid Dissolving Microneedles for Effective Photodynamic Therapy of Superficial Tumors with Enhanced Long-Term Stability. *Adv. Healthc. Mater.* **2019**, *8*, 1900896. [CrossRef]
92. Xu, Q.; Li, X.; Zhang, P.; Wang, Y. Rapidly Dissolving Microneedle Patch for Synergistic Gene and Photothermal Therapy of Subcutaneous Tumor. *J. Mater. Chem. B* **2020**, *8*, 4331–4339. [CrossRef]
93. Hao, Y.; Chen, Y.; He, X.; Yang, F.; Han, R.; Yang, C.; Li, W.; Qian, Z. Near-Infrared Responsive 5-Fluorouracil and Indocyanine Green Loaded MPEG-PCL Nanoparticle Integrated with Dissolvable Microneedle for Skin Cancer Therapy. *Bioact. Mater.* **2020**, *5*, 542–552. [CrossRef] [PubMed]
94. Hao, Y.; Li, W.; Zhou, X.; Yang, F.; Qian, Z. Microneedles-Based Transdermal Drug Delivery Systems: A Review. *J. Biomed. Nanotechnol.* **2017**, *13*, 1581–1597. [CrossRef] [PubMed]
95. Fukushima, K.; Ise, A.; Morita, H.; Hasegawa, R.; Ito, Y.; Sugioka, N.; Takada, K. Two-Layered Dissolving Microneedles for Percutaneous Delivery of Peptide/Protein Drugs in Rats. *Pharm. Res.* **2011**, *28*, 7–21. [CrossRef] [PubMed]
96. Poirier, D.; Renaud, F.; Dewar, V.; Strodiot, L.; Wauters, F.; Janimak, J.; Shimada, T.; Nomura, T.; Kabata, K.; Kuruma, K.; et al. Hepatitis B Surface Antigen Incorporated in Dissolvable Microneedle Array Patch Is Antigenic and Thermostable. *Biomaterials* **2017**, *145*, 256–265. [CrossRef] [PubMed]
97. Shokri, J.; Adibkia, K. *Application of Cellulose and Cellulose Derivatives in Pharmaceutical Industries*; IntechOpen: London, UK, 2013; ISBN 978-953-51-1191-7.
98. Falo, L.D., Jr.; Erdos, G.; Ozdoganlar, O.B. Microneedle Arrays for Cancer Therapy Applications. Patent 14/934,927, 19 May 2016.
99. Lan, X.; Zhu, W.; Huang, X.; Yu, Y.; Xiao, H.; Jin, L.; Jane Pu, J.; Xie, X.; She, J.; Yan Lui, V.W.; et al. Microneedles Loaded with Anti-PD-1–Cisplatin Nanoparticles for Synergistic Cancer Immuno-Chemotherapy. *Nanoscale* **2020**, *12*, 18885–18898. [CrossRef]
100. Ye, C.; Zhang, R. Semiconductor Microneedle Assembly Based on Gene Therapy, Manufacturing Method and Manufacturing Mold. Chinese Patent CN106426729A, 17 February 2022.
101. Bacterial Nanocellulose-Hyaluronic Acid Microneedle Patches for Skin Applications: In Vitro and in Vivo Evaluation. Available online: https://www.sciencedirect.com/science/article/pii/S0928493120332689 (accessed on 8 March 2022).
102. Chen, M.C.; Huang, S.F.; Lai, K.Y.; Ling, M.H. Fully Embeddable Chitosan Microneedles as a Sustained Release Depot for Intradermal Vaccination. *Biomaterials* **2013**, *34*, 3077–3086. [CrossRef]
103. Cavalu, S.; Simon, V. Microstructure and bioactivity of acrylic bone cements for prosthetic surgery. *J. Optoelectron. Adv. Mater.* **2006**, *8*, 1520–1523.
104. Moreira, A.F.; Rodrigues, C.F.; Jacinto, T.A.; Miguel, S.P.; Costa, E.C.; Correia, I.J. Poly (Vinyl Alcohol)/Chitosan Layer-by-Layer Microneedles for Cancer Chemo-Photothermal Therapy. *Int. J. Pharm.* **2020**, *576*, 118907. [CrossRef]
105. Ahmad, Z.; Khan, M.I.; Siddique, M.I.; Sarwar, H.S.; Shahnaz, G.; Hussain, S.Z.; Bukhari, N.I.; Hussain, I.; Sohail, M.F. Fabrication and Characterization of Thiolated Chitosan Microneedle Patch for Transdermal Delivery of Tacrolimus. *AAPS PharmSciTech* **2020**, *21*, 68. [CrossRef]
106. Chen, M.C.; Ling, M.H.; Lai, K.Y.; Pramudityo, E. Chitosan Microneedle Patches for Sustained Transdermal Delivery of Macromolecules. *Biomacromolecules* **2012**, *13*, 4022–4031. [CrossRef]
107. Zhang, Y.; Wu, M.; Tan, D.; Liu, Q.; Xia, R.; Chen, M.; Liu, Y.; Xue, L.; Lei, Y. A Dissolving and Glucose-Responsive Insulin-Releasing Microneedle Patch for Type 1 Diabetes Therapy. *J. Mater. Chem. B* **2021**, *9*, 648–657. [CrossRef]

108. Pineda-Álvarez, R.A.; Bernad-Bernad, M.J.; Rodríguez-Cruz, I.M.; Escobar-Chávez, J.J. Development and Characterization of Starch/Gelatin Microneedle Arrays Loaded with Lecithin–Gelatin Nanoparticles of Losartan for Transdermal Delivery. *J. Pharm. Innov.* **2020**. [CrossRef]
109. Li, J.; Zeng, M.; Shan, H.; Tong, C. Microneedle Patches as Drug and Vaccine Delivery Platform. *Curr. Med. Chem.* **2017**, *24*, 2413–2422. [CrossRef]
110. Donnelly, R.F.; Singh, T.R.R.; Morrow, D.I.; Woolfson, A.D. *Microneedle-Mediated Transdermal and Intradermal Drug Delivery*; Wiley-Blackwell: Hoboken, NJ, USA, 2012; Volume 17, pp. 71–84.
111. Sivamani, R.K.; Liepmann, D.; Maibach, H.I. Microneedles and Transdermal Applications. *Expert Opin. Drug Deliv.* **2007**, *4*, 19–25. [CrossRef]
112. Donnelly, R.F.; Singh, T.R.R.; Garland, M.J.; Migalska, K.; Majithiya, R.; McCrudden, C.M.; Kole, P.L.; Mahmood, T.M.T.; McCarthy, H.O.; Woolfson, A.D. Hydrogel-Forming Microneedle Arrays for Enhanced Transdermal Drug Delivery. *Adv. Funct. Mater.* **2012**, *22*, 4879–4890. [CrossRef]
113. Ashraf, M.W.; Tayyaba, S.; Afzulpurkar, N. Micro Electromechanical Systems (MEMS) Based Microfluidic Devices for Biomedical Applications. *Int. J. Mol. Sci.* **2011**, *12*, 3648–3704. [CrossRef]
114. Singh, T.R.R.; Mcmillan, H.; Mooney, K.; Alkilani, A.Z.; Donnelly, R.F. Microneedles for Drug Delivery and Monitoring. In *Microfluidic Devices for Biomedical Applications*; Li, X., Zhou, Y., Eds.; Woodhead Publishing Series in Biomaterials; Woodhead Publishing: Sawston, UK, 2013; pp. 185–230. ISBN 978-0-85709-697-5.
115. Roh, H.; Yoon, Y.J.; Park, J.S.; Kang, D.-H.; Kwak, S.M.; Lee, B.C.; Im, M. Fabrication of High-Density Out-of-Plane Microneedle Arrays with Various Heights and Diverse Cross-Sectional Shapes. *Nano-Micro Lett.* **2021**, *14*, 24. [CrossRef]
116. Influence of the Delivery Systems Using a Microneedle Array on the Permeation of a Hydrophilic Molecule, Calcein. Available online: https://www.sciencedirect.com/science/article/abs/pii/S0939641108000532 (accessed on 12 March 2022).
117. Chircov, C.; Grumezescu, A.M. Microelectromechanical Systems (MEMS) for Biomedical Applications. *Micromachines* **2022**, *13*, 164. [CrossRef] [PubMed]
118. 3D and 4D Lithography of Untethered Microrobots. Available online: https://www.sciencedirect.com/science/article/pii/S0079642521000323 (accessed on 12 March 2022).
119. Madou, M.J. *Fundamentals of Microfabrication*; CRC Press: Boca Raton, FL, USA, 1997.
120. Banks, D. *Microengineering, MEMS, and Interfacing: A Practical Guide*; CRC Press: Boca Raton, FL, USA, 2006.
121. Bariya, S.H.; Gohel, M.C.; Mehta, T.A.; Sharma, O.P. Microneedles: An Emerging Transdermal Drug Delivery System. *J. Pharm. Pharmacol.* **2012**, *64*, 11–29. [CrossRef] [PubMed]
122. El-Eskandarany, M.S. *Mechanical Alloying: Energy Storage, Protective Coatings, and Medical Applications*; William Andrew: Norwich, NY, USA, 2020.
123. Microfabrication Technologies Used for Creating Smart Devices for Industrial Applications. Available online: https://www.sciencedirect.com/science/article/pii/B9780081020555000115 (accessed on 8 March 2022).
124. What Is an Ion Plating?—Definition from Corrosionpedia. Available online: https://www.corrosionpedia.com/definition/685/ion-plating (accessed on 8 March 2022).
125. Nuxoll, E. BioMEMS in Drug Delivery. *Adv. Drug Deliv. Rev.* **2013**, *65*, 1611–1625. [CrossRef] [PubMed]
126. Madou, M.J. *Fundamentals of Microfabrication and Nanotechnology*; CRC Press: Boca Raton, FL, USA, 2012; ISBN 978-1-4822-7466-0.
127. Ji, Y.J.; Kim, K.S.; Kim, K.H.; Byun, J.Y.; Yeom, G.Y. A Brief Review of Plasma Enhanced Atomic Layer Deposition of Si3N4. *Appl. Sci. Converg. Technol.* **2019**, *28*, 142–147. [CrossRef]
128. Tran, K.T.M.; Nguyen, T.D. Lithography-Based Methods to Manufacture Biomaterials at Small Scales. *J. Sci. Adv. Mater. Devices* **2017**, *2*, 1–14. [CrossRef]
129. Madou, M.J. *Fundamentals of Microfabrication: The Science of Miniaturization*, 1st ed.; CRC Press: Boca Raton, FL, USA, 2002; ISBN 978-1-315-27422-5.
130. Madou, M.J. *Fundamentals of Microfabrication: The Science of Miniaturization*, 2nd ed.; CRC Press: Boca Raton, FL, USA, 2017.
131. Moreau, W.M. *Semiconductor Lithography: Principles, Practices, and Materials*; Springer Science & Business Media: Berlin, Germany, 2012.
132. Larrañeta, E.; Lutton, R.E.M.; Woolfson, A.D.; Donnelly, R.F. Microneedle Arrays as Transdermal and Intradermal Drug Delivery Systems: Materials Science, Manufacture and Commercial Development. *Mater. Sci. Eng. R Rep.* **2016**, *104*, 1–32. [CrossRef]
133. Bellah, M.M.; Christensen, S.M.; Iqbal, S.M. Nanostructures for Medical Diagnostics. *J. Nanomater.* **2012**, *2012*, e486301. [CrossRef]
134. Molecular Sensors and Nanodevices—2nd Edition. Available online: https://www.elsevier.com/books/molecular-sensors-and-nanodevices/zhang/978-0-12-814862-4 (accessed on 8 March 2022).
135. Deng, Z.; Yang, Q.; Chen, F.; Meng, X.; Bian, H.; Yong, J.; Shan, C.; Hou, X. Fabrication of Large-Area Concave Microlens Array on Silicon by Femtosecond Laser Micromachining. *Opt. Lett.* **2015**, *40*, 1928–1931. [CrossRef]
136. Garín, M.; Khoury, R.; Martín, I.; Johnson, E.V. Direct Etching at the Nanoscale through Nanoparticle-Directed Capillary Condensation. *Nanoscale* **2020**, *12*, 9240–9245. [CrossRef]
137. Virji, M.; Stefaniak, A. A Review of Engineered Nanomaterial Manufacturing Processes and Associated Exposure. In *Comprehensive Materials Processing*; Elsevier: Amsterdam, The Netherlands, 2014; Volume 8, pp. 103–125. ISBN 978-0-08-096533-8.
138. Holker, J.D.; Calle, G.A.; Branch, K.D.; Mastrototaro, J.J.; Antwerp, W.P.V. Analyte Sensor and Method of Making the Same. U.S. Patent US09502204, 19 November 2002.

139. Textile-Based Micro Electro Mechanical System (MEMS) Accelerometer for Pelvic Tilt Mesurement. Available online: https://www.sciencedirect.com/science/article/pii/S1877705812026082 (accessed on 12 March 2022).
140. Acid Etching of Human Enamel in Clinical Applications: A Systematic Review. Available online: https://www.sciencedirect.com/science/article/abs/pii/S002239131300379X (accessed on 12 March 2022).
141. Diéguez, L.; Winter, M.A.; Pocock, K.J.; Bremmell, K.E.; Thierry, B. Efficient Microfluidic Negative Enrichment of Circulating Tumor Cells in Blood Using Roughened PDMS. *Analyst* **2015**, *140*, 3565–3572. [CrossRef]
142. Kuo, J.T.W.; Li, C.; Meng, E. Fabrication and Characterization of a Microfluidic Module for Chemical Gradient Generation Utilizing Passive Pumping. In Proceedings of the 2014 36th Annual International Conference of the IEEE Engineering in Medicine and Biology Society, Chicago, IL, USA, 26–30 August 2014; pp. 4415–4418.
143. Kim, J.H.; Chang, W.S.; Kim, D.; Yang, J.R.; Han, J.T.; Lee, G.W.; Kim, J.T.; Seol, S.K. 3D Printing of Reduced Graphene Oxide Nanowires. *Adv. Mater.* **2015**, *27*, 157–161. [CrossRef]
144. Jung, J.H.; Jin, S.G. Microneedle for Transdermal Drug Delivery: Current Trends and Fabrication. *J. Pharm. Investig.* **2021**, *51*, 503–517. [CrossRef]
145. Ahmad, Z.; Rahman, A.M.N.A.A. Plastics in Waveguide Application. In *Reference Module in Materials Science and Materials Engineering*; Elsevier: Amsterdam, The Netherlands, 2021; ISBN 978-0-12-803581-8.
146. Hu, X.; Lu, C.; Wang, Q.; Xu, J.; Cui, Y. A High-Precision, Template-Assisted, Anisotropic Wet Etching Method for Fabricating Perovskite Microstructure Arrays. *RSC Adv.* **2020**, *10*, 38220–38226. [CrossRef]
147. Plummer, J.D. *Silicon VLSI Technology: Fundamentals, Practice and Modeling*; Pearson Education India: Noida, India, 2009.
148. Wu, W.I.; Rezai, P.; Hsu, H.H.; Selvaganapathy, P.R. Materials and Methods for the Microfabrication of Microfluidic Biomedical Devices. In *Microfluidic Devices for Biomedical Applications*; Li, X., Zhou, Y., Eds.; Woodhead Publishing Series in Biomaterials; Woodhead Publishing: Sawston, UK, 2013; pp. 3–62. ISBN 978-0-85709-697-5.
149. Lee, E.R. *Microdrop Generation*; CRC Press: Boca Raton, FL, USA, 2018; ISBN 978-1-315-22030-7.
150. Materials and Methods for the Microfabrication of Microfluidic Biomedical Devices. Available online: https://www.sciencedirect.com/science/article/pii/B9780857096975500013 (accessed on 16 March 2022).
151. Rodriguez, A.; Molinero, D.; Valera, E.; Trifonov, T.; Marsal, L.F.; Pallarès, J.; Alcubilla, R. Fabrication of Silicon Oxide Microneedles from Macroporous Silicon. *Sens. Actuators B: Chem.* **2005**, *109*, 135–140. [CrossRef]
152. Unraveling the Selective Etching Mechanism of Silicon Nitride over Silicon Dioxide by Phosphoric Acid: First-Principles Study. Available online: https://www.sciencedirect.com/science/article/abs/pii/S0169433221004529 (accessed on 16 March 2022).
153. Jivani, R.R.; Lakhtaria, G.J.; Patadiya, D.D.; Patel, L.D.; Jivani, N.P.; Jhala, B.P. RETRACTED: Biomedical Microelectromechanical Systems (BioMEMS): Revolution in Drug Delivery and Analytical Techniques. *Saudi Pharm. J.* **2016**, *24*, 1–20. [CrossRef]
154. Bonabi, A.; Tähkä, S.; Ollikainen, E.; Jokinen, V.; Sikanen, T. Metallization of Organically Modified Ceramics for Microfluidic Electrochemical Assays. *Micromachines* **2019**, *10*, 605. [CrossRef]
155. Process Optimization and Characterization of Silicon Microneedles Fabricated by Wet Etch Technology. Available online: https://www.sciencedirect.com/science/article/abs/pii/S0026269205001825 (accessed on 16 March 2022).
156. Dutta, S.; Imran, M.; Kumar, P.; Pal, R.; Datta, P.; Chatterjee, R. Comparison of Etch Characteristics of KOH, TMAH and EDP for Bulk Micromachining of Silicon (110). *Microsyst. Technol.* **2011**, *17*, 1621. [CrossRef]
157. Tanaka, H.; Abe, Y.; Inoue, K.; Shikida, M.; Sato, K. Effects of Ppb-Level Metal Impurities in Aqueous Potassium Hydroxide Solution on the Etching of Si {110} and {100}. *Sens. Mater.* **2003**, *15*, 43–51.
158. Laconte, J.; Flandre, D.; Raskin, J.P. *Micromachined Thin-Film Sensors for SOI-CMOS Co-Integration*; Springer Science & Business Media: Berlin, Germany, 2006.
159. Pal, P.; Swarnalatha, V.; Rao, A.V.N.; Pandey, A.K.; Tanaka, H.; Sato, K. High Speed Silicon Wet Anisotropic Etching for Applications in Bulk Micromachining: A Review. *Micro Nano Syst. Lett.* **2021**, *9*, 4. [CrossRef]
160. Pal, P.; Sato, K. A Comprehensive Review on Convex and Concave Corners in Silicon Bulk Micromachining Based on Anisotropic Wet Chemical Etching. *Micro Nano Syst. Lett.* **2015**, *3*, 6. [CrossRef]
161. Ekinci, H. *Plasma and Reactive Ion Etching*; Elsevier: Amsterdam, The Netherlands, 2016.
162. Gosálvez, M.A.; Ferrando, N.; Fedoryshyn, Y.; Leuthold, J.; McPeak, K.M. Evidence for Faster Etching at the Mask-Substrate Interface: Atomistic Simulation of Complex Cavities at the Micron-/Submicron-Scale by the Continuous Cellular Automaton. *J. Micromech. Microeng.* **2016**, *26*, 045013. [CrossRef]
163. Composition Tailored Isotropic and Anisotropic Wet Etching of Glass. Available online: https://www.sciencedirect.com/science/article/pii/S2214785320406704 (accessed on 16 March 2022).
164. Shayan, M.; Merati, A.R.; Arezoo, B.; Rezvankhah, M.A. Study on Atomistic Model for Simulation of Anisotropic Wet Etching. *J. Micro/Nanolithography* **2011**, *10*, 029701. [CrossRef]
165. Rezvankhah, M.A.; Shayan, M.; Merati, A.R.; Pahlevani, M. Step Flow Model in Continuous Cellular Automata Method for Simulation of Anisotropic Etching of Silicon. *J. Micro/Nanolithography* **2013**, *12*, 023004. [CrossRef]
166. Narasimha Rao, A.V.; Swarnalatha, V.; Pandey, A.K.; Pal, P. Determination of Precise Crystallographic Directions on Si{111} Wafers Using Self-Aligning Pre-Etched Pattern. *Micro Nano Syst. Lett.* **2018**, *6*, 4. [CrossRef]
167. Differences in Anisotropic Etching Properties of KOH and TMAH Solutions. Available online: https://www.sciencedirect.com/science/article/abs/pii/S0924424799002642 (accessed on 16 March 2022).

168. Cavalu, S.; Banica, F.; Simon, V.; Akin, I.; Goller, G. Surface Modification of Alumina/Zirconia Ceramics Upon Different Fluoride-Based Treatments. *Int. J. Appl. Ceram. Technol.* **2014**, *11*, 402–411. [CrossRef]
169. Efremov, A.M.; Murin, D.B.; Kwon, K.H. Concerning the Effect of Type of Fluorocarbon Gas on the Output Characteristics of the Reactive-Ion Etching Process. *Russ. Microelectron* **2020**, *49*, 157–165. [CrossRef]
170. Vähänissi, J. Xenon Difluoride Etching of Sacrificial Layers for Fabrication of Microelectromechanical Devices. Master's Thesis, Aalto University, Espoo, Finland, 2019. Available online: https://aaltodoc.aalto.fi/handle/123456789/37148 (accessed on 30 March 2022).
171. Ekinci, H.; Jahed, N.M.S.; Soltani, M.; Cui, B. The Role of Oxygen on Anisotropy in Chromium Oxide Hard Mask Etching for Sub-Micron Fabrication. *IEEE Trans. Nanotechnol.* **2021**, *20*, 33–38. [CrossRef]
172. Andrianov, N. Boron Trichloride Dry Etching. In *Boron Trichloride Dry Etching*; Shohet, J.L., Ed.; Taylor and Francis Ltd.: Boca Raton, FL, USA, 2016; Volume 1, pp. 193–202. ISBN 978-1-351-20495-8.
173. Li, X.J.; Zhou, Y. *Microfluidic Devices for Biomedical Applications*; Woodhead Publishing: Sawston, UK, 2021.
174. Pinto, R.M.R.; Gund, V.; Calaza, C.; Nagaraja, K.K.; Vinayakumar, K.B. Piezoelectric Aluminum Nitride Thin-Films: A Review of Wet and Dry Etching Techniques. *Microelectron. Eng.* **2022**, *257*, 111753. [CrossRef]
175. Ohmi, H.; Sato, J.; Shirasu, Y.; Hirano, T.; Kakiuchi, H.; Yasutake, K. Significant Improvement of Copper Dry Etching Property of a High-Pressure Hydrogen-Based Plasma by Nitrogen Gas Addition. *ACS Omega* **2019**, *4*, 4360–4366. [CrossRef]
176. Takahashi, H. Method and System for Dry Etching a Metal Nitride. U.S. Patent No. 7,815,814, 19 October 2010.
177. Puliyalil, H.; Cvelbar, U. Selective Plasma Etching of Polymeric Substrates for Advanced Applications. *Nanomaterials* **2016**, *6*, 108. [CrossRef]
178. Hill, S.; Qian, W.; Chen, W.; Fu, J. Surface Micromachining of Polydimethylsiloxane for Microfluidics Applications. *Biomicrofluidics* **2016**, *10*, 054114. [CrossRef]
179. Ortigoza-Diaz, J.; Scholten, K.; Larson, C.; Cobo, A.; Hudson, T.; Yoo, J.; Baldwin, A.; Weltman Hirschberg, A.; Meng, E. Techniques and Considerations in the Microfabrication of Parylene C Microelectromechanical Systems. *Micromachines* **2018**, *9*, 422. [CrossRef]
180. Comparison of Dry Etching of PMMA and Polycarbonate in Diffusion Pump-Based $O_2$ Capacitively Coupled Plasma and Inductively Coupled Plasma. Available online: https://www.sciencedirect.com/science/article/abs/pii/S0040609010002476 (accessed on 16 March 2022).
181. Joo, Y.W.; Park, Y.H.; Noh, H.S.; Kim, J.K.; Lee, S.H.; Cho, G.S.; Song, H.J.; Jeon, M.H.; Lee, J.W. Dry etching of polycarbonate using $O_2/SF_6$, $O_2/N_2$ and $O_2/CH_4$ plasmas. *J. Korean Vac. Soc.* **2008**, *17*, 16–22. [CrossRef]
182. Chen, Y.; Mao, H.; Tan, Q.; Xue, C.; Ou, W.; Liu, J.; Chen, D. Fabrication of Polyimide Sacrificial Layers with Inclined Sidewalls Based on Reactive Ion Etching. *AIP Adv.* **2014**, *4*, 031328. [CrossRef]
183. Han, J.; Yin, Z.; Zou, H.; Wang, W.; Feng, J. A New Dry Etching Method with the High Etching Rate for Patterning Cross–Linked SU–8 Thick Films. *J. Electr. Eng.* **2016**, *67*, 212–216. [CrossRef]
184. Veselov, D.S.; Bakun, A.D.; Voronov, Y.A. Reactive Ion Etching of Silicon Using Low-Power Plasma Etcher. *J. Phys. Conf. Ser.* **2016**, *748*, 012017. [CrossRef]
185. Huff, M. Recent Advances in Reactive Ion Etching and Applications of High-Aspect-Ratio Microfabrication. *Micromachines* **2021**, *12*, 991. [CrossRef]
186. Lin, L.; Zhang, M.; Qiu, D.; Jing, X.; Jiang, F.; Yu, D. Dry Etching of Fused Silica Glass in C4F8/Ar Inductively Coupled Plasmas for through Glass via (TGV) Applications. In Proceedings of the 2014 15th International Conference on Electronic Packaging Technology, Chengdu, China, 12–15 August 2014; pp. 334–339.
187. Franz, G. Plasma Etch Processes. In *Low Pressure Plasmas and Microstructuring Technology*; Franz, G., Ed.; Springer: Berlin, Heidelberg, 2009; pp. 439–515. ISBN 978-3-540-85849-2.
188. Tucak, A.; Sirbubalo, M.; Hindija, L.; Rahić, O.; Hadžiabdić, J.; Muhamedagić, K.; Čekić, A.; Vranić, E. Microneedles: Characteristics, Materials, Production Methods and Commercial Development. *Micromachines* **2020**, *11*, 961. [CrossRef]
189. Zant, P.V. *Microchip Fabrication*; McGraw-Hill Education: New York, NY, USA, 2014.
190. Lee, J.; Li, P.C.H. Development of Immunoassays for Protein Analysis on Nanobioarray Chips. In *Microfluidic Devices for Biomedical Applications*; Li, X., Zhou, Y., Eds.; Woodhead Publishing Series in Biomaterials; Woodhead Publishing: Sawston, UK, 2013; pp. 445–464. ISBN 978-0-85709-697-5.
191. Mao, P. Ultra-High-Aspect-Ratio Nanofluidic Channels for High-Throughput Biological Applications. Ph.D. Thesis, Massachusetts Institute of Technology, Cambridge, MA, USA, 2009.
192. Liu, Y.; Eng, P.F.; Guy, O.J.; Roberts, K.; Ashraf, H.; Knight, N. Advanced Deep Reactive-Ion Etching Technology for Hollow Microneedles for Transdermal Blood Sampling and Drug Delivery. *IET Nanobiotechnol.* **2013**, *7*, 59–62. [CrossRef]
193. Microfabricated Microneedles: A Novel Approach to Transdermal Drug Delivery. Available online: https://www.sciencedirect.com/science/article/abs/pii/S0022354915506242 (accessed on 16 March 2022).
194. Howells, O.; Blayney, G.J.; Gualeni, B.; Birchall, J.C.; Eng, P.F.; Ashraf, H.; Sharma, S.; Guy, O.J. Design, Fabrication, and Characterisation of a Silicon Microneedle Array for Transdermal Therapeutic Delivery Using a Single Step Wet Etch Process. *Eur. J. Pharm. Biopharm.* **2022**, *171*, 19–28. [CrossRef]
195. Madou, M.J. *Fundamentals of Microfabrication: The Science of Miniaturization*, 3rd ed.; CRC Press: Boca Raton, FL, USA, 2011; ISBN 978-0-8493-0826-0.

196. Bachmann, M.D. *Manipulating Anisotropic Transport and Superconductivity by Focused Ion Beam Microstructuring;* Springer Nature: Berlin, Germany, 2020.
197. Madou, M.J. *Manufacturing Techniques for Microfabrication and Nanotechnology;* CRC Press: Boca Raton, FL, USA, 2011; ISBN 978-0-429-11246-1.
198. Li, S.; Li, W.; Prausnitz, M. Individually Coated Microneedles for Co-Delivery of Multiple Compounds with Different Properties. *Drug Deliv. Transl. Res.* **2018**, *8*, 1043–1052. [CrossRef]
199. Moffatt, K.; Donnelly, R.F. Microneedle Technology. In *Drug Delivery Devices and Therapeutic Systems;* Chappel, E., Ed.; Developments in Biomedical Engineering and Bioelectronics; Academic Press: Cambridge, MA, USA, 2021; pp. 345–366.
200. Yang, S.J.; Jeong, J.O.; Lim, Y.M.; Park, J.S. Synthesis and Characterization of PVP Microneedle Patch Using Metal Bioelectrodes for Novel Drug Delivery System. *Mater. Des.* **2021**, *201*, 109485. [CrossRef]
201. Microchannels Created by Sugar and Metal Microneedles: Characterization by Microscopy, Macromolecular Flux and Other Techniques. Available online: https://www.sciencedirect.com/science/article/abs/pii/S0022354916305123 (accessed on 10 March 2022).
202. Amer, R.I.; El-Osaily, G.H.; Bakr, R.O.; El Dine, R.S.; Fayez, A.M. Characterization and Pharmacological Evaluation of Anti-Cellulite Herbal Product(s) Encapsulated in 3D-Fabricated Polymeric Microneedles. *Sci. Rep.* **2020**, *10*, 6316. [CrossRef]
203. Arshad, M.S.; Zafar, S.; Zahra, A.T.; Zaman, M.H.; Akhtar, A.; Kucuk, I.; Farhan, M.; Chang, M.W.; Ahmad, Z. Fabrication and Characterisation of Self-Applicating Heparin Sodium Microneedle Patches. *J. Drug Target.* **2021**, *29*, 60–68. [CrossRef] [PubMed]
204. Kim, S.J.; Park, S.J.; Kim, S.I. Swelling Behavior of Interpenetrating Polymer Network Hydrogels Composed of Poly(Vinyl Alcohol) and Chitosan. *React. Funct. Polym.* **2003**, *55*, 53–59. [CrossRef]
205. Shrestha, P.; Stoeber, B. Imaging Fluid Injections into Soft Biological Tissue to Extract Permeability Model Parameters. *Phys. Fluids* **2020**, *32*, 011905. [CrossRef]
206. Development of SiRNA-Loaded Chitosan Nanoparticles Targeting Galectin-1 for the Treatment of Glioblastoma Multiforme via Intranasal Administration. Available online: https://www.sciencedirect.com/science/article/abs/pii/S0168365916300955 (accessed on 10 March 2022).
207. Multiscale Simulations of Drug Distributions in Polymer Dissolvable Microneedles. Available online: https://www.sciencedirect.com/science/article/abs/pii/S0927776520300746 (accessed on 10 March 2022).
208. Baert, B.; Vansteelandt, S.; De Spiegeleer, B. Ion Mobility Spectrometry as a High-Throughput Technique for in Vitro Transdermal Franz Diffusion Cell Experiments of Ibuprofen. *J. Pharm. Biomed. Anal.* **2011**, *55*, 472–478. [CrossRef]
209. Widera, G.; Johnson, J.; Kim, L.; Libiran, L.; Nyam, K.; Daddona, P.E.; Cormier, M. Effect of Delivery Parameters on Immunization to Ovalbumin Following Intracutaneous Administration by a Coated Microneedle Array Patch System. *Vaccine* **2006**, *24*, 1653–1664. [CrossRef]
210. Kochhar, J.S.; Zou, S.; Chan, S.Y.; Kang, L. Protein Encapsulation in Polymeric Microneedles by Photolithography. *Int. J. Nanomed.* **2012**, *7*, 3143–3154. [CrossRef]
211. Park, J.H.; Allen, M.G.; Prausnitz, M.R. Biodegradable Polymer Microneedles: Fabrication, Mechanics and Transdermal Drug Delivery. *J. Control. Release* **2005**, *104*, 51–66. [CrossRef]
212. Huang, S.; Liu, H.; Huang, S.; Fu, T.; Xue, W.; Guo, R. Dextran Methacrylate Hydrogel Microneedles Loaded with Doxorubicin and Trametinib for Continuous Transdermal Administration of Melanoma. *Carbohydr. Polym.* **2020**, *246*, 116650. [CrossRef]
213. Zhang, Y.; Brown, K.; Siebenaler, K.; Determan, A.; Dohmeier, D.; Hansen, K. Development of Lidocaine-Coated Microneedle Product for Rapid, Safe, and Prolonged Local Analgesic Action. *Pharm. Res.* **2012**, *29*, 170–177. [CrossRef]
214. Kumar, A.; Wonganan, P.; Sandoval, M.; Li, X.; Zhu, S.; Cui, Z. Microneedle-Mediated Transcutaneous Immunization with Plasmid DNA Coated on Cationic PLGA Nanoparticle. *J. Control. Release* **2012**, *23*, 230–239. [CrossRef]
215. Kennedy, J.; Larrañeta, E.; McCrudden, M.T.C.; McCrudden, C.M.; Brady, A.J.; Fallows, S.J.; McCarthy, H.O.; Kissenpfennig, A.; Donnelly, R.F. In Vivo Studies Investigating Biodistribution of Nanoparticle-Encapsulated Rhodamine B Delivered via Dissolving Microneedles. *J. Control. Release* **2017**, *265*, 57–65. [CrossRef]
216. Zhou, C.P.; Liu, Y.L.; Wang, H.L.; Zhang, P.X.; Zhang, J.L. Transdermal Delivery of Insulin Using Microneedle Rollers in Vivo. *Int. J. Pharm.* **2010**, *392*, 127–133. [CrossRef]
217. Halder, J.; Gupta, S.; Kumari, R.; Gupta, G.D.; Rai, V.K. Microneedle Array: Applications, Recent Advances, and Clinical Pertinence in Transdermal Drug Delivery. *J. Pharm. Innov.* **2021**, *16*, 558–565. [CrossRef]
218. Langer, R. Transdermal Drug Delivery: Past Progress, Current Status, and Future Prospects. *Adv. Drug Deliv. Rev.* **2004**, *56*, 557–558. [CrossRef]
219. Choy, Y.B.; Prausnitz, M.R. The Rule of Five for Non-Oral Routes of Drug Delivery: Ophthalmic, Inhalation and Transdermal. *Pharm. Res.* **2011**, *28*, 943–948. [CrossRef]
220. Rojekar, S.; Vora, L.K.; Tekko, I.A.; Volpe-Zanutto, F.; McCarthy, H.O.; Vavia, P.R.; Donnelly, R.F. Etravirine-Loaded Dissolving Microneedle Arrays for Long-Acting Delivery. *Eur. J. Pharm. Biopharm.* **2021**, *165*, 41–51. [CrossRef]
221. Zhu, L.; Yu, X.; Li, Q.; Zhang, Y.; Jin, Y.; Du, L. Estriol Dissolving Microneedle Patches for Protection against Ionizing Radiation-Induced Injury. *Eur. J. Pharm. Sci.* **2021**, *163*, 105881. [CrossRef]
222. Albadr, A.A.; Tekko, I.A.; Vora, L.K.; Ali, A.A.; Laverty, G.; Donnelly, R.F.; Thakur, R.R.S. Rapidly Dissolving Microneedle Patch of Amphotericin B for Intracorneal Fungal Infections. *Drug Deliv. Transl. Res.* **2022**, *12*, 931–943. [CrossRef]

223. Tekko, I.A.; Vora, L.K.; Volpe-Zanutto, F.; Moffatt, K.; Jarrahian, C.; McCarthy, H.O.; Donnelly, R.F. Novel Bilayer Microarray Patch-Assisted Long-Acting Micro-Depot Cabotegravir Intradermal Delivery for HIV Pre-Exposure Prophylaxis. *Adv. Funct. Mater.* **2022**, *32*, 2106999. [CrossRef]
224. Paredes, A.J.; Volpe-Zanutto, F.; Vora, L.K.; Tekko, I.A.; Permana, A.D.; Picco, C.J.; McCarthy, H.O.; Donnelly, R.F. Systemic Delivery of Tenofovir Alafenamide Using Dissolving and Implantable Microneedle Patches. *Mater. Today Biol.* **2022**, *13*, 100217. [CrossRef]
225. Mc Crudden, M.T.C.; Larrañeta, E.; Clark, A.; Jarrahian, C.; Rein-Weston, A.; Lachau-Durand, S.; Niemeijer, N.; Williams, P.; Haeck, C.; McCarthy, H.O.; et al. Design, Formulation and Evaluation of Novel Dissolving Microarray Patches Containing a Long-Acting Rilpivirine Nanosuspension. *J. Control. Release* **2018**, *292*, 119–129. [CrossRef]
226. Li, M.; Vora, L.K.; Peng, K.; Donnelly, R.F. Trilayer Microneedle Array Assisted Transdermal and Intradermal Delivery of Dexamethasone. *Int. J. Pharm.* **2022**, *612*, 121295. [CrossRef]
227. Jamaledin, R.; Di Natale, C.; Onesto, V.; Taraghdari, Z.; Zare, E.; Makvandi, P.; Vecchione, R.; Netti, P. Progress in Microneedle-Mediated Protein Delivery. *J. Clin. Med.* **2020**, *9*, 542. [CrossRef]
228. Liu, T.; Chen, M.; Fu, J.; Sun, Y.; Lu, C.; Quan, G.; Pan, X.; Wu, C. Recent Advances in Microneedles-Mediated Transdermal Delivery of Protein and Peptide Drugs. *Acta Pharm. Sin. B* **2021**, *11*, 2326–2343. [CrossRef]
229. Liu, S.; Yeo, D.C.; Wiraja, C.; Tey, H.L.; Mrksich, M.; Xu, C. Peptide Delivery with Poly(Ethylene Glycol) Diacrylate Microneedles through Swelling Effect. *Bioeng. Transl. Med.* **2017**, *2*, 258–267. [CrossRef]
230. Jeong, H.R.; Kim, J.Y.; Kim, S.N.; Park, J.H. Local Dermal Delivery of Cyclosporin A, a Hydrophobic and High Molecular Weight Drug, Using Dissolving Microneedles. *Eur. J. Pharm. Biopharm.* **2018**, *127*, 237–243. [CrossRef]
231. Damiri, F.; Bachra, Y.; Berrada, M. Synthesis and Characterization of 4-Formylphenylboronic Acid Cross-Linked Chitosan Hydrogel with Dual Action: Glucose-Sensitivity and Controlled Insulin Release. *Chin. J. Anal. Chem.* **2022**, *50*, 100092. [CrossRef]
232. McAllister, D.V.; Wang, P.M.; Davis, S.P.; Park, J.H.; Canatella, P.J.; Allen, M.G.; Prausnitz, M.R. Microfabricated Needles for Transdermal Delivery of Macromolecules and Nanoparticles: Fabrication Methods and Transport Studies. *Proc. Natl. Acad. Sci. USA* **2003**, *100*, 13755–13760. [CrossRef]
233. Chen, H.; Zhu, H.; Zheng, J.; Mou, D.; Wan, J.; Zhang, J.; Shi, T.; Zhao, Y.; Xu, H.; Yang, X. Iontophoresis-Driven Penetration of Nanovesicles through Microneedle-Induced Skin Microchannels for Enhancing Transdermal Delivery of Insulin. *J. Control. Release* **2009**, *139*, 63–72. [CrossRef]
234. Ye, Y.; Yu, J.; Wang, C.; Nguyen, N.Y.; Walker, G.M.; Buse, J.B.; Gu, Z. Microneedles Integrated with Pancreatic Cells and Synthetic Glucose-Signal Amplifiers for Smart Insulin Delivery. *Adv. Mater.* **2016**, *28*, 3115–3121. [CrossRef] [PubMed]
235. Daddona, P.E.; Matriano, J.A.; Mandema, J.; Maa, Y.F. Parathyroid Hormone (1-34)-Coated Microneedle Patch System: Clinical Pharmacokinetics and Pharmacodynamics for Treatment of Osteoporosis. *Pharm. Res.* **2011**, *28*, 159–165. [CrossRef] [PubMed]
236. Noh, G.; Keum, T.; Seo, J.E.; Bashyal, S.; Eum, N.S.; Kweon, M.J.; Lee, S.; Sohn, D.H.; Lee, S. Iontophoretic Transdermal Delivery of Human Growth Hormone (HGH) and the Combination Effect of a New Type Microneedle, Tappy Tok Tok®. *Pharmaceutics* **2018**, *10*, 153. [CrossRef] [PubMed]
237. Dissolving Polymer Microneedle Patches for Rapid and Efficient Transdermal Delivery of Insulin to Diabetic Rats. Available online: https://www.sciencedirect.com/science/article/abs/pii/S174270611300322X (accessed on 31 March 2022).
238. Yu, J.; Zhang, Y.; Ye, Y.; DiSanto, R.; Sun, W.; Ranson, D.; Ligler, F.S.; Buse, J.B.; Gu, Z. Microneedle-Array Patches Loaded with Hypoxia-Sensitive Vesicles Provide Fast Glucose-Responsive Insulin Delivery. *Proc. Natl. Acad. Sci. USA* **2015**, *112*, 8260–8265. [CrossRef]
239. Damiri, F.; Rahman, M.H.; Zehravi, M.; Awaji, A.A.; Nasrullah, M.Z.; Gad, H.A.; Bani-Fwaz, M.Z.; Varma, R.S.; Germoush, M.O.; Al-malky, H.S.; et al. MXene (Ti3C2Tx)-Embedded Nanocomposite Hydrogels for Biomedical Applications: A Review. *Materials* **2022**, *15*, 1666. [CrossRef]
240. Prausnitz, M.R. Engineering Microneedle Patches for Vaccination and Drug Delivery to Skin. *Annu. Rev. Chem. Biomol. Eng.* **2017**, *8*, 177–200. [CrossRef]
241. Mikszta, J.A.; Alarcon, J.B.; Brittingham, J.M.; Sutter, D.E.; Pettis, R.J.; Harvey, N.G. Improved Genetic Immunization via Micromechanical Disruption of Skin-Barrier Function and Targeted Epidermal Delivery. *Nat. Med.* **2002**, *8*, 415–419. [CrossRef]
242. Development of a Thermostable Microneedle Patch for Influenza Vaccination. Available online: https://www.sciencedirect.com/science/article/abs/pii/S0022354915302306 (accessed on 11 March 2022).
243. Ogai, N.; Nonaka, I.; Toda, Y.; Ono, T.; Minegishi, S.; Inou, A.; Hachiya, M.; Fukamizu, H. Enhanced Immunity in Intradermal Vaccination by Novel Hollow Microneedles. *Skin Res. Technol.* **2018**, *24*, 630–635. [CrossRef]
244. Kim, N.W.; Kim, S.Y.; Lee, J.E.; Yin, Y.; Lee, J.H.; Lim, S.Y.; Kim, E.S.; Duong, H.T.T.; Kim, H.K.; Kim, S.; et al. Enhanced Cancer Vaccination by In Situ Nanomicelle-Generating Dissolving Microneedles. *ACS Nano* **2018**, *12*, 9702–9713. [CrossRef]
245. Caffarel-Salvador, E.; Brady, A.J.; Eltayib, E.; Meng, T.; Alonso-Vicente, A.; Gonzalez-Vazquez, P.; Torrisi, B.M.; Vicente-Perez, E.M.; Mooney, K.; Jones, D.S.; et al. Hydrogel-Forming Microneedle Arrays Allow Detection of Drugs and Glucose in Vivo: Potential for Use in Diagnosis and Therapeutic Drug Monitoring. *PLoS ONE* **2015**, *10*, e0145644. [CrossRef]
246. Chang, H.; Zheng, M.; Yu, X.; Than, A.; Seeni, R.Z.; Kang, R.; Tian, J.; Khanh, D.P.; Liu, L.; Chen, P.; et al. A Swellable Microneedle Patch to Rapidly Extract Skin Interstitial Fluid for Timely Metabolic Analysis. *Adv. Mater.* **2017**, *29*, 1702243. [CrossRef]
247. Jin, J.; Reese, V.; Coler, R.; Carter, D.; Rolandi, M. Chitin Microneedles for an Easy-to-Use Tuberculosis Skin Test. *Adv. Healthc. Mater.* **2014**, *3*, 349–353. [CrossRef]

248. El-Laboudi, A.; Oliver, N.S.; Cass, A.; Johnston, D. Use of Microneedle Array Devices for Continuous Glucose Monitoring: A Review. *Diabetes Technol. Ther.* **2013**, *15*, 101–115. [CrossRef]
249. Pires, L.R.; Vinayakumar, K.B.; Turos, M.; Miguel, V.; Gaspar, J. A Perspective on Microneedle-Based Drug Delivery and Diagnostics in Paediatrics. *J. Pers. Med.* **2019**, *9*, 49. [CrossRef]
250. Singh, V.; Kesharwani, P. Recent Advances in Microneedles-Based Drug Delivery Device in the Diagnosis and Treatment of Cancer. *J. Control. Release* **2021**, *338*, 394–409. [CrossRef]
251. Ventrelli, L.; Marsilio Strambini, L.; Barillaro, G. Microneedles for Transdermal Biosensing: Current Picture and Future Direction. *Adv. Healthc. Mater.* **2015**, *4*, 2606–2640. [CrossRef]
252. Strambini, L.M.; Longo, A.; Scarano, S.; Prescimone, T.; Palchetti, I.; Minunni, M.; Giannessi, D.; Barillaro, G. Self-Powered Microneedle-Based Biosensors for Pain-Free High-Accuracy Measurement of Glycaemia in Interstitial Fluid. *Biosens. Bioelectron.* **2015**, *66*, 162–168. [CrossRef]
253. Dardano, P.; Rea, I.; De Stefano, L. Microneedles-Based Electrochemical Sensors: New Tools for Advanced Biosensing. *Curr. Opin. Electrochem.* **2019**, *17*, 121–127. [CrossRef]
254. Zhao, L.; Wen, Z.; Jiang, F.; Zheng, Z.; Lu, S. Silk/Polyols/GOD Microneedle Based Electrochemical Biosensor for Continuous Glucose Monitoring. *RSC Adv.* **2020**, *10*, 6163–6171. [CrossRef] [PubMed]
255. Bollella, P.; Sharma, S.; Cass, A.E.G.; Antiochia, R. Microneedle-Based Biosensor for Minimally-Invasive Lactate Detection. *Biosens. Bioelectron.* **2019**, *123*, 152–159. [CrossRef] [PubMed]
256. Wang, M.; Hu, L.; Xu, C. Recent Advances in the Design of Polymeric Microneedles for Transdermal Drug Delivery and Biosensing. *Lab Chip* **2017**, *17*, 1373–1387. [CrossRef] [PubMed]
257. Caliò, A.; Dardano, P.; Di Palma, V.; Bevilacqua, M.F.; Di Matteo, A.; Iuele, H.; De Stefano, L. Polymeric Microneedles Based Enzymatic Electrodes for Electrochemical Biosensing of Glucose and Lactic Acid. *Sens. Actuators B Chem.* **2016**, *236*, 343–349. [CrossRef]
258. Jin, Q.; Chen, H.J.; Li, X.; Huang, X.; Wu, Q.; He, G.; Hang, T.; Yang, C.; Jiang, Z.; Li, E.; et al. Reduced Graphene Oxide Nanohybrid–Assembled Microneedles as Mini-Invasive Electrodes for Real-Time Transdermal Biosensing. *Small* **2019**, *15*, 1804298. [CrossRef]
259. Duarah, S.; Sharma, M.; Wen, J. Recent Advances in Microneedle-Based Drug Delivery: Special Emphasis on Its Use in Paediatric Population. *Eur. J. Pharm. Biopharm.* **2019**, *136*, 48–69. [CrossRef]
260. Moreira, A.F.; Rodrigues, C.F.; Jacinto, T.A.; Miguel, S.P.; Costa, E.C.; Correia, I.J. Microneedle-Based Delivery Devices for Cancer Therapy: A Review. *Pharmacol. Res.* **2019**, *148*, 104438. [CrossRef]
261. Hao, Y.; Chen, Y.; Lei, M.; Zhang, T.; Cao, Y.; Peng, J.; Chen, L.; Qian, Z. Near-Infrared Responsive PEGylated Gold Nanorod and Doxorubicin Loaded Dissolvable Hyaluronic Acid Microneedles for Human Epidermoid Cancer Therapy. *Adv. Ther.* **2018**, *1*, 1800008. [CrossRef]
262. Gadag, S.; Narayan, R.; Nayak, A.S.; Catalina Ardila, D.; Sant, S.; Nayak, Y.; Garg, S.; Nayak, U.Y. Development and Preclinical Evaluation of Microneedle-Assisted Resveratrol Loaded Nanostructured Lipid Carriers for Localized Delivery to Breast Cancer Therapy. *Int. J. Pharm.* **2021**, *606*, 120877. [CrossRef]
263. Wang, C.; Ye, Y.; Hochu, G.M.; Sadeghifar, H.; Gu, Z. Enhanced Cancer Immunotherapy by Microneedle Patch-Assisted Delivery of Anti-PD1 Antibody. *Nano Lett.* **2016**, *16*, 2334–2340. [CrossRef]
264. Patel, S.R.; Lin, A.S.P.; Edelhauser, H.F.; Prausnitz, M.R. Suprachoroidal Drug Delivery to the Back of the Eye Using Hollow Microneedles. *Pharm. Res.* **2011**, *28*, 166–176. [CrossRef]
265. Jiang, J.; Gill, H.S.; Ghate, D.; McCarey, B.E.; Patel, S.R.; Edelhauser, H.F.; Prausnitz, M.R. Coated Microneedles for Drug Delivery to the Eye. *Investig. Ophthalmol. Vis. Sci.* **2007**, *48*, 4038–4043. [CrossRef]
266. Liu, P.; Du, H.; Chen, Y.; Wang, H.; Mao, J.; Zhang, L.; Tao, J.; Zhu, J. Polymer Microneedles with Interconnected Porous Structures: Via a Phase Inversion Route for Transdermal Medical Applications. *J. Mater. Chem. B* **2020**, *8*, 2032–2039. [CrossRef]
267. Gao, Y.; Hou, M.; Yang, R.; Zhang, L.; Xu, Z.; Kang, Y.; Xue, P. Transdermal Delivery of Therapeutics through Dissolvable Gelatin/Sucrose Films Coated on PEGDA Microneedle Arrays with Improved Skin Permeability. *J. Mater. Chem. B* **2019**, *7*, 7515–7524. [CrossRef]
268. Machekposhti, S.A.; Soltani, M.; Najafizadeh, P.; Ebrahimi, S.A.; Chen, P. Biocompatible Polymer Microneedle for Topical/Dermal Delivery of Tranexamic Acid. *J. Control. Release* **2017**, *261*, 87–92. [CrossRef]
269. Lutton, R.E.M.; Moore, J.; Larrañeta, E.; Ligett, S.; Woolfson, A.D.; Donnelly, R.F. Microneedle Characterisation: The Need for Universal Acceptance Criteria and GMP Specifications when Moving towards Commercialisation. *Drug Deliv. Transl. Res.* **2015**, *5*, 313–331. [CrossRef]
270. Richter-Johnson, J.; Kumar, P.; Choonara, Y.E.; du Toit, L.C.; Pillay, V. Therapeutic Applications and Pharmacoeconomics of Microneedle Technology. *Expert Rev. Pharm. Outcomes Res.* **2018**, *18*, 359–369. [CrossRef]
271. Fluzone, Fluzone High-Dose and Fluzone Intradermal. Available online: https://www.fda.gov/vaccines-blood-biologics/vaccines/fluzone-fluzone-high-dose-and-fluzone-intradermal (accessed on 29 May 2021).
272. Intanza—European Medicines Agency. Available online: https://www.ema.europa.eu/en/medicines/human/EPAR/intanza (accessed on 29 May 2021).
273. Singh, A.; Yadav, S. Microneedling: Advances and Widening Horizons. *Indian Dermatol. Online J.* **2016**, *7*, 244. [CrossRef]
274. Dugam, S.; Tade, R.; Dhole, R.; Nangare, S. Emerging Era of Microneedle Array for Pharmaceutical and Biomedical Applications: Recent Advances and Toxicological Perspectives. *Futur. J. Pharm. Sci.* **2021**, *7*, 19. [CrossRef]

*pharmaceutics*

MDPI

*Review*

# Silk Fibroin Microneedles for Transdermal Drug Delivery: Where Do We Stand and How Far Can We Proceed?

**Zhenzhen Qi [1], Zheng Yan [1], Guohongfang Tan [1], Tianshuo Jia [1], Yiyu Geng [1], Huiyan Shao [1], Subhas C. Kundu [2] and Shenzhou Lu [1,*]**

1 National Engineering Laboratory for Modern Silk, College of Textile and Clothing Engineering, Soochow University, Suzhou 215123, China
2 3Bs Research Group, I3Bs Research Institute on Biomaterials, Biodegrabilities, and Biomimetics, Headquarters of the European Institute of Excellence on Tissue Engineering and Regenerative Medicine, University of Minho, AvePark, Guimaraes, 4805-017 Barco, Portugal
* Correspondence: lushenzhou@suda.edu.cn; Tel.: +86-512-67061152

**Abstract:** Microneedles are a patient-friendly technique for delivering drugs to the site of action in place of traditional oral and injectable administration. Silk fibroin represents an interesting polymeric biomaterial because of its mechanical properties, thermal stability, biocompatibility and possibility of control via genetic engineering. This review focuses on the critical research progress of silk fibroin microneedles since their inception, analyzes in detail the structure and properties of silk fibroin, the types of silk fibroin microneedles, drug delivery applications and clinical trials, and summarizes the future development trend in this field. It also proposes the future research direction of silk fibroin microneedles, including increasing drug loading doses and enriching drug loading types as well as exploring silk fibroin microneedles with stimulation-responsive drug release functions. The safety and effectiveness of silk fibroin microneedles should be further verified in clinical trials at different stages.

**Keywords:** silk fibroin microneedles; transdermal delivery; intelligently responsive; clinical transformation

## 1. Introduction

Skin is the first line of defense against infection and injury to protect the human body from harmful environments [1,2]; it plays a pivotal role in maintaining essential functions of host physiology. According to rough estimates, skin covers an area of about 1.5–2.0 $m^2$ in the human body [3], accounting for nearly one-fifth of the total weight of people, making it the largest organ in the human body. Skin comprises the epidermis, dermis and subcutaneous tissue [4]. As the outermost layer of skin, the epidermis is generally 100–240 μm [3,5]. Local and systemic drug administration with the skin as the primary organ can be found in the oldest surviving medical records [6], now known as transdermal drug delivery. As early as 3000 BC, descriptions of ancient Babylon note ointments and perfumes containing plant and mineral extracts to treat diseases [6]. The key to transdermal drug delivery is to understand the skin's structure, function and composition, which is also a crucial point in the design of transdermal drug delivery-related drugs and the form of administration [7].

Drug penetration through the skin can be divided into three main types: intercellular, intracellular and follicular [8]. Small molecule drugs are transported to the continuous subcutaneous tissue through the intercellular pathway. The polar/non-polar solute assigned by the appropriate O/W coefficient can diffuse the drug into water and keratinocytes via intracellular pathways [5,9,10] but with reduced bioavailability. The most primitive transdermal drug delivery is a patch, in which the required drug is used as a paste, wrapped with bandages or gauze, and then applied to the affected area for local treatment [11]. The drugs suitable for this type have small molecular weight and low availability [12,13], which leads to the large number of drugs needed for treatment and the possibility of excessive waste.

To improve drug availability and permeability, different methods are used to improve skin permeability. Commonly used methods include chemical substances, iontophoresis, ultrasound, etc. [14,15]. However, these methods commonly cause irreversible physiological damage to human tissues, and repeated use in the same place may cause skin ulceration; thus, they are not suitable for long-term use. The latest and most used methods include new chemical enhancers, electroporation, thermal ablation, microcrystalline rejuvenation and microneedles. These technologies enable macromolecular drugs and biological drugs to better penetrate the cuticle to the dermis, improve the efficiency of transdermal delivery, and enhance drug availability. However, the use of additional chemical reagents as well as lasers and heat will cause certain damage to the skin and can cause discomfort for patients [16].

Microneedles are a new transdermal method obtained by combining a transdermal patch with a hypodermic needle [17]. The length of the microneedle can be controlled to easily puncture the cuticle of the skin without touching the dermis and subcutaneous tissues with pain nerves, and the drug can be released without pain [18], thus achieving high drug availability. In addition, microneedles can be easily removed and provide better drug slow-release function, further reducing patients' dependence on drugs [19–21]. At the same time, microneedles, as drug carriers, are extremely helpful for releasing macromolecular medications [22,23].

The synthetic polymer material used as microneedles' substrate has the problems of a complex preparation process and poor biocompatibility [24]. Collagen, hyaluronic acid, polysaccharide, silk fibroin and other natural polymer materials have good biosafety and are a source of environmental protection. However, due to the mechanical properties, the application of collagen, hyaluronic acid and polysaccharide in microneedles is limited. Silk fibroin has highly elastic mechanical properties [25], a significant raw material source, and many unique advantages, such as good biological stability of enzymes [26,27], antioxidant activity stability [28,29], and biological stability in biomolecular drugs [30] and vaccines [31,32]. Silk fibroin is often prepared into films, hydrogels, nanoparticles and microneedles, which can be used in various fields such as medical cosmetology, tissue engineering and drug delivery. In particular, the preparation of microneedles plays a pivotal role in drug delivery [18,33–35]. This review focuses on the latest research progress of silk fibroin in the field of microneedles, analyzes in detail the structure and properties of silk fibroins, the types of silk fibroin microneedles, drug delivery applications and the clinical transformation of silk fibroin microneedles, and summarizes the current research focus and future development trend in this field.

## 2. Structure and Properties of Silk Fibroin

### 2.1. Structure of Silk Fibroin

Silk is composed of silk sericin and silk fibroin [36]. Silk sericin is a kind of globulin with the characteristics of anti-oxidation, bacteriostasis and biocompatibility. Silk sericin can effectively reduce free radicals and reduce sun and air pollutants. Based on the above features, silk sericin is mainly used in medical cosmetology and other fields [37,38]. Silk fibroin is a kind of fibrous protein containing 18 types of amino acids, primarily glycine (Gly), alanine (Ala) and serine (Ser), accounting for more than 80% of the total content [39].

Silk fibroin protein is composed of three proteins, including a heavy chain (H chain), a light chain (L chain) and p25 glycoprotein, whose molecular weights are 390 kDa, 26 kDa and 28 kDa, respectively. In the silk fibroin secreted by the mature silkworm, the H and L chains are covalently connected by a pair of disulfide bonds [40]. An aggregate of six H-L chains and a p25 glycoprotein are assembled by hydrophobic action to form a basic unit, that is, H chain:L chain:p25 glycoprotein = 6:6:1 [41,42]. From the composition perspective, the H chain of silk fibroin is a highly ordered polymer formed by 11 hydrophilic regions through 12 hydrophobic regions [43] (Figure 1). Studies have found that the core part of the H chain is a β-folded structure formed by the orderly arrangement of the highly repeated sequence GAGAGX (X is mainly tyrosine or serine), which plays a significant role in the crystallization process of silk fibroin and is primarily distributed in the crystallization region [44,45]. In the amorphous region, there are essentially amorphous amino acids, such as tryptophan (Trp), phenylalanine (Phe) and tyrosine (Tyr), which have large side chain groups [46].

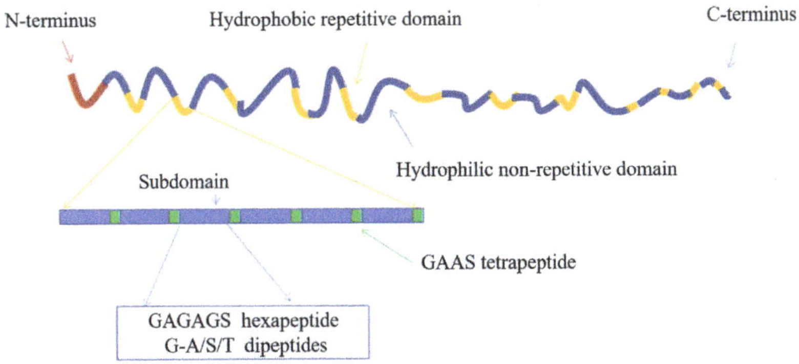


**Figure 1.** Diagram of H chain of silk fibroin. Image used with permission of [47].

The secondary structure of proteins is mainly composed of the random coil, α-helix, β-sheet and β-turning [48,49]. Among them, the β-sheet includes the parallel β-sheet and antiparallel β-sheet. The latter structure is more stable in energy and produces shorter hydrogen bonds [50]. The random coil is unstable and will be transformed into the β-sheet under specific external forces, such as temperature, humidity, pH change and others. The β-sheet can generate physical crosslinking points under intermolecular force and hydrogen bonding, thus improving the mechanical properties of silk fibroin materials [25]. Amino acid repeating polypeptide fragments (GAGAGS) with minor or no side groups in the silk fibroin molecular chain are arranged in regular order to form hydrophobic β-sheet, which creates the possibility for further accumulation of hydrophobic β-sheet into silk II crystals [51,52]. Silk fibroin mainly contains two molecular conformations, Silk I and Silk II, among which Silk I is a β-turning conformation of II, and Silk II is an antiparallel β-sheet layered structure, which is stable and insoluble in water and most solvents, including strong acids and weak bases [53]. Silk I is easily transformed into Silk II under the influence of different solution conditions and temperatures, which some scientists have considered. Still, our recent study found that porous materials with the structure of Silk I show good long-term stability, thermal stability and chemical stability [54,55].

*2.2. Biocompatibility of Silk Fibroin*

One of the oldest natural polymers, silk has been successfully used for surgical sutures. Silk fibroin was purified by degumming. It was found that it was highly biocompatible and degraded slowly in vivo [56]. Since most of the amino acid residues in silk fibroin are non-polar, and the polar amino acid residues are in the crystallization region, the silk fibroin can be modified by chemical modification, and the modified silk fibroin has good blood compatibility [57].

Compared with other types of polymers, such as collagen and polylactic acid, silk fibroin-derived materials have better biocompatibility due to the β-sheet structure. Meinel [58] verified that the inflammatory response in vivo caused by silk fibroin film was equal to or smaller than that observed on collagen film and far smaller than that of polylactic acid film. $TiO_2$ microspheres decorated with silk fibroin in situ showed enhanced biocompatibility compared with $TiO_2$ microspheres [59].

### 2.3. The Advantages and Disadvantages of Silk Fibroin for Drug Release

In recent years, more and more researchers have found that silk fibroin has better characteristics for drug delivery than other biological materials, such as good biological stability of enzymes [26,27], antioxidant activity stability [28,29], biological stability in biomacromolecular drugs [30] and application in vaccines [31,32]. These unique advantages gradually improve the application prospect and irreplaceability of silk fibroin. Silk fibroin is often prepared into films, hydrogels, nanoparticles, microneedles and other forms according to its uses, which can be used in various fields such as medical cosmetology, tissue engineering, drug delivery and others.

The most common method of loading drugs with silk fibroin protein is to dissolve or blend the medicine directly into silk fibroin solution. This method is commonly used to prepare films [60] and hydrogels [61,62]. However, it is necessary to ensure that the structure and activity of the drug will not be affected during the manufacturing process. In addition, drugs can also be adsorbed or covalently crosslinked to the prepared silk fibroin matrix. Peroxidase can be covalently coupled to the silk fibroin scaffold using water-soluble carbodiimide [63]. Of course, whether a drug can be covalently crosslinked with silk fibroin or form a conjugate depends on the physical and chemical properties of the drug, and the use of this method is subject to certain restrictions [64]. Loading drugs into nanoparticles and microspheres is also a viable option. This enables targeted drug delivery and controlled drug release. Drug-loaded microspheres or nanoparticles can be blended with silk fibroin or coated on the surface of the silk matrix. However, the safety of nanoparticles is controversial, and they also face the challenges of low drug loading and wide size distribution.

Silk fibroin has a unique structure and can be adjusted to form different carrier forms. Among them, the secondary structure of silk fibroin protein has other characteristics and can be changed by external stimuli. The loading, release kinetics and stability of drugs can be processed by reversing the preparation and post-treatment methods of materials [65]. The loading efficiency and release curve of heparin-loaded silk fibroin nanofilm is controlled by the β-fold content after treatment with simple solvents (glycerol and methanol). The nanofilm can be used as a carrier to achieve continuous release of epirubicin [66]. The anion side group is increased by diazo coupling to modify the tyrosine side chain in silk fibroin, and the drug loading quantity is improved [67].

As an excellent biomaterial, silk fibroin has been prepared in many forms under mild processing conditions, including microspheres, films, hydrogels, liposomes, microneedles and microcapsules. However, these standard production techniques usually produce particles with a large distribution due to the irregular forces involved, resulting in low bioactivity of loaded enzymes, cells and growth factors [68]. At the same time, the degumming process not only reduces the mechanical strength of silk but also affects the structure, size, surface potential and drug release efficiency of microspheres in the process of silk fibroin purification due to the difference in molecular weight [69]. In addition, untreated silk fibroin microneedles are prone to fracture during insertion, and their rapid dissolution may lead to the sudden release of drugs, causing hypoglycemia and other side effects [70].

## 3. Types of Silk Fibroin Microneedles

According to the microneedle substrate and drug delivery mechanism, microneedles can be roughly divided into five different types [71] (Figure 2): (1) Solid microneedles can puncture the skin to improve drug transport rate and penetration rate, but their poke-patch delivery mode is inefficient, and it is difficult to control drug dosage [72,73]; (2) Drugs can be coated on microneedles on the surface of the needle tip. This coat-poke method often fails to meet the dose requirements and the dose is not easy to control [74–77]; (3) Hollow microneedles inject liquid drug preparation through internal holes. This poke-flow method overcomes the dose limitation, and the drug delivery velocity and dose can be controlled through free diffusion, external pressure or electronic control of external pressure. However, the structure of hollow microneedles is relatively complex. There are problems such as blockage, drug leakage, structural fragility and poor insertion [78–80]. (4) Dissolving microneedles are made of soluble polymers and encapsulated drugs. The disadvantages of hollow microneedles, such as high cost and a low dose of coating microneedles, are eliminated here. However, the method of poke-dissolve also has its disadvantages, including low mechanical strength and deposit of needle tip material in the cortex after dissolution [81–83]; (5) Swelling microneedles, also known as hydrogel microneedles, are a kind of microneedle that absorbs water and swells to form hydrogel after penetrating the skin, thus completing drug release. The drug release rate of the microneedles can be comparable to that of dissolved microneedles by regulating the change speed and degree of swelling. The tip material of this microneedle will not dissolve and deposit in the cortex, which solves the potential biocompatibility problem of dissolving microneedles and provides the possibility for the realization of a microneedle intelligent drug delivery system.

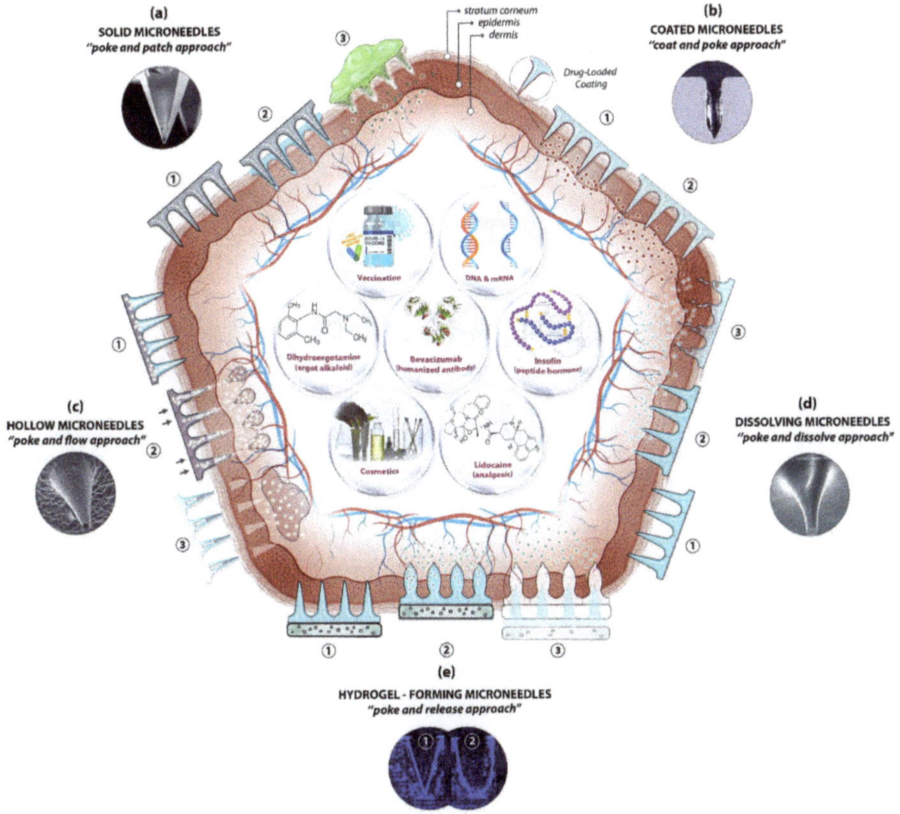


**Figure 2.** Schematic diagram of drug delivery method based on microneedles (MN): (**a**) solid MN; (**b**) coated MN; (**c**) hollow MN; (**d**) dissolving MN; (**e**) swelling MN. The step-by-step process for each delivery method is numbered from 1 to 3. It shows representative microscopic images of MN types and examples of deliverable substances, such as insulin, vaccines, DNA and RNA. Image used with permission of [72].

### *3.1. Dissolving Silk Fibroin Microneedles*

Dissolving microneedles are used as a peridermal drug delivery system for drug and vaccine delivery [82], which not only avoids the shortcomings of conventional drug delivery methods but also uses biocompatible and biodegradable materials. This overcomes the problem of microneedles breaking in vivo. Recently, silk fibroin, as a natural biological material, has been used to manufacture dissolving microneedles due to its excellent biocompatibility and good mechanical properties [25,84].

The preparation method of dissolving silk fibroin microneedles is mainly mold casting, which is a method to prepare microneedles by mold casting and demolding [85]. As shown in the figure below, Cao et al. [86] described this method. First, the silk fibroin solution was mixed with the drug in a certain ratio, and then the mixed solution was evenly smeared on the polydimethylsiloxane (PDMS) microneedle mold. Finally, the PDMS mold filled with silk fibroin protein solution was sent to a constant temperature and humidity room for drying, and the microneedles could be detached after drying completely. Because the mold casting method is prepared at room temperature, the preparation conditions are mild, the cost is low, the shape is easy to control; thus, it is widely used in the preparation of soluble silk fibroin microneedles (Figure 3).

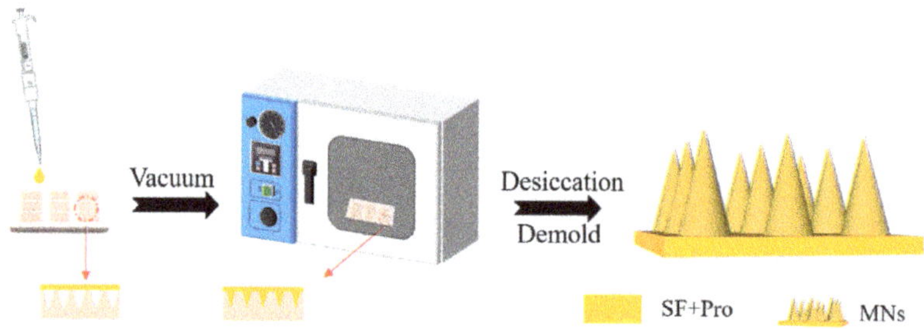


**Figure 3.** Preparation of microneedles by template pouring. Image used with permission of [86].

Although dissolving microneedles prepared with pure silk fibroin protein have many advantages, they are not accessible for piercing the skin in clinical application. In the actual operation process, there are different requirements for the tip and base of soluble microneedles. The end of the needle needs to be able to penetrate the cuticle, which requires sufficient strength, and the needle holder needs to be able to act as a platform to apply force. Silk fibroin is mechanically strong enough to be used as a needle tip. However, silk fibroin as a base is easily broken [82]. To solve this problem, Lau et al. [82] prepared a composite dissolving microneedle by using silk fibroin as the tip and polyvinyl alcohol (PVA) as the base. The process is shown in Figure 4a. Comparing the skin insertion conditions of pure silk fibroin microneedles and composite dissolved microneedles, the results showed that the composite microneedles could pierce the skin more effectively than pure silk fibroin microneedles because the PVA flexible base provided enough skin attachment and stress dispersion. In addition, Lin et al. [87] also proposed a method of preparing double-layer silk fibroin microneedles. They enhanced the mechanical strength of silk fibroin microneedles through glutaryl alcohol crosslinking and water vapor annealing. They then coated the enhanced microneedles with a mixture of silk fibroin and drug to obtain double-layer silk fibroin microneedles (Figure 4b). This method also facilitates skin piercing.

In addition to the mold casting method, Shin et al. [88] used riboflavin as a photoinitiator to prepare silk fibroin microneedles using digital light processing 3D printing technology. The mechanical properties of this method are good. A single needle can withstand the compression force of over 1000 mN and can successfully pierce pig skin. However, compared with the mold pouring method (Figure 5b), the microneedles prepared by 3D printing (Figure 5a) have poorer morphology and are limited by materials.

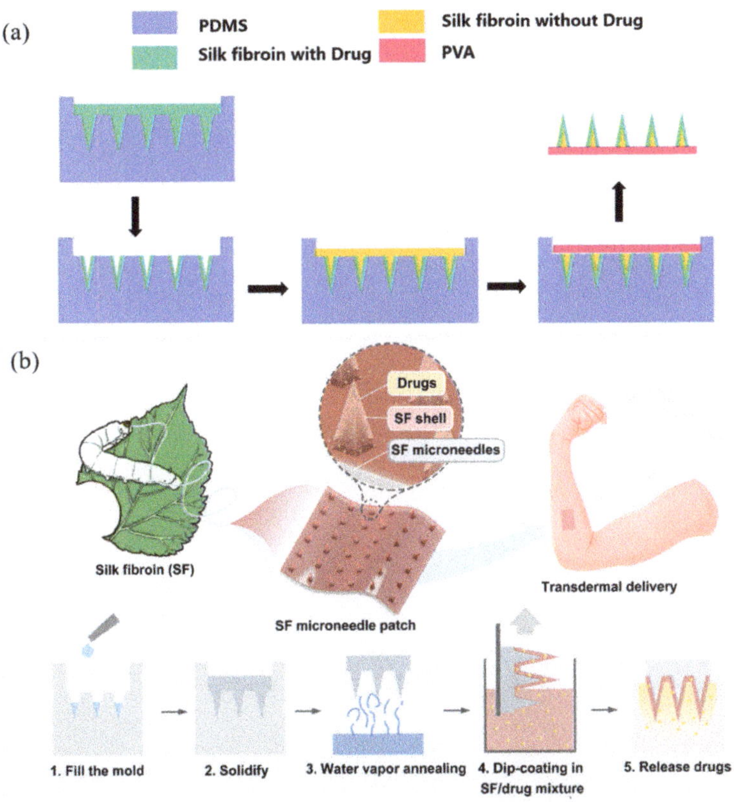


**Figure 4.** (**a**) Schematic diagram of composite dissolved microneedles: drug-loaded silk fibroin protein is used as the tip of the outermost layer, drug-free silk fibroin protein as the second layer, and PVA as the base; (**b**) Schematic diagram of the production of double-layer silk fibroin microneedles: the silk fibroin solution containing glutaraldehyde is poured into the PDMS mold, and after drying, steam annealing treatment takes place, and the silk fibroin solution is soaked in medicine on the surface of the dry microneedles. Image used with permission of [82,87].

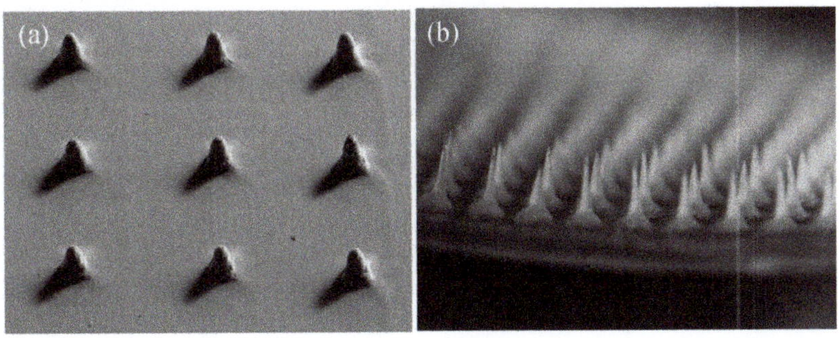


**Figure 5.** Morphologies of microneedles prepared by different methods: (**a**) 3D printing; (**b**) Formwork pouring method. Image used with permission of [30,88].

### 3.2. Swelling Silk Fibroin Microneedles

The drug release mechanism of swelling microneedles is as follows: when body fluid (the main component is water) penetrates the polymer skeleton, the molecular chains of polymer materials will stretch and expand [89,90]. By reducing the entanglement degree between polymers, the mesh size will be larger than the kinetic size of the drug, thus promoting drug release [91,92]. Its advantage is that the drug release rate can be adjusted by controlling the swelling degree of microneedles [30,35]. When harmful drug reactions or excessive drug release occurs, the microneedles can be controlled by timely removal [93].

Microneedles can be divided into two categories according to the solution: one is where the solution of the tip and the base is the same. Yin et al. [18] mixed small molecules with regenerated silk fibroin solution at different mass ratios, centrifuged repeatedly to ensure that the tip was filled entirely, and continued to add liquid and obtained uniform swelling of silk fibroin microneedles after air drying. Under the optimal ratio, the swelling degree of microneedles reached 650% (Figure 6a). Wang et al. [17] prepared silk fibroin swelling microneedles by adding proline to silk fibroin solution. The swelling tip was observed by an electron microscope. With the increase in proline dosage, the swelling degree decreased from 200% to 80%, and the solubility of the tip was less than 3%, which is an ideal release microneedle with swelling without dissolution. With this preparation method, microneedles with uniform drug distribution can be obtained. When the solution enters the microneedles, the overall structure will swell and the mesh size will become larger.

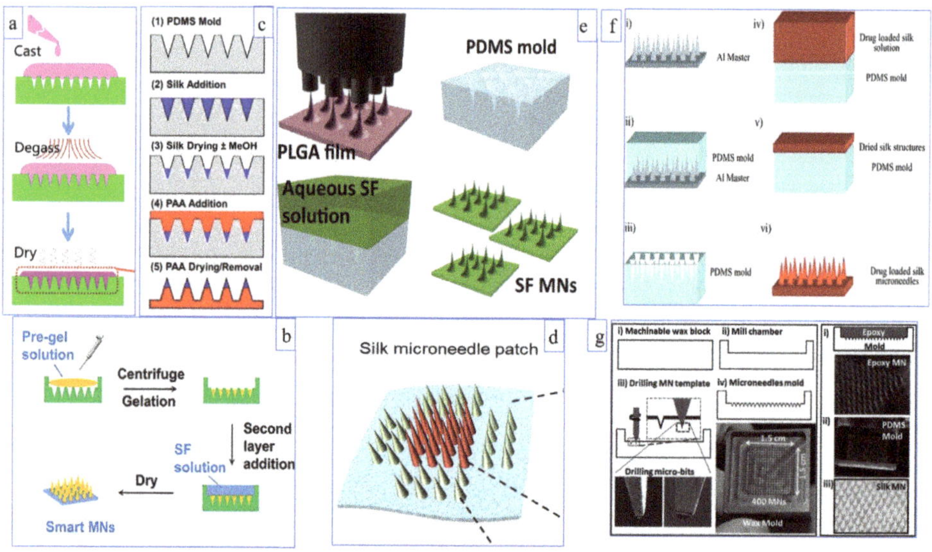


**Figure 6.** (**a**) The tip and the base are the same solution; (**b**,**c**) Different solution between tip and base; (**d**) Different microneedles in different positions; (**e**) Negative mold for hot-drawn material; (**f**) Aluminum needle master plates prepared by high-speed micro-milling; (**g**) Wax plate drilling for template preparation. Image used with permission of [18,32,33,94–97].

The other category is when the solution of the needle tip and the substrate are not the exact solutions, including but not limited to pure silk fibroin solution, functional silk fibroin solution and other polymer solutions. As shown in Figure 6b, Chen et al. [94,98] used the pre-gel of silk fibroin protein to form a tip with a semi-interpenetrating structure, with pure silk fibroin solution as the base. The internal phase presents the hydration phase, while the external phase presents the dehydration phase. The microneedles show channels under a hydration state under external stimulation. DeMuth and Boopathy et al. [32,99] used silk fibroin as the tip and polyacrylic acid as the base, as shown in Figure 6c. The drug was stored in the needle tip and annealed with methanol. The needle tip fell off in the body, and body fluids controlled the swelling and slow release. The slow swelling of the silk fibroin part from the tip and the complete release within a few days characterizes this preparation method. Moreover, silk fibroin has good biocompatibility and will not cause adverse reactions in the body.

In the above discussion, all PDMS molds are used, but there are differences in the solution configuration. Next, different molds and methods are discussed. One uses inkjet technology to precisely design various microneedles at other locations. As shown in Figure 6d, Wang et al. [33] filled the central $4 \times 4$ array with a drug solution, and the peripheral $4 \times 2$ displayed a functional silk fibroin solution. The peripheral microneedles would release quickly within a few minutes, while the inner peripheral drug solution would release slowly. The other method is hot drawing or using an inverted mold to make the master plate, pouring PDMS for a negative mold. Lee et al. [95] used a spatial discrete thermal stretching system to manufacture a microneedle template of poly (lactic acid-glycolic acid) copolymer with various geometric shapes and an inverted mold using PDMS (Figure 6e). The swelling fibroin microneedles prepared by this method can effectively pierce the skin and control drug release. In addition, high-speed micro-milling ([96], Figure 6f) and drilling on the wax plate ([97], Figure 6g) can also be used to prepare the positive mode of microneedles.

### 3.3. *Intelligently Responsive Silk Fibroin Microneedles*

Stimulation-responsive materials are generally considered intelligent; although they cannot perform advanced complex functions, they are the cornerstone of building advanced complex, intelligent systems [100]. Stimulus-responsive materials can change their size under specific stimulus conditions, which makes them widely used in drug delivery, disease diagnosis and substance detection [101,102]. Figure 7 shows the physical changes (such as expansion/contraction, assembly/dissociation, sol/gel, etc.), chemical changes (such as degradation, crosslinking, etc.) or a combination of the two after stimulation of the stimulation-responsive materials. These basic modules build the cornerstone of stimulus-responsive materials, and drugs can be integrated into the materials to respond to stimuli and test the intelligent delivery of drugs [103].

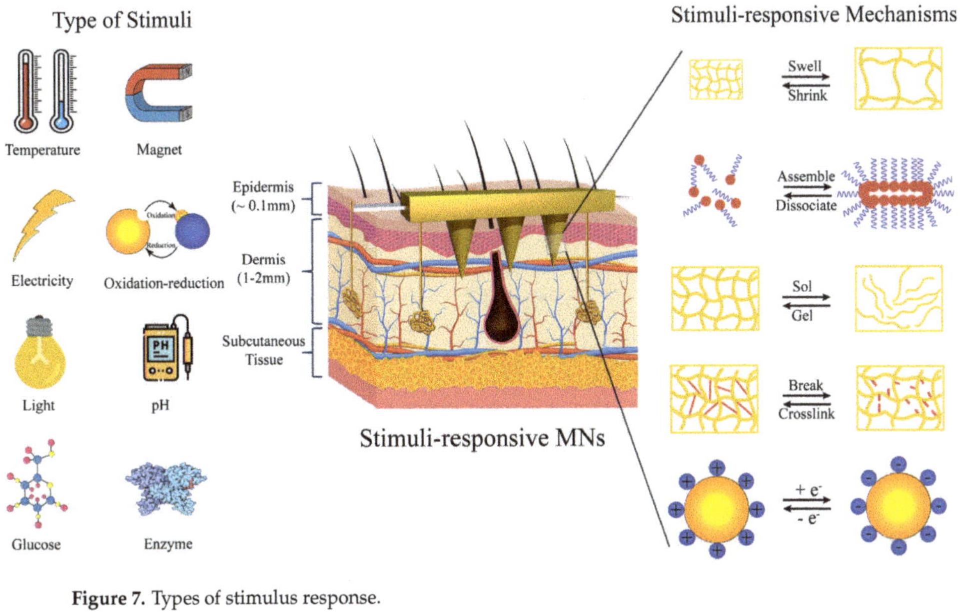


**Figure 7.** Types of stimulus response.

Dissolved microneedles and swelling microneedles can only release drugs spontaneously according to the established design procedures, which cannot meet the complex requirements of the human internal environment. Based on this, some researchers began to develop silk fibroin microneedles with the intelligent response for drug-controlled release. Compared with traditional drug delivery systems, smart drug delivery systems have more advantages: (1) the blood drug concentration is relatively stable; (2) drug efficacy is improved and drug dosage is reduced; (3) responsive delivery; (4) the number of drugs used is reduced [104,105]. Intelligent drug delivery refers to the responsive delivery of drugs to organisms by drug-carrying innovative response materials based on changes in physiological stimuli (pH value, temperature, enzymes and different biological molecules, etc.) or external stimuli (electric field, current, magnetic field, light and external mechanical force, etc.) [106,107]. The release mechanism based on physiological stimuli in organisms is primarily passive, which can respond to changes in the microenvironment in organisms to achieve intelligent drug delivery. Chen [94] reported a semi-interpenetrating network of hydrogel microneedles prepared from silk fibroin and phenylboric acid/acrylamide for glucose-responsive insulin delivery. 4-(2-acrylamide ethyl aminoformyl)-3-fluorophenylboric acid/N-isopropylacrylamide with a molar ratio of 7.5/92.5 was selected to synthesize phenylboric acid to ensure the highest glucose sensitivity. Hydrogels containing borate and silk fibroin with network structure were prepared by polymerization and catalysis of ammonium persulfate/tetramethylethylenediamine. A two-layer strategy was adopted to manufacture an intelligent microneedle composed of a semi-interpenetrating hydrogel containing silk fibroin and a needle body composed of silk fibroin, thus showing different swelling degrees under different glucose concentrations and achieving responsive insulin delivery. Due to the complexity of the physiological environment in vivo, it is often difficult to accurately control the release rate of such passive drug release, so active and targeted drug release mechanisms should be adopted to improve the overall therapeutic effect. Gao et al. [35] reported an intelligent origami silk fibroin microneedle dressing with innovative drug release, biochemical sensing, epidermal sensing, and wound healing monitoring capabilities. The microneedles were prepared by mixing silica colloidal solution with SF solution. After demolding, the microneedles were immersed in hydrofluoric acid to obtain the filament microneedles with inverse opal photonic crystal (IO PC) structure. The drug-laden N-isopropylacrylamide was poured into a microneedle with many pores and an IO PC structure. The volume phase transformation temperature of N-isopropylacrylamide is 37 °C, and when the temperature exceeds 37 °C, the microneedles produce volume shrinkage, so as to achieve drug release. Wang et al. [33] reported designing, manufacturing and applying a hetero-fibroin microneedle (SMN) patch to bypass the blood–brain barrier and deliver multiple drugs directly to the tumor site. SMN can induce rapid drug delivery by remote infrared triggering.

The above intelligent response of silk fibroin microneedles based on physiological or external stimuli has dramatically expanded the application of silk fibroin. However, the stimulation-responsive elements of these smart microneedles are not derived from the silk fibroin substrate; additional responsive features are added. Although introducing these stimulus-responsive elements brings more prosperous functions to the microneedles, it is also accompanied by many disadvantages, such as complex processing, low intelligent responsiveness and poor biological security.

Dissolving microneedles are made from a soluble polymer and encapsulated drugs. The method of poke-dissolve has some disadvantages, including poor mechanical properties and depositing of the needle in the cortex. At the same time, dissolving microneedles are not suitable for applications that require frequent dosing, such as insulin, which is the value of non-injectable dosing. In addition, microneedle dissolution allows the needle material to enter the dermis, which requires strict sterility throughout the process, resulting in higher costs for microneedle use, which negates its usefulness. Due to the rapid release of drugs, the dissolving microneedles have an effect similar to that of injection, which can cause a sudden rise in blood drug concentration in the body within a short period of time, which often leads to certain sequelae (such as hypoglycemia). For drugs with a short half-life, dissolving microneedles have difficulty maintaining effective blood concentration in vivo for a long period, which affects the therapeutic effect. Swelling microneedles, also known as hydrogel microneedles, are a kind of microneedle that absorbs water and swells to form a hydrogel after penetrating the skin, thus completing drug release. The microneedles can control the drug release rate by regulating the change speed and degree of swelling. The tip part of the microneedle will not be deposited in the cortex, which solves the potential biosafety hazard of dissolving microneedles, and also provides the possibility for the realization of microneedle intelligent drug delivery systems. The above two types of microneedles can only release drugs spontaneously according to established design procedures and cannot meet the complex needs of the human internal environment. Based on the basic platform of swelling microneedles, a microenvironment can be formed inside the swelling microneedles. Stimulation-responsive materials such as microgels and micelles in the microenvironment will undergo responsive intelligent changes under the stimulation of various external or internal physiological signals, especially structural changes (such as contraction, expansion and dissociation) or unique response pathways to control drug release.

## 4. Silk Fibroin Microneedles for Drug Delivery

The molecular weight is the most significant difference between biomacromolecule drugs and traditional small-molecule drugs [108,109]. In general, small molecule drugs refer to compounds with molecular weights less than 1000 Da, and most small molecule drugs have molecular weights less than 500 Da. However, biologic drugs are mostly proteins with huge molecular weights, usually more than 5000 Da, and complex structures.

### *4.1. Transdermal Delivery of Small Molecule Drugs*

Temozolomide (TMZ), with a relative molecular mass of 194.15, is one of the drugs used to treat glioblastoma. It can be converted into the active product 5-(3-methyl-1-triazeno)imidazole-4-carboxamide, which promotes tumor cell apoptosis through the mismatched repair of methylation add-ons. Regarding the administration of TMZ, some researchers also adopted the method of percutaneous administration. Zhao et al. [110] loaded TMZ and paclitaxel with polyethylene glycol dimethacrylate (PEG-DMA) hydrogel to inhibit the growth of postoperative glioma. PEG-DMA gel is non-degradable and requires secondary surgical removal. By combining TMZ with other drugs, Wang et al. [33] prepared a microneedle patch using silk fibroin as material. The biosafety of silk fibroin prevents secondary clearance after surgery. Lee et al. [111] proposed a highly flexible microneedle device for vascular drug delivery. It comprises a highly porous silk fibroin membrane and silk fibroin tip. The microneedle device successfully wrapped around the outer surface of blood vessels and delivered the anti-proliferative drug Sirolimus to the injured vascular tissue. Melatonin is mostly an amine hormone used to regulate the sleep quality of people with insomnia. Currently, patients are often given oral medication, but the half-life of melatonin is very short, so it is difficult to maintain sufficient drug concentration in the body [112]. Qi et al. [34] used small molecular additives to change the silk fibroin protein's crystalline structure and control melatonin's release rate. In vitro drug release results showed that effective drug concentrations were quickly obtained during early administration. Melatonin is released continuously to maintain a stable concentration of the drug. The use of microneedles to deliver small molecule drugs not only supports the long-term stability of blood drug concentration in vivo but also avoids the liver first-pass effect caused by oral administration and improves the bioavailability of drugs.

### *4.2. Transdermal Delivery of Macromolecule Drugs*

In terms of molecular weight, compared with traditional oral, subcutaneous injection and transdermal patches, microneedles can significantly improve the delivery of drugs with high-fat solubility, small effective dose and strong pharmacological effect, so as to achieve transdermal absorption of water-soluble drugs and biomacromolecules, especially for antigens or biomacromolecules [113,114]. The transdermal delivery of macromolecule drugs by silk fibroin microneedles is briefly described for the example of taking insulin for the treatment of diabetes.

Insulin, a protein drug with a simple spatial structure, comprises two peptide chains connected by disulfide bonds [115]. As a biological peptide, Insulin has poor stability and needs to be kept between 2–8 °C during distribution and storage [116].

The microneedles used for transdermal insulin delivery mainly include hollow microneedles [117,118], swelling microneedles [119] and dissolving microneedles [120,121]. The preparation process of hollow microneedles is complex and expensive [122], and the pinhole is easily blocked, thus affecting drug delivery [123]. In recent years, dissolving microneedles have attracted more and more attention due to their apparent advantages, such as simple preparation, high drug loading and one-step application, and they have been widely used for insulin delivery in studies. Silk fibroin has recently been used to manufacture dissolved microneedles due to its better mechanical properties, toughness and biocompatibility. Liu et al. [82] reported a multi-layer conical microneedle patch prepared from insulin-loaded pure silk fibroin solution as the outer layer and drug-free silk fibroin solution as the inner layer. The multi-layer microneedles showed good penetrating performance and hypoglycemic ability. However, untreated microneedles prepared with pure silk fibroin are prone to break and dissolve rapidly, which can lead to a burst of insulin release and hypoglycemia. Zhu et al. [30] reported a composite silk fibroin microneedle patch to solve this problem. The microneedle patch was prepared at 25 °C using a two-step microforming method. Unmixed silk fibroin was used for the dissolved tip, and the swelling backing was prepared using silk fibroin with proline modification. After the microneedle patch penetrates the skin, the tip is quickly dissolved by body fluids, and insulin is released. At the same time, body fluids contact the backing through microchannels formed by the tip of the needle, causing it to expand and subsequently release insulin continuously. Drug administration results in diabetic rats showed that blood glucose reached the lowest level within 3 h and recovered to the initial level 6 h later. The structure showed obvious hypoglycemic effects and could meet the need of rapid hypoglycemic reduction after meals. At the same time, continuous insulin release can be achieved without the risk of hypoglycemia. Insulin has good stability in this solid substrate, maintaining more than 90% of its biological activity after 30 days at room temperature. As a protein, silk fibroin can be hydrolyzed under the action of enzymes and thus eliminated from the body [124]. Cao et al. [86] selected silk fibroin modified by proline to prepare a swelling microneedle, whose microneedle structure was mainly Silk I crystalline structure. The drug loading of the microneedle patch is 20 IU/0.5 $cm^2$, which can provide insulin sustained release for 12 h and control the blood glucose of diabetic rats to maintain normal levels, avoiding frequent administration.

### *4.3. Silk Fibroin Microneedles for Transdermal Administration of Vaccines*

Vaccine administration by subcutaneous (SC) or intramuscular (IM) injection is the most commonly prescribed route for inoculation [125–127]. Vaccine activity and efficacy require strict requirements for vaccine distribution and transportation, which is also a significant challenge for developing countries [125,128]. Compared with IM/SC injection, transdermal vaccination with microneedles, as an emerging technology, could reduce the required amount of vaccines and further improve immunogenicity with the potential of lowering the cost of vaccination, expanding a promising administration route [129,130]. At the same time, commonly used vaccines are composed of antigens or antibodies, and their molecular weight is too large for transdermal delivery through traditional methods [131]. An interesting approach to dealing with this obstacle is the use of microneedles [125]. The acceptance of patients is improved, and the antigen/antibody activity can be stable in the dry environment, thus saving the cost of transportation and distribution.

Jordan et al. [128] evaluated the ability of microneedles prepared from silk fibroin to deliver vaccines against influenza, Shigella and Clostridium difficile infection. The microneedle carrier uses silk fibroin protein and has high biocompatibility. The stability and mechanical strength of the vaccine are also guaranteed. By inoculating the mice with separate antigens, it was found that a large amount of Shigella-protective invasion plasmid antigen (Ipa) was found in the mice, and no redness and swelling appeared on the skin where the microneedles were applied. The experiment proved that the microneedles had good biological safety and that the internal vaccine could be released smoothly. Archana et al. [32] focused on the study of stabilized recombinant HIV-1 envelope glycoprotein antibody variants. After the vaccine was mixed with silk solution, it was evenly poured into the PDMS mold and dried. Polyacrylic acid was used as microneedle base material. When applied to the skin, the polyacrylic acid backing will dissolve rapidly, and the silk fibroin tip containing the vaccine will be implanted into the epidermis/epithelium. The crystallinity of the silk fibroin will significantly improve the release rate of the vaccine. Blood epidermis/dermis was collected and analyzed 7, 14, and 21 days after the skin was punctured. Tip sequences containing labeled trimer were observed in the epidermis, and the total antigen signal decreased steadily within 14 days, which was longer lasting and more effective than the injection form. Peter et al. [99] also designed an implantable silk fibroin hydrogel composite microneedle with polyacrylic acid as the backing to obtain mixed microneedles, successfully achieving sustained skin vaccine release at a low level within 1–2 weeks. The implantable microneedle platform has the ability to optimize vaccine release dynamics, resulting in a more than 10-fold increase in antigen-specific T-cell and humoral immune responses compared to traditional parenteral needle immunization.

## 5. Clinical Transformation of Microneedles and Silk Fibroin Materials

### 5.1. Commercial Application of Silk Fibroin Medical Apparatus

Silk is a natural protein polymer that has been approved by the US Food and Drug Administration (FDA) for medical use. From a conversion perspective, to our knowledge, only a few silk fibroin-based medical products have received regulatory approval for clinical use worldwide to date (Table 1), including SERI scaffold with SILK VOIVE injectable implant (Sofregen Medical Inc., Framingham, MA, USA) and Silk Protein Wound Dressing (Suzhou Soho Biomaterial Science and Technology Co., Ltd., Suzhou, China). In 1995, AST-1 Silk Fibroin Wound Protective Dressing developed by Soochow University obtained a registration certificate, and clinical application began in 1996. On the basis of AST-1 Silk Fibroin Wound Protective Dressing, the product was adjusted according to clinical conditions, and Silk Protein Wound Dressing was launched and put on the market in 2012. Silk Protein Wound Dressing is indicated for second-degree burn wound healing. Detailed clinical data on Silk Protein Wound Dressing has not yet been published. In 2019, Zhejiang Xingyue Biotechnology Co., Ltd. (Yongkang, China) developed a silk fibroin regeneration and repair membrane. The full-layer skin defect experiment using New Zealand rabbits showed that the silk fibroin membrane could significantly reduce the wound healing time and improve the wound healing quality, which was superior to the control products on the market. In a 71-patient randomized controlled clinical trial (NCT01993030), the silk fibroin membrane significantly accelerated wound healing and reduced the incidence of adverse reactions compared with marketed controls. The SERI surgical scaffold was commercialized in 2013 for soft tissue support and repair. The current SERI is suitable for abdominal wall reconstruction and investigational plastic surgery applications, including total body molding, humeroplasty, abdominoplasty, mastexy, and breast reconstruction [132–134]. Some clinical reports indicate that SERI may cause side effects such as infection and poor stent integration in the later stage, requiring surgical removal. Silk Voice, developed by Sofregen, is the only approved natural silk protein injection. Silk Voice was approved in 2018 for the treatment of vocal cord mediation and vocal cord insufficiency.

**Table 1.** Commercially available silk fibroin products.

| Official Title | Type | Company | Application | Announced Date | Registration Certificate Number |
|---|---|---|---|---|---|
| AST-1 Silk Fibroin Wound Protective Dressing | Single-layer dressing | Soochow University (Suzhou Institute of Silk Technology) | It is used to prevent bacterial infection of the wound. It presents no irritation to the skin, can promote the growth of wound cells, and has good permeable steam. | 1995 | Su1995-95264098 |
| Silk Protein Wound Dressing | Double-layer dressing | Suzhou Soho Biomaterial Science and Technology Co., Ltd. | It is used for clinical second-degree wound healing; is suitable for mild and severe acne, skin allergies and laser photon treatment of early postoperative pigmentation; and reduces the formation of fatigue marks. | 2012 | Su2012-2640182 |
| SILK VOICE® Injectable Implant | Injectable implant | SOFREGEN MEDICAL Inc. | It is used for clinical second-degree wound healing; is suitable for mild and severe acne, skin allergies and laser photon treatment of early postoperative pigmentation; and reduces the formation of fatigue marks. | 2012 | - |
| Silk fibroin membrane dressing | Single-layer dressing | Zhejiang Xingyue Biotechnology Co., Ltd. | It covers the skin wound, blocks the external bacteria, and prevents the granulation tissue from growing into the dressing. At the same time, the water in the wound blood and exudate is discharged as water vapor to provide a healing environment for the wound, and the blood cells and other visible components left behind form a scab. | 2020 | SFDA2020-3140593 |
| SERI® Surgical Scaffold | Scaffold | SOFREGEN MEDICAL Inc. | A temporary brace used for soft tissue support and repair to strengthen defects where weaknesses or gaps exist. This includes soft tissue reinforcement in plastic and reconstructive surgery, as well as soft tissue reconstruction in general. | 2021 | - |

### 5.2. Clinical Application of Silk Fibroin Medical Apparatus

Over the past 20 years, there has been a resurgence of interest in silk for biomedical use, which has led to many clinical trials. Table 2 shows the clinical trials of silk fibroin medical devices. Nowadays, silk fibroin is widely used in wound repair dressings and orthopedic repair materials. The primary application forms are dressing, film, stents, etc.

Silk fibroin materials show excellent application prospects in skin wound healing due to their hemostatic properties, low inflammatory potential, air permeability and antibacterial ability. Silk Protein Wound Dressing is a silk fibroin sponge-silicone double-layer scaffold for skin wound healing and has received regulatory approval worldwide for clinical use. However, this silk fibroin-based medical product is not widely used in clinical trials today. Zhang et al. [135] compared the wound healing ability of Silk Protein Wound Dressing in a preclinical animal model and then conducted a randomized, single-blind phase I clinical trial. The silk fibroin film was dried for 100 min at 65 °C and RH90%. It is a waterproof film with a thickness of 64.9 µm. In a rabbit model of full-layer wound healing, wounds treated with silk fibroin film showed better epidermal remodeling and granulation tissue than those treated with Silk Protein Wound Dressing. The clinical trial enrolled 71 patients (36 randomly assigned to the membrane group and 35 randomly assigned to the Silk Protein Wound Dressing group). The wound healing rate of patients in the silk fibroin film group was significantly faster than that in the Silk Protein Wound Dressing group, and 100% wound healing was achieved in the silk fibroin film group by day 14 after injury. As the wound heals, the silk fibroin film spontaneously detaches from the regenerated skin area. The exact mechanism of the improved clinical performance in the silk fibroin film group compared to the Silk Protein Wound Dressing group is unclear.

This study demonstrated the ability to manufacture silk fibroin membranes as wound dressings for successful skin repair and regeneration under good manufacturing practices. The potential for relatively simple modifications to silk membranes for additional functions, such as binding pores or the introduction of bioactive molecules [136], makes silk membranes particularly attractive as wound dressings.

**Table 2.** Clinical trials of silk fibroin medical devices.

| Official Title | Type | Condition | Primary Purpose | Status | Start Date /Completion Date | Trial ID |
|---|---|---|---|---|---|---|
| A Multi-Center Open Study to Evaluate the SeriACL™ Device for Primary Anterior Cruciate Ligament Repair | ACL Reconstruction (SeriACL™ Device) | Phase 1 | Treatment | Unknown | 2007.6/ 2008.10 | NCT00490594 |
| Randomized, Active-controlled, Single-blind, Parallel Two-group Trial of HQ® Matrix Medical Wound Dressing and Sidaiyi® Wound Dressing for the Treatment of Donor Site Wounds | HQ® Matrix Medical Wound Dressing | Not Applicable | Treatment | Completed | 2013.8/ 2015.6 | NCT01993030 CQZ1800141 |
| Efficacy and Safety of Wound Dressing Containing Silk Fibroin with Bioactive Coating Layer Versus Medicated Paraffin Gauze Dressing in the Treatment of Split-thickness Skin Graft Donor Sites | Silk fibroin with bioactive coating layer dressing | Phase 1/2 | Treatment | Completed | 2014.3/ 2015.5 | NCT02091076 |
| A Prospective Open-Label Study to Evaluate the Safety of the Meniscal Repair Scaffold, FibroFix™ Meniscus, in the Treatment of Meniscal Defects | FibroFix™ Meniscus scaffold | Not Applicable | Treatment | Terminated (Safety devices explanted. 12 m post-explant safety f/u as agreed with UK MHRA) | 2015.4/ 2017.10 | NCT02205645 |
| Multi-center, Randomized, Active-controlled, Single-blind, Parallel Two-group Trial of HQ® Matrix Soft Tissue Mesh and ULTRAPRO® Partially Absorbable Lightweight Mesh for the Treatment of Inguinal Hernia | HQ® Matrix Soft Tissue Mesh | Not Applicable | Treatment | Unknown | 2015.7/ 2016.12 (estimated) | NCT02487628 |
| Comparison of Microbial Adherence to Various Sutures in Patients Undergoing Oral Surgery | Silk suture | Not Applicable | Treatment | Unknown | 2016.1/ 2017.1 (estimated) | NCT02653924 |
| A Pilot Feasibility Randomized Controlled Trial to Assess the Clinical and Cost Effectiveness of Dialkylcarbamoylchloride (DACC)-Coated Postoperative Dressings Versus Standard Care in the Prevention of Surgical Site Infection in Clean or Clean-contaminated Vascular and Cardiothoracic Surgery | DACC-Coated Post-Operative Dressing | Not Applicable | Treatment | Recruiting | 2017.1/ 2025.1 (estimated) | NCT02992951 |
| Silk Scaffold Surgical Incision Dressing Interventional Study | Experimental silk/adhesive prototype | Phase 1 | Assessment | Recruiting | 2022.8/ 2023.5 (estimated) | NCT05508945 |
| Safety and efficacy of absorbable silk fibroin film for alveolar ridge preservation after extraction | Absorbable silk fibroin film | Phase 3/4 | Assessment | Completed | - | CQZ1900597 ChiCTR-IOR-17025031 |

### *5.3. Clinical Application of Microneedle Devices*

This paper searched and sorted the clinical applications of silk fibroin medical devices and microneedle devices of other materials [137]. We listed completed and ongoing clinical trials based on information provided at www.clinicaltrials.gov. In clinical trials, researchers mainly verified the clinical safety and efficacy of microneedles for drug delivery systems, as shown in Table 3. These clinical data indicate that microneedles for drug delivery are effective quickly and with less insertion pain. This mainly includes dissolving microneedles, hollow microneedles, coated microneedles and microdetectors used for administering vaccines, macromolecular drugs and monitoring human physiological conditions.

**Table 3.** Clinical research progress in microneedle devices.

| Official Title | Type | Phase | Primary Purpose | Status | Start Date /Completion Date | Trial ID |
|---|---|---|---|---|---|---|
| Insulin Delivery Using Microneedles in Type 1 Diabetes | Hollow | Phase 2/3 | Treatment | Completed | 2009.2/ 2014.1 | NCT00837512 |
| Clinical Assessment of a Novel Microprobe Array Continuous Glucose Monitor for Type 1 Diabetes | Microprobe glucose sensor | Phase 1/2/3/4 | Diagnostic | Completed | 2013.11/ 2018.6 | NCT01908530 |
| A Phase I Study of the Safety, Reactogenicity, Acceptability and Immunogenicity of Inactivated Influenza Vaccine Delivered by Microneedle Patch or by Hypodermic Needle | Dissolving microneedle | Phase 1 | Prevention | Completed | 2015.5/ 2019.7 | NCT02438423 |
| Microneedle Sensing of Beta-lactam Antibiotic Concentrations in Human Interstitial Fluid | Biosensors | Phase 1 | Device Feasibility | Completed | 2019.2/ 2020.12 | NCT03847610 |
| A clinical trial of dose-response using a microneedle array containing Japanese encephalitis vaccine in healthy adult individuals | Dissolving microneedle | Phase 1/2 | Prevention | Completed | 2019.7/ 2020.2 | jRCTs011190004 |
| A Phase I/II, Double-blind, Randomized, Active-controlled, Age De-escalation Trial to Assess the safety and Immunogenicity of a Measles Rubella Vaccine (MRV) Microneedle Patch (MRV-MNP) in Adults, MRV-primed Toddlers, and MRV-naïve Infants | Dissolving microneedle | Phase 1/2 | Assessment | Recruiting | 2021.5/ 2022.6 (estimated) | NCT04394689 |

## 6. Future Development Trends

This article reviewed the characteristics of silk fibroin and the preparation methods of different microneedle types. More importantly, the development of silk fibroin microneedles for drug delivery is introduced in detail.

Currently, most of the drugs on the market are small-molecule drugs prepared by chemical synthesis. However, the number of new drugs such as proteins, peptides and antibodies is on the rise. The market is estimated to exceed US $217 billion, accounting for 10% of the pharmaceutical market [138]. These biomacromolecules differ from chemically synthesized small molecules and have a relatively large molecular size and conformational flexibility. Peptides and proteins are considered multi-domain biopolymers, consisting of residues with rich cation, polarity and hydrophobicity differences [139]. Unlike many materials, silk fibroin is inherently stable to changes in temperature and humidity. The unique block copolymerization structure enables it to assemble into a nanometer crystalline domain. As a result, silk fibroin has better characteristics in drug delivery than other biological materials, such as good biological stability of enzymes, antioxidant activity, and biological stability for biomolecular drugs and vaccines. These unique advantages gradually improve the application prospect and position of silk fibroin [27,140–142]. Therefore, silk fibroin is an excellent candidate material for preparing microneedles. Silk fibroin microneedles have developed from soluble microneedles and swelling microneedles to intelligent responsive microneedles, which can effectively carry small molecule drugs, large molecule drugs and vaccines. Silk fibroin microneedles have achieved the same or even more powerful effects as needle injection in terms of form and function. Despite these encouraging results, more efforts are needed to accelerate the entry of silk fibroin microneedles into the medical market.

The first issue is safety. Although the biosafety of silk fibroin has widely been recognized, basic studies remain necessary, including those involving cytotoxicity, acute/chronic systemic toxicity, hemolysis testing, stimulation testing, implantation testing, implant testing, intradermal reaction testing, biodegradation testing, carcinogenic testing, etc. The safety of silk fibroin microneedles still needs further thorough verification in different animal or preclinical models.

The second is the drug-carrying dose and type. Although some active biological enzymes (horseradish peroxidase, glucose oxidase [143]) and some vaccines (influenza vaccine, HIV vaccine, adenovirus vaccine [144] and others) have been successfully used, it is still worth studying how to increase the carrying dose, which will provide effective dose support for the transformation from experimental animals to human beings. At the same time, about 40% of research drugs are hydrophobic, among which there are many macromolecular drugs. Further study is required to improve the carrying dose and conform to the water-soluble environmental processing of silk fibroin microneedles. Of course, this must be carried out according to the specific drug. Another possible solution is to extend the current microneedle manufacturing method. The existing template method has shortcomings in the large-scale preparation of microneedles and the delivery of large doses of drugs. The extended microneedle manufacturing method is expected to solve this problem.

The third is intelligence. Traditional microneedle drug delivery can only spontaneously slow-release drugs according to pre-set procedures. With the development of personalized medicine, the traditional way cannot meet the needs of the complex environment in the human body. The silk fibroin microneedles with stimulatory response function are expected to play a significant role in the drug-controlled release. This can help improve the effectiveness of treatment and reduce the risk of inappropriate drug use. Intelligent responsive silk fibroin microneedles can be realized in two ways: one is to chemically modify the microneedle substrate to obtain stimulation-responsive silk fibroin material; the other is to add stimulation-responsive elements (such as stimulation-responsive nanoparticles, microspheres, vesicles or supramolecular aggregates) to pure silk fibroin protein. This will help the silk fibroin microneedles achieve intelligent responsiveness.

The current regulatory approval process based on the microneedle patch is not ideal, mainly due to the advanced technology. For future market applications, standardized regulation of sterilization methods, durability, safety and disposal of microneedles after use is also required. The ultimate sterilization of microneedle patches can save most of the cost compared to aseptic manufacturing. Several microneedle-based sterilizations have been studied. According to the requirements of the European Pharmacopoeia, the sterilization of microneedle patches is based on steam sterilization, dry heat sterilization and ionizing radiation. According to the different properties of microneedle substrates, the sterilization process has different effects. Wet and dry heat sterilization can damage the morphology and penetration ability of silk fibroin microneedles, but gamma irradiation sterilization seems to be the only viable option. After gamma ray sterilization, the activity and release of drugs contained in microneedles did not change significantly [145,146].

In addition, there is insufficient data on the side effects of microneedles (e.g., skin irritation, microneedle substrate deposition), and more research is needed to select polymers that minimize skin irritation. Silk fibroin protein has incomparable advantages in biosecurity. However, it is still necessary to determine the specific amount of silk fibroin remaining in the skin after removal of microneedles and the removal of residues in the later stage. Deposition of the substrate may not be an important problem in the case of a single microneedle administration but may be significant if the microneedles are used frequently over a long period of time.

## 7. Conclusions

This review focuses on the critical research progress of silk fibroin microneedles since inception, analyzes in detail the structure and properties of silk fibroin, types of silk fibroin microneedles, drug delivery application and clinical transformation progress, and summarizes the future development trend in this field. It also proposes future research directions for silk fibroin microneedles in increasing drug loading dose and enriching drug loading types as well as exploring silk fibroin microneedles with stimulation-responsive drug release functions. The safety and effectiveness of silk fibroin microneedles should be adequately verified in clinical trials at different stages. What we have achieved determines where we stand, and what we will do in the future determines how far we can proceed.

**Funding:** National Natural Science Foundation of China (Grant No. 51973144), College Nature Science Research Project of Jiangsu Province, China (Grant No. 20KJA540002), PAPD and Six Talent Peaks Project in Jiangsu Province (Grant No. SWYY-038) supported this work.

**Institutional Review Board Statement:** Not applicable.

**Informed Consent Statement:** Not applicable.

**Data Availability Statement:** Not applicable.

**Conflicts of Interest:** The authors declare no conflict of interest.

## References

1. Adolphe, C.; Wainwright, B. pathways to improving skin regeneration. *Expert Rev. Mol. Med.* **2005**, *7*, 1–14. [CrossRef] [PubMed]
2. Elias, P.M. Stratum Corneum Defensive Functions: An Integrated View. *J. Gen. Intern. Med.* **2005**, *20*, 183–200. [CrossRef] [PubMed]
3. Ahmed Saeed Al-Japairai, K.; Mahmood, S.; Hamed Almurisi, S.; Reddy Venugopal, J.; Rebhi Hilles, A.; Azmana, M.; Raman, S. Current trends in polymer microneedle for transdermal drug delivery. *Int. J. Pharm.* **2020**, *587*, 119673. [CrossRef] [PubMed]
4. Yang, D.; Chen, M.; Sun, Y.; Jin, Y.; Lu, C.; Pan, X.; Quan, G.; Wu, C. Microneedle-mediated transdermal drug delivery for treating diverse skin diseases. *Acta Biomater.* **2021**, *121*, 119–133. [CrossRef] [PubMed]
5. Karim, Z.; Karwa, P.; Hiremath, S.R.R. Polymeric microneedles for transdermal drug delivery—A review of recent studies. *J. Drug Deliv. Sci. Technol.* **2022**, *77*, 103760. [CrossRef]
6. Pastore, M.N.; Kalia, Y.N.; Horstmann, M.; Roberts, M.S. Transdermal patches: History, development and pharmacology. *Br. J. Pharmacol.* **2015**, *172*, 2179–2209. [CrossRef]
7. Ruan, S.; Zhang, Y.; Feng, N. Microneedle-mediated transdermal nanodelivery systems: A review. *Biomater. Sci.* **2021**, *9*, 8065–8089. [CrossRef]
8. Thomas, B.J.; Finnin, B.C. The transdermal revolution. *Drug Discov. Today* **2004**, *9*, 697–703. [CrossRef]
9. Haque, T.; Talukder, M.M.U. Chemical Enhancer: A Simplistic Way to Modulate Barrier Function of the Stratum Corneum. *Adv. Pharm. Bull.* **2018**, *8*, 169–179. [CrossRef]
10. Ye, Y.; Yu, J.; Wen, D.; Kahkoska, A.R.; Gu, Z. Polymeric microneedles for transdermal protein delivery. *Adv. Drug Deliv. Rev.* **2018**, *127*, 106–118. [CrossRef]
11. Mahmood, S.; Mandal, U.K.; Chatterjee, B. Transdermal delivery of raloxifene HCl via ethosomal system: Formulation, advanced characterizations and pharmacokinetic evaluation. *Int. J. Pharm.* **2018**, *542*, 36–46. [CrossRef]
12. Economidou, S.N.; Lamprou, D.A.; Douroumis, D. 3D printing applications for transdermal drug delivery. *Int. J. Pharm.* **2018**, *544*, 415–424. [CrossRef]
13. Lim, D.-J.; Kim, H.-J. Microneedles in Action: Microneedling and Microneedles-Assisted Transdermal Delivery. *Polymers* **2022**, *14*, 1608. [CrossRef]
14. Lee, H.; Song, C.; Baik, S.; Kim, D.; Hyeon, T.; Kim, D.-H. Device-assisted transdermal drug delivery. *Adv. Drug Deliv. Rev.* **2018**, *127*, 35–45. [CrossRef]
15. Waghule, T.; Singhvi, G.; Dubey, S.K.; Pandey, M.M.; Gupta, G.; Singh, M.; Dua, K. Microneedles: A smart approach and increasing potential for transdermal drug delivery system. *Biomed. Pharmacother.* **2019**, *109*, 1249–1258. [CrossRef]
16. Nayak, A.; Babla, H.; Han, T.; Das, D.B. Lidocaine carboxymethylcellulose with gelatine co-polymer hydrogel delivery by combined microneedle and ultrasound. *Drug Deliv.* **2016**, *23*, 658–669. [CrossRef]
17. Wang, S.; Zhu, M.; Zhao, L.; Kuang, D.; Kundu, S.C.; Lu, S. Insulin-Loaded Silk Fibroin Microneedles as Sustained Release System. *ACS Biomater. Sci. Eng.* **2019**, *5*, 1887–1894. [CrossRef]
18. Yin, Z.P.; Kuang, D.J.; Wang, S.Y.; Zheng, Z.Z.; Yadavalli, V.K.; Lu, S.Z. Swellable silk fibroin microneedles for transdermal drug delivery. *Int. J. Biol. Macromol.* **2018**, *106*, 48–56. [CrossRef]
19. Gill, H.S.; Prausnitz, M.R. Coated microneedles for transdermal delivery. *J. Control. Release* **2007**, *117*, 227–237. [CrossRef]
20. Zhao, J.; Xu, G.; Yao, X.; Zhou, H.; Lyu, B.; Pei, S.; Wen, P. Microneedle-based insulin transdermal delivery system: Current status and translation challenges. *Drug Deliv. Transl. Res.* **2022**, *12*, 2403–2427. [CrossRef]
21. Li, X.; Zhao, Z.; Zhang, M.; Ling, G.; Zhang, P. Research progress of microneedles in the treatment of melanoma. *J. Control. Release* **2022**, *348*, 631–647. [CrossRef] [PubMed]
22. Sabri, A.H.; Kim, Y.; Marlow, M.; Scurr, D.J.; Segal, J.; Banga, A.K.; Kagan, L.; Lee, J.B. Intradermal and transdermal drug delivery using microneedles—Fabrication, performance evaluation and application to lymphatic delivery. *Adv. Drug Deliv. Rev.* **2020**, *153*, 195–215. [CrossRef] [PubMed]
23. Freiherr, J.; Hallschmid, M.; Frey, W.H.; Brünner, Y.F.; Chapman, C.D.; Hölscher, C.; Craft, S.; De Felice, F.G.; Benedict, C. Intranasal Insulin as a Treatment for Alzheimer's Disease: A Review of Basic Research and Clinical Evidence. *CNS Drugs* **2013**, *27*, 505–514. [CrossRef]

24. Gera, A.K.; Burra, R.K. The Rise of Polymeric Microneedles: Recent Developments, Advances, Challenges, and Applications with Regard to Transdermal Drug Delivery. *J. Funct. Biomater.* **2022**, *13*, 81. [CrossRef] [PubMed]
25. Johari, N.; Khodaei, A.; Samadikuchaksaraei, A.; Reis, R.L.; Kundu, S.C.; Moroni, L. Ancient fibrous biomaterials from silkworm protein fibroin and spider silk blends: Biomechanical patterns. *Acta Biomater.* **2022**, *153*, 38–67. [CrossRef] [PubMed]
26. Lu, S.-z.; Wang, X.-q.; Uppal, N.; Kaplan, D.L.; Li, M.-z. Stabilization of horseradish peroxidase in silk materials. *Front. Mater. Sci. China* **2009**, *3*, 367–411. [CrossRef]
27. Lu, S.; Wang, X.; Lu, Q.; Hu, X.; Uppal, N.; Omenetto, F.G.; Kaplan, D.L. Stabilization of Enzymes in Silk Films. *Biomacromolecules* **2009**, *10*, 1032–1042. [CrossRef]
28. Lozano-Pérez, A.A.; Rivero, H.C.; Pérez Hernández, M.d.C.; Pagán, A.; Montalbán, M.G.; Víllora, G.; Cénis, J.L. Silk fibroin nanoparticles: Efficient vehicles for the natural antioxidant quercetin. *Int. J. Pharm.* **2017**, *518*, 11–19. [CrossRef]
29. Luo, T.; Yang, L.; Wu, J.; Zheng, Z.; Li, G.; Wang, X.; Kaplan, D.L. Stabilization of Natural Antioxidants by Silk Biomaterials. *ACS Appl. Mater. Interfaces* **2016**, *8*, 13573–13582. [CrossRef]
30. Zhu, M.; Liu, Y.; Jiang, F.; Cao, J.; Kundu, S.C.; Lu, S. Combined Silk Fibroin Microneedles for Insulin Delivery. *ACS Biomater. Sci. Eng.* **2020**, *6*, 3422–3429. [CrossRef]
31. Pritchard, E.M.; Kaplan, D.L. Silk fibroin biomaterials for controlled release drug delivery. *Expert Opin. Drug Deliv.* **2011**, *8*, 797–811. [CrossRef] [PubMed]
32. Boopathy, A.V.; Mandal, A.; Kulp, D.W.; Menis, S.; Bennett, N.R.; Watkins, H.C.; Wang, W.; Martin, J.T.; Thai, N.T.; He, Y.; et al. Enhancing humoral immunity via sustained-release implantable microneedle patch vaccination. *Proc. Natl. Acad. Sci. USA* **2019**, *116*, 16473–16478. [CrossRef]
33. Wang, Z.; Yang, Z.; Jiang, J.; Shi, Z.; Mao, Y.; Qin, N.; Tao, T.H. Silk Microneedle Patch Capable of On-Demand Multidrug Delivery to the Brain for Glioblastoma Treatment. *Adv. Mater.* **2022**, *34*, 2106606–2106688. [CrossRef] [PubMed]
34. Qi, Z.; Cao, J.; Tao, X.; Wu, X.; Kundu, S.C.; Lu, S. Silk Fibroin Microneedle Patches for the Treatment of Insomnia. *Pharmaceutics* **2021**, *13*, 2198. [CrossRef] [PubMed]
35. Gao, B.; Guo, M.; Lyu, K.; Chu, T.; He, B. Intelligent Silk Fibroin Based Microneedle Dressing (i-SMD). *Adv. Funct. Mater.* **2021**, *31*, 2006839–2006897. [CrossRef]
36. Altman, G.H.; Diaz, F.; Jakuba, C.; Calabro, T.; Horan, R.L.; Chen, J.; Lu, H.; Richmond, J.; Kaplan, D.L. Silk-based biomaterials. *Biomaterials* **2003**, *24*, 401–416. [CrossRef]
37. Hess, S.; van Beek, J.; Pannell, L.K. Acid hydrolysis of silk fibroins and determination of the enrichment of isotopically labeled amino acids using precolumn derivatization and high-performance liquid chromatography–electrospray ionization–mass spectrometry. *Anal. Biochem.* **2002**, *311*, 19–26. [CrossRef]
38. Kurihara, H.; Sezutsu, H.; Tamura, T.; Yamada, K. Production of an active feline interferon in the cocoon of transgenic silkworms using the fibroin H-chain expression system. *Biochem. Biophys. Res. Commun.* **2007**, *355*, 976–980. [CrossRef]
39. Zhou, C.-Z.; Confalonieri, F.; Jacquet, M.; Perasso, R.; Li, Z.-G.; Janin, J. Silk fibroin: Structural implications of a remarkable amino acid sequence. *Proteins Struct. Funct. Bioinform.* **2001**, *44*, 119–122. [CrossRef]
40. Zhou, C.-Z.; Confalonieri, F.; Medina, N.; Zivanovic, Y.; Esnault, C.; Yang, T.; Jacquet, M.; Janin, J.; Duguet, M.; Perasso, R.; et al. Fine organization of Bombyx mori fibroin heavy chain gene. *Nucleic Acids Res.* **2000**, *28*, 2413–2419. [CrossRef]
41. Rockwood, D.N.; Preda, R.C.; Yücel, T.; Wang, X.; Lovett, M.L.; Kaplan, D.L. Materials fabrication from Bombyx mori silk fibroin. *Nat. Protoc.* **2011**, *6*, 1612–1631. [CrossRef]
42. Bai, S.; Zhang, X.; Lu, Q.; Sheng, W.; Liu, L.; Dong, B.; Kaplan, D.L.; Zhu, H. Reversible Hydrogel–Solution System of Silk with High Beta-Sheet Content. *Biomacromolecules* **2014**, *15*, 3044–3051. [CrossRef]
43. Inoue, S.; Tanaka, K.; Arisaka, F.; Kimura, S.; Ohtomo, K.; Mizuno, S. Silk Fibroin of Bombyx mori Is Secreted, Assembling a High Molecular Mass Elementary Unit Consisting of H-chain, L-chain, and P25, with a 6:6:1 Molar Ratio*. *J. Biol. Chem.* **2000**, *275*, 40517–40528. [CrossRef]
44. Yang, Y.; Shao, Z.; Chen, X.; Zhou, P. Optical Spectroscopy to Investigate the Structure of Regenerated Bombyx mori Silk Fibroin in Solution. *Biomacromolecules* **2004**, *5*, 773–779. [CrossRef]
45. Koide, S.; Huang, X.; Link, K.; Koide, A.; Bu, Z.; Engelman, D.M. Design of single-layer β-sheets without a hydrophobic core. *Nature* **2000**, *403*, 456–460. [CrossRef]
46. Kyte, J.; Doolittle, R.F. A simple method for displaying the hydropathic character of a protein. *J. Mol. Biol.* **1982**, *157*, 105–132. [CrossRef]
47. Koh, L.-D.; Cheng, Y.; Teng, C.-P.; Khin, Y.-W.; Loh, X.-J.; Tee, S.-Y.; Low, M.; Ye, E.; Yu, H.-D.; Zhang, Y.-W.; et al. Structures, mechanical properties and applications of silk fibroin materials. *Prog. Polym. Sci.* **2015**, *46*, 86–110. [CrossRef]
48. Lammel, A.S.; Hu, X.; Park, S.-H.; Kaplan, D.L.; Scheibel, T.R. Controlling silk fibroin particle features for drug delivery. *Biomaterials* **2010**, *31*, 4583–4591. [CrossRef]
49. Nova, A.; Keten, S.; Pugno, N.M.; Redaelli, A.; Buehler, M.J. Molecular and Nanostructural Mechanisms of Deformation, Strength and Toughness of Spider Silk Fibrils. *Nano Lett.* **2010**, *10*, 2626–2634. [CrossRef]
50. Marsh, R.E.; Corey, R.B.; Pauling, L. An investigation of the structure of silk fibroin. *Biochim. Et Biophys. Acta* **1955**, *16*, 1–34. [CrossRef]
51. Vepari, C.; Kaplan, D.L. Silk as a biomaterial. *Prog. Polym. Sci.* **2007**, *32*, 991–1007. [CrossRef] [PubMed]

52. Yin, Z.; Wu, F.; Xing, T.; Yadavalli, V.K.; Kundu, S.C.; Lu, S. A silk fibroin hydrogel with reversible sol–gel transition. *RSC Adv.* **2017**, *7*, 24085–24096. [CrossRef]
53. Rusa, C.C.; Bridges, C.; Ha, S.-W.; Tonelli, A.E. Conformational Changes Induced in Bombyx mori Silk Fibroin by Cyclodextrin Inclusion Complexation. *Macromolecules* **2005**, *38*, 5640–5646. [CrossRef]
54. Lu, S.; Li, J.; Zhang, S.; Yin, Z.; Xing, T.; Kaplan, D.L. The influence of the hydrophilic–lipophilic environment on the structure of silk fibroin protein. *J. Mater. Chem. B* **2015**, *3*, 2599–2606. [CrossRef] [PubMed]
55. Zhao, M.; Qi, Z.; Tao, X.; Newkirk, C.; Hu, X.; Lu, S. Chemical, Thermal, Time, and Enzymatic Stability of Silk Materials with Silk I Structure. *Int. J. Mol. Sci.* **2021**, *22*, 4136. [CrossRef]
56. Wray, L.S.; Hu, X.; Gallego, J.; Georgakoudi, I.; Omenetto, F.G.; Schmidt, D.; Kaplan, D.L. Effect of processing on silk-based biomaterials: Reproducibility and biocompatibility. *J. Biomed. Mater. Res. Part B Appl. Biomater.* **2011**, *99B*, 89–101. [CrossRef]
57. Liu, X.; Xia, Q.; Zhou, J.; Zhang, Y.; Ju, H.; Deng, Z. Chemical Modification of Silk Fibroin through Serine Amino Acid Residues. *Materials* **2022**, *15*, 4399. [CrossRef]
58. Meinel, L.; Hofmann, S.; Karageorgiou, V.; Kirker-Head, C.; McCool, J.; Gronowicz, G.; Zichner, L.; Langer, R.; Vunjak-Novakovic, G.; Kaplan, D.L. The inflammatory responses to silk films in vitro and in vivo. *Biomaterials* **2005**, *26*, 147–155. [CrossRef]
59. Zhang, C.; Zhang, X.; Chen, S.; Zhang, J.; Li, S.; Li, X.; Ikoma, T.; Chen, W. In situ decoration of $TiO_2$ nanowire microspheres with silk fibroin for enhanced biocompatibility. *Mater. Lett.* **2022**, *324*, 132688. [CrossRef]
60. Hofmann, S.; Wong Po Foo, C.T.; Rossetti, F.; Textor, M.; Vunjak-Novakovic, G.; Kaplan, D.L.; Merkle, H.P.; Meinel, L. Silk fibroin as an organic polymer for controlled drug delivery. *J. Control. Release* **2006**, *111*, 219–227. [CrossRef]
61. Zhang, W.; Wang, X.; Wang, S.; Zhao, J.; Xu, L.; Zhu, C.; Zeng, D.; Chen, J.; Zhang, Z.; Kaplan, D.L.; et al. The use of injectable sonication-induced silk hydrogel for VEGF165 and BMP-2 delivery for elevation of the maxillary sinus floor. *Biomaterials* **2011**, *32*, 9415–9424. [CrossRef]
62. Sakunpongpitiporn, P.; Naeowong, W.; Sirivat, A. Enhanced transdermal insulin basal release from silk fibroin (SF) hydrogels via iontophoresis. *Drug Deliv.* **2022**, *29*, 2234–2244. [CrossRef]
63. Vepari, C.P.; Kaplan, D.L. Covalently immobilized enzyme gradients within three-dimensional porous scaffolds. *Biotechnol. Bioeng.* **2006**, *93*, 1130–1137. [CrossRef]
64. Wenk, E.; Merkle, H.P.; Meinel, L. Silk fibroin as a vehicle for drug delivery applications. *J. Control. Release* **2011**, *150*, 128–141. [CrossRef]
65. Yavuz, B.; Chambre, L.; Kaplan, D.L. Extended release formulations using silk proteins for controlled delivery of therapeutics. *Expert Opin. Drug Deliv.* **2019**, *16*, 741–756. [CrossRef]
66. Choi, M.; Choi, D.; Hong, J. Correction to "Multilayered Controlled Drug Release Silk Fibroin Nanofilm by Manipulating Secondary Structure". *Biomacromolecules* **2018**, *19*, 3902–3903. [CrossRef]
67. Coburn, J.M.; Na, E.; Kaplan, D.L. Modulation of vincristine and doxorubicin binding and release from silk films. *J. Control. Release* **2015**, *220*, 229–238. [CrossRef]
68. Pandey, V.; Haider, T.; Jain, P.; Gupta, P.N.; Soni, V. Silk as a leading-edge biological macromolecule for improved drug delivery. *J. Drug Deliv. Sci. Technol.* **2020**, *55*, 101294. [CrossRef]
69. Wang, Z.; Li, X.; Cui, Y.; Cheng, K.; Dong, M.; Liu, L. Effect of molecular weight of regenerated silk fibroin on silk-based spheres for drug delivery. *Korean J. Chem. Eng.* **2020**, *37*, 1732–1742. [CrossRef]
70. Zhang, L.; Guo, R.; Wang, S.; Yang, X.; Ling, G.; Zhang, P. Fabrication, evaluation and applications of dissolving microneedles. *Int. J. Pharm.* **2021**, *604*, 120749. [CrossRef]
71. Avcil, M.; Çelik, A. Microneedles in Drug Delivery: Progress and Challenges. *Micromachines* **2021**, *12*, 1321. [CrossRef] [PubMed]
72. Hashmi, S.; Ling, P.; Hashmi, G.; Reed, M.; Gaugler, R.; Trimmer, W. Genetic transformation of nematodes using arrays of micromechanical piercing structures. *Biotechniques* **1995**, *19*, 766–770. [PubMed]
73. Henry, S.; McAllister, D.V.; Allen, M.G.; Prausnitz, M.R. Microfabricated Microneedles: A Novel Approach to Transdermal Drug Delivery. *J. Pharm. Sci.* **1998**, *87*, 922–925. [CrossRef] [PubMed]
74. Daddona, P.E.; Matriano, J.A.; Mandema, J.; Maa, Y.-F. Parathyroid Hormone (1-34)-Coated Microneedle Patch System: Clinical Pharmacokinetics and Pharmacodynamics for Treatment of Osteoporosis. *Pharm. Res.* **2011**, *28*, 159–165. [CrossRef] [PubMed]
75. Ross, S.; Scoutaris, N.; Lamprou, D.; Mallinson, D.; Douroumis, D. Inkjet printing of insulin microneedles for transdermal delivery. *Drug Deliv. Transl. Res.* **2015**, *5*, 451–461. [CrossRef]
76. Meyer, B.K.; Kendall, M.A.F.; Williams, D.M.; Bett, A.J.; Dubey, S.; Gentzel, R.C.; Casimiro, D.; Forster, A.; Corbett, H.; Crichton, M.; et al. Immune response and reactogenicity of an unadjuvanted intradermally delivered human papillomavirus vaccine using a first generation Nanopatch™ in rhesus macaques: An exploratory, pre-clinical feasibility assessment. *Vaccine X* **2019**, *2*, 100030–100083. [CrossRef]
77. Wang, Z.; Luan, J.; Seth, A.; Liu, L.; You, M.; Gupta, P.; Rathi, P.; Wang, Y.; Cao, S.; Jiang, Q.; et al. Microneedle patch for the ultrasensitive quantification of protein biomarkers in interstitial fluid. *Nat. Biomed. Eng.* **2021**, *5*, 64–76. [CrossRef]
78. McAllister, D.V.; Wang, P.M.; Davis, S.P.; Park, J.-H.; Canatella, P.J.; Allen, M.G.; Prausnitz, M.R. Microfabricated needles for transdermal delivery of macromolecules and nanoparticles: Fabrication methods and transport studies. *Proc. Natl. Acad. Sci. USA* **2003**, *100*, 13755–13760. [CrossRef]
79. Nicholas, D.; Logan, K.A.; Sheng, Y.; Gao, J.; Farrell, S.; Dixon, D.; Callan, B.; McHale, A.P.; Callan, J.F. Rapid paper based colorimetric detection of glucose using a hollow microneedle device. *Int. J. Pharm.* **2018**, *547*, 244–249. [CrossRef]

80. Lim, D.-J.; Vines, J.B.; Park, H.; Lee, S.-H. Microneedles: A versatile strategy for transdermal delivery of biological molecules. *Int. J. Biol. Macromol.* **2018**, *110*, 30–38. [CrossRef]
81. Ita, K. Dissolving microneedles for transdermal drug delivery: Advances and challenges. *Biomed. Pharmacother.* **2017**, *93*, 1116–1127. [CrossRef]
82. Lau, S.; Fei, J.; Liu, H.; Chen, W.; Liu, R. Multilayered pyramidal dissolving microneedle patches with flexible pedestals for improving effective drug delivery. *J. Control. Release* **2017**, *265*, 113–119. [CrossRef]
83. Rouphael, N.G.; Lai, L.; Tandon, S.; McCullough, M.P.; Kong, Y.; Kabbani, S.; Natrajan, M.S.; Xu, Y.; Zhu, Y.; Wang, D.; et al. Immunologic mechanisms of seasonal influenza vaccination administered by microneedle patch from a randomized phase I trial. *NPJ Vaccines* **2021**, *6*, 89–139. [CrossRef]
84. You, X.; Pak, J.J.; Chang, J.H. Rapidly dissolving silk protein microneedles for transdermal drug delivery. In Proceedings of the 2010 IEEE International Conference on Nano/Molecular Medicine and Engineering, Hung Hom, China, 5–9 December 2010; pp. 144–147.
85. Jung, J.H.; Jin, S.G. Microneedle for transdermal drug delivery: Current trends and fabrication. *J. Pharm. Investig.* **2021**, *51*, 503–517. [CrossRef]
86. Cao, J.; Liu, Y.; Qi, Z.; Tao, X.; Kundu, S.C.; Lu, S. Sustained release of insulin from silk microneedles. *J. Drug Deliv. Sci. Technol.* **2022**, *74*, 103611. [CrossRef]
87. Lin, Z.; Li, Y.; Meng, G.; Hu, X.; Zeng, Z.; Zhao, B.; Lin, N.; Liu, X.Y. Reinforcement of Silk Microneedle Patches for Accurate Transdermal Delivery. *Biomacromolecules* **2021**, *22*, 5319–5326. [CrossRef]
88. Shin, D.; Hyun, J. Silk fibroin microneedles fabricated by digital light processing 3D printing. *J. Ind. Eng. Chem.* **2021**, *95*, 126–133. [CrossRef]
89. Courtenay, A.J.; McAlister, E.; McCrudden, M.T.C.; Vora, L.; Steiner, L.; Levin, G.; Levy-Nissenbaum, E.; Shterman, N.; Kearney, M.-C.; McCarthy, H.O.; et al. Hydrogel-forming microneedle arrays as a therapeutic option for transdermal esketamine delivery. *J. Control. Release* **2020**, *322*, 177–186. [CrossRef]
90. Ranjan Yadav, P.; Iqbal Nasiri, M.; Vora, L.K.; Larrañeta, E.; Donnelly, R.F.; Pattanayek, S.K.; Bhusan Das, D. Super-swelling hydrogel-forming microneedle based transdermal drug delivery: Mathematical modelling, simulation and experimental validation. *Int. J. Pharm.* **2022**, *622*, 121835. [CrossRef]
91. Jin, X.; Zhu, D.D.; Chen, B.Z.; Ashfaq, M.; Guo, X.D. Insulin delivery systems combined with microneedle technology. *Adv. Drug Deliv. Rev.* **2018**, *127*, 119–137. [CrossRef]
92. Donnelly, R.F.; Singh, T.R.R.; Garland, M.J.; Migalska, K.; Majithiya, R.; McCrudden, C.M.; Kole, P.L.; Mahmood, T.M.T.; McCarthy, H.O.; Woolfson, A.D. Hydrogel-Forming Microneedle Arrays for Enhanced Transdermal Drug Delivery. *Adv. Funct. Mater.* **2012**, *22*, 4879–4890. [CrossRef] [PubMed]
93. Migdadi, E.M.; Courtenay, A.J.; Tekko, I.A.; McCrudden, M.T.C.; Kearney, M.-C.; McAlister, E.; McCarthy, H.O.; Donnelly, R.F. Hydrogel-forming microneedles enhance transdermal delivery of metformin hydrochloride. *J. Control. Release* **2018**, *285*, 142–151. [CrossRef] [PubMed]
94. Chen, S.; Matsumoto, H.; Moro-oka, Y.; Tanaka, M.; Miyahara, Y.; Suganami, T.; Matsumoto, A. Microneedle-Array Patch Fabricated with Enzyme-Free Polymeric Components Capable of On-Demand Insulin Delivery. *Adv. Funct. Mater.* **2019**, *29*, 1807369. [CrossRef]
95. Lee, J.; Park, S.H.; Seo, I.H.; Lee, K.J.; Ryu, W. Rapid and repeatable fabrication of high A/R silk fibroin microneedles using thermally-drawn micromolds. *Eur. J. Pharm. Biopharm.* **2015**, *94*, 11–19. [CrossRef] [PubMed]
96. Tsioris, K.; Raja, W.K.; Pritchard, E.M.; Panilaitis, B.; Kaplan, D.L.; Omenetto, F.G. Fabrication of Silk Microneedles for Controlled-Release Drug Delivery. *Adv. Funct. Mater.* **2012**, *22*, 330–335. [CrossRef]
97. Raja, W.K.; MacCorkle, S.; Diwan, I.M.; Abdurrob, A.; Lu, J.; Omenetto, F.G.; Kaplan, D.L. Transdermal Delivery Devices: Fabrication, Mechanics and Drug Release from Silk. *Small* **2013**, *9*, 3704–3713. [CrossRef]
98. Chen, S.; Matsumoto, H.; Moro-oka, Y.; Tanaka, M.; Miyahara, Y.; Suganami, T.; Matsumoto, A. Smart Microneedle Fabricated with Silk Fibroin Combined Semi-interpenetrating Network Hydrogel for Glucose-Responsive Insulin Delivery. *ACS Biomater. Sci. Eng.* **2019**, *5*, 5781–5789. [CrossRef]
99. DeMuth, P.C.; Min, Y.; Irvine, D.J.; Hammond, P.T. Implantable Silk Composite Microneedles for Programmable Vaccine Release Kinetics and Enhanced Immunogenicity in Transcutaneous Immunization. *Adv. Healthc. Mater.* **2014**, *3*, 47–58. [CrossRef]
100. Zhang, X.; Chen, L.; Lim, K.H.; Gonuguntla, S.; Lim, K.W.; Pranantyo, D.; Yong, W.P.; Yam, W.J.T.; Low, Z.; Teo, W.J.; et al. The Pathway to Intelligence: Using Stimuli-Responsive Materials as Building Blocks for Constructing Smart and Functional Systems. *Adv. Mater.* **2019**, *31*, 1804540. [CrossRef]
101. Klajn, R. Immobilized azobenzenes for the construction of photoresponsive materials. *Pure Appl. Chem.* **2010**, *82*, 2247–2279. [CrossRef]
102. Chen, L.; Wang, W.; Su, B.; Wen, Y.; Li, C.; Zhou, Y.; Li, M.; Shi, X.; Du, H.; Song, Y.; et al. A Light-Responsive Release Platform by Controlling the Wetting Behavior of Hydrophobic Surface. *ACS Nano* **2014**, *8*, 744–751. [CrossRef]
103. Lu, Y.; Aimetti, A.A.; Langer, R.; Gu, Z. Bioresponsive materials. *Nat. Rev. Mater.* **2016**, *2*, 16075. [CrossRef]
104. Patra, D.; Sengupta, S.; Duan, W.; Zhang, H.; Pavlick, R.; Sen, A. Intelligent, self-powered, drug delivery systems. *Nanoscale* **2013**, *5*, 1273–1283. [CrossRef]

105. Gao, S.; Tang, G.; Hua, D.; Xiong, R.; Han, J.; Jiang, S.; Zhang, Q.; Huang, C. Stimuli-responsive bio-based polymeric systems and their applications. *J. Mater. Chem. B* **2019**, *7*, 709–729. [CrossRef]
106. Karimi, M.; Ghasemi, A.; Sahandi Zangabad, P.; Rahighi, R.; Moosavi Basri, S.M.; Mirshekari, H.; Amiri, M.; Shafaei Pishabad, Z.; Aslani, A.; Bozorgomid, M.; et al. Smart micro/nanoparticles in stimulus-responsive drug/gene delivery systems. *Chem. Soc. Rev.* **2016**, *45*, 1457–1501. [CrossRef]
107. Di, J.; Yu, J.; Wang, Q.; Yao, S.; Suo, D.; Ye, Y.; Pless, M.; Zhu, Y.; Jing, Y.; Gu, Z. Ultrasound-triggered noninvasive regulation of blood glucose levels using microgels integrated with insulin nanocapsules. *Nano Res.* **2017**, *10*, 1393–1402. [CrossRef]
108. Gao, Y.; Hou, M.; Yang, R.; Zhang, L.; Xu, Z.; Kang, Y.; Xue, P. Highly Porous Silk Fibroin Scaffold Packed in PEGDA/Sucrose Microneedles for Controllable Transdermal Drug Delivery. *Biomacromolecules* **2019**, *20*, 1334–1345. [CrossRef]
109. Chen, J.; Ren, H.; Zhou, P.; Zheng, S.; Du, B.; Liu, X.; Xiao, F. Microneedle-Mediat. *Drug Deliv. Cutan. Dis.* **2022**, *10*, 1032041.
110. Zhao, M.; Bozzato, E.; Joudiou, N.; Ghiassinejad, S.; Danhier, F.; Gallez, B.; Préat, V. Codelivery of paclitaxel and temozolomide through a photopolymerizable hydrogel prevents glioblastoma recurrence after surgical resection. *J. Control. Release* **2019**, *309*, 72–81. [CrossRef]
111. Lee, J.; Jang, E.H.; Kim, J.H.; Park, S.; Kang, Y.; Park, S.; Lee, K.; Kim, J.-H.; Youn, Y.-N.; Ryu, W. Highly flexible and porous silk fibroin microneedle wraps for perivascular drug delivery. *J. Control. Release* **2021**, *340*, 125–135. [CrossRef]
112. Cardinali, D.P.; Srinivasan, V.; Brzezinski, A.; Brown, G.M. Melatonin and its analogs in insomnia and depression. *J. Pineal Res.* **2012**, *52*, 365–375. [CrossRef] [PubMed]
113. Li, J.; Zeng, M.; Shan, H.; Tong, C. Microneedle Patches as Drug and Vaccine Delivery Platform. *Curr. Med. Chem.* **2017**, *24*, 2413–2422. [CrossRef] [PubMed]
114. Ma, G.; Wu, C. Microneedle, bio-microneedle and bio-inspired microneedle: A review. *J. Control. Release* **2017**, *251*, 11–23. [CrossRef] [PubMed]
115. Alpert, J.S. An Amazing Story: The Discovery of Insulin. *Am. J. Med.* **2016**, *129*, 231–232. [CrossRef]
116. Heinemann, L.; Braune, K.; Carter, A.; Zayani, A.; Krämer, L.A. Insulin Storage: A Critical Reappraisal. *J. Diabetes Sci. Technol.* **2020**, *15*, 147–159. [CrossRef]
117. Mishra, R.; Maiti, T.K.; Bhattacharyya, T.K. Feasibility Studies on Nafion Membrane Actuated Micropump Integrated with Hollow Microneedles for Insulin Delivery Device. *J. Microelectromechanical Syst.* **2019**, *28*, 987–996. [CrossRef]
118. Economidou, S.N.; Uddin, M.J.; Marques, M.J.; Douroumis, D.; Sow, W.T.; Li, H.; Reid, A.; Windmill, J.F.C.; Podoleanu, A. A novel 3D printed hollow microneedle microelectromechanical system for controlled, personalized transdermal drug delivery. *Addit. Manuf.* **2021**, *38*, 101815. [CrossRef]
119. Seong, K.-Y.; Seo, M.-S.; Hwang, D.Y.; O'Cearbhaill, E.D.; Sreenan, S.; Karp, J.M.; Yang, S.Y. A self-adherent, bullet-shaped microneedle patch for controlled transdermal delivery of insulin. *J. Control. Release* **2017**, *265*, 48–56. [CrossRef]
120. Fakhraei Lahiji, S.; Jang, Y.; Ma, Y.; Dangol, M.; Yang, H.; Jang, M.; Jung, H. Effects of dissolving microneedle fabrication parameters on the activity of encapsulated lysozyme. *Eur. J. Pharm. Sci.* **2018**, *117*, 290–296. [CrossRef]
121. Liu, D.; Yu, B.; Jiang, G.; Yu, W.; Zhang, Y.; Xu, B. Fabrication of composite microneedles integrated with insulin-loaded CaCO3 microparticles and PVP for transdermal delivery in diabetic rats. *Mater. Sci. Eng. C* **2018**, *90*, 180–188. [CrossRef]
122. Ita, K. Transdermal Delivery of Drugs with Microneedles—Potential and Challenges. *Pharmaceutics* **2015**, *7*, 90–105. [CrossRef]
123. Martanto, W.; Moore, J.S.; Couse, T.; Prausnitz, M.R. Mechanism of fluid infusion during microneedle insertion and retraction. *J. Control. Release* **2006**, *112*, 357–361. [CrossRef]
124. Cao, Y.; Wang, B. Biodegradation of Silk Biomaterials. *Int. J. Mol. Sci.* **2009**, *10*, 1514–1524. [CrossRef]
125. Sheng, T.; Luo, B.; Zhang, W.; Ge, X.; Yu, J.; Zhang, Y.; Gu, Z. Microneedle-Mediated Vaccination: Innovation and Translation. *Adv. Drug Deliv. Rev.* **2021**, *179*, 113919. [CrossRef]
126. Giudice, E.L.; Campbell, J.D. Needle-free vaccine delivery. *Adv. Drug Deliv. Rev.* **2006**, *58*, 68–89. [CrossRef]
127. Kim, Y.-C.; Park, J.-H.; Prausnitz, M.R. Microneedles for drug and vaccine delivery. *Adv. Drug Deliv. Rev.* **2012**, *64*, 1547–1568. [CrossRef]
128. Stinson, J.A.; Raja, W.K.; Lee, S.; Kim, H.B.; Diwan, I.; Tutunjian, S.; Panilaitis, B.; Omenetto, F.G.; Tzipori, S.; Kaplan, D.L. Silk Fibroin Microneedles for Transdermal Vaccine Delivery. *ACS Biomater. Sci. Eng.* **2017**, *3*, 360–369. [CrossRef]
129. Menon, I.; Bagwe, P.; Gomes, K.B.; Bajaj, L.; Gala, R.; Uddin, M.N.; D'Souza, M.J.; Zughaier, S.M. Microneedles: A New Generation Vaccine Delivery System. *Micromachines* **2021**, *12*, 435. [CrossRef]
130. Shin, C.I.; Jeong, S.D.; Rejinold, N.S.; Kim, Y.-C. Microneedles for vaccine delivery: Challenges and future perspectives. *Ther. Deliv.* **2017**, *8*, 447–460. [CrossRef]
131. Ita, K. Transdermal delivery of drugs with microneedles: Strategies and outcomes. *J. Drug Deliv. Sci. Technol.* **2015**, *29*, 16–23. [CrossRef]
132. Kornstein, A.N. SERI Surgical Scaffold as an Adjunct to Conventional Brachioplasty. *Plast. Reconstr. Surg. Glob. Open* **2014**, *2*, e190. [CrossRef] [PubMed]
133. Holland, C.; Numata, K.; Rnjak-Kovacina, J.; Seib, F.P. The Biomedical Use of Silk: Past, Present, Future. *Adv. Healthc. Mater.* **2019**, *8*, 1800465. [CrossRef] [PubMed]
134. Crowley, T.P.; Collin, T. Re: 'Seri™: A surgical scaffold for breast reconstruction or for bacterial ingrowth?'. *J. Plast. Reconstr. Aesthetic Surg.* **2015**, *68*, 1629.

135. Zhang, W.; Chen, L.; Chen, J.; Wang, L.; Gui, X.; Ran, J.; Xu, G.; Zhao, H.; Zeng, M.; Ji, J.; et al. Wound Healing: Silk Fibroin Biomaterial Shows Safe and Effective Wound Healing in Animal Models and a Randomized Controlled Clinical. *Adv. Healthc. Mater.* **2017**, *6*, 1700121. [CrossRef]
136. Gil, E.S.; Panilaitis, B.; Bellas, E.; Kaplan, D.L. Functionalized Silk Biomaterials for Wound Healing. *Adv. Healthcare Mater.* **2013**, *2*, 206–217. [CrossRef]
137. Smith, F.; Sabri, A.H.; Heppel, M.; Fonseca, I.; Chowdhury, F.; Cheung, K.; Willmor, S.; Rawson, F.; Marlow, M. The clinical and translational prospects of microneedle devices, with a focus on insulin therapy for diabetes mellitus as a case study. *Int. J. Pharm.* **2022**, *628*, 122234. [CrossRef]
138. Wu, J.; Sahoo, J.K.; Li, Y.; Xu, Q.; Kaplan, D.L. Challenges in delivering therapeutic peptides and proteins: A silk-based solution. *J. Control. Release* **2022**, *345*, 176–189. [CrossRef]
139. Bruno, B.J.; Miller, G.D.; Lim, C.S. Basics and recent advances in peptide and protein drug delivery. *Ther. Deliv.* **2013**, *4*, 1443–1467. [CrossRef]
140. Guo, C.; Li, C.; Kaplan, D.L. Enzymatic Degradation of Bombyx mori Silk Materials: A Review. *Biomacromolecules* **2020**, *21*, 1678–1686. [CrossRef]
141. Numata, K.; Kaplan, D.L. Silk-based delivery systems of bioactive molecules. *Adv. Drug Deliv. Rev.* **2010**, *62*, 1497–1508. [CrossRef]
142. Lu, Q.; Wang, X.; Hu, X.; Cebe, P.; Omenetto, F.; Kaplan, D.L. Stabilization and Release of Enzymes from Silk Films. *Macromol. Biosci.* **2010**, *10*, 359–368. [CrossRef]
143. Kuzuhara, A.; Asakura, T.; Tomoda, R.; Matsunaga, T. Use of silk fibroin for enzyme membrane. *J. Biotechnol.* **1987**, *5*, 199–207. [CrossRef]
144. Zhang, J.; Pritchard, E.; Hu, X.; Valentin, T.; Panilaitis, B.; Omenetto, F.G.; Kaplan, D.L. Stabilization of vaccines and antibiotics in silk and eliminating the cold chain. *Proc. Natl. Acad. Sci. USA* **2012**, *109*, 11981–11986. [CrossRef]
145. McCrudden, M.T.C.; Alkilani, A.Z.; Courtenay, A.J.; McCrudden, C.M.; McCloskey, B.; Walker, C.; Alshraiedeh, N.; Lutton, R.E.M.; Gilmore, B.F.; Woolfson, A.D.; et al. Considerations in the sterile manufacture of polymeric microneedle arrays. *Drug Deliv. Transl. Res.* **2015**, *5*, 3–14. [CrossRef]
146. Mistilis, M.J.; Joyce, J.C.; Esser, E.S.; Skountzou, I.; Compans, R.W.; Bommarius, A.S.; Prausnitz, M.R. Long-term stability of influenza vaccine in a dissolving microneedle patch. *Drug Deliv. Transl. Res.* **2017**, *7*, 195–205. [CrossRef]

pharmaceutics

MDPI

*Systematic Review*

# Microneedles in Advanced Microfluidic Systems: A Systematic Review throughout Lab and Organ-on-a-Chip Applications

**Renata Maia [1,2], Violeta Carvalho [1,2,3,4], Rui Lima [4,5,6], Graça Minas [1,2] and Raquel O. Rodrigues [1,2,7,8,*]**

1 Center for MicroElectromechanical Systems (CMEMS-UMinho), University of Minho, Campus de Azurém, 4800-058 Guimarães, Portugal
2 LABBELS—Associate Laboratory, 4806-909 Braga/Guimarães, Portugal
3 ALGORITMI Center, University of Minho, Campus de Azurém, 4800-058 Guimarães, Portugal
4 MEtRICs, Mechanical Engineering Department, University of Minho, Campus de Azurém, 4800-058 Guimarães, Portugal
5 CEFT—Transport Phenomena Research Center, Faculty of Engineering, University of Porto, Rua Dr. Roberto Frias, 4200-465 Porto, Portugal
6 ALiCE—Associate Laboratory in Chemical Engineering, Faculty of Engineering, University of Porto, Rua Dr. Roberto Frias, 4200-465 Porto, Portugal
7 Advanced (Magnetic) Theranostic Nanostructures Lab, Nanomedicine Unit, INL–International Iberian Nanotechnology Laboratory, Av. Mestre José Veiga, 4715-330 Braga, Portugal
8 Division of Engineering in Medicine, Brigham and Women's Hospital, Department of Medicine, Harvard Medical School, Cambridge, MA 02139, USA
* Correspondence: raquel.rodrigues@dei.uminho.pt

**Abstract:** Microneedles (MNs) have been widely used in biomedical applications for drug delivery and biomarker detection purposes. Furthermore, MNs can also be used as a stand-alone tool to be combined with microfluidic devices. For that purpose, lab- or organ-on-a-chip are being developed. This systematic review aims to summarize the most recent progress in these emerging systems, to identify their advantages and limitations, and discuss promising potential applications of MNs in microfluidics. Therefore, three databases were used to search papers of interest, and their selection was made following the guidelines for systematic reviews proposed by PRISMA. In the selected studies, the MNs type, fabrication strategy, materials, and function/application were evaluated. The literature reviewed showed that although the use of MNs for lab-on-a-chip has been more explored than for organ-on-a-chip, some recent studies have explored this applicability with great potential for the monitoring of organ models. Overall, it is shown that the presence of MNs in advanced microfluidic devices can simplify drug delivery and microinjection, as well as fluid extraction for biomarker detection by using integrated biosensors, which is a promising tool to precisely monitor, in real-time, different kinds of biomarkers in lab- and organ-on-a-chip platforms.

**Keywords:** microfluidic; microneedles; organ-on-a-chip; lab-on-a-chip; drug screening; biomarkers detection

## 1. Introduction

Microfluidic technology is present in lab-on-a-chip and organ-on-a-chip platforms. In order to enable high-throughput screening and automation, lab-on-a-chip (LoC) devices—also known as multitasking devices—combine many (bio)chemical laboratory operations in a single integrated chip that ranges in size from a few millimeters to a few square centimeters [1]. The most alluring benefits of these platforms are their capacity to autonomously and efficiently execute a number of lab processes on a single chip with minimal external inputs [2], as well as with low reagent consumption and high-throughput analysis [3]. To offer an in-situ and quick result for an immediate diagnosis and treatment, point-of-care testing (POCT) is required. For modern POCT diagnostic systems, sample-to-answer format, high sensitivity, and a short analysis time are the most crucial qualities. Since LoC can miniaturize and combine the majority of the functional modules used in central labs into a tiny chip, LoC technologies have been regarded as one of the potential options that can satisfy the needs of POCT [4]. For example, Samper et al., 2019, describe a 3D printed chip to create a microfluidic biosensing portable system, where the data is transmitted via Bluetooth [5]. Another example is the study of Zhang et al., 2020, which demonstrated the integration of a smartphone detection into a microfluidic device (acoustofluidic platform) for hemoglobin measurement. To detect the fluorescent signal, the researchers created a quantum dot-based fluorescence test for hemoglobin and paired it with an integrated UV irradiation source and a commercial smartphone [6].

Organ-on-a-chip (OoC) platforms replicate tissue and miniaturized organs, while preserving tissue/organ-level function and homeostasis [7]. They are found on microfluidic devices with perfused chambers that range from micrometers to millimeters in size, and are fed by continuous media flow [8]. As a result of the continuous flow of cellular media, shear flow conditions and nutrient/gas exchanges, OoC can be mimicked as in vivo, extending the cell culture's lifetime compared to static in vitro cultures [9]. Therefore, OoC can reproduce important features of the complexity of organs and biosystems [10]. Several studies in the literature use OoC to examine specific target organs, including the liver [11], heart [12], brain [13], and kidneys [14], among others. The aim of many of the OoC is to facilitate drug toxicity detection in healthy and diseased organ models. Because OoC can include patient primary human cells or stem-cell-derived cells, the OoC system has the potential to be designed as a model platform capable of predicting optimized and personalized drug treatments [15]. However, important hurdles must be overcome to create a valid and robust preclinical organ model. For that, appropriate organ scaling, tissue vascularization, recapitulation of the immunological response, repeatability, organ monitoring, oxygenation, pH, shear rate, cell viability, and cell density, are some of the parameters that need to be considered when designing an OoC [16]. Among all these features, monitoring the OoC platforms is a huge step to guarantee reproducibility and appropriate chemical, physical, and cell analysis. Therefore, OoC and LoC can be combined, especially regarding the integration of micro (bio)sensors of LoC into OoC, bringing advanced microfluidic devices into a new era.

Microneedles (MNs), which are based on the concept of miniaturized needles, are increasingly used in biomedical technology. These have the ability to assess biological information with minimal invasion, and are frequently used as a strategy to deliver drugs [17], biomolecules such as proteins [18], RNA, or DNA [19] into cells with temporal and spatial precision [20,21]. The dimensions of MNs may vary depending on the application. The most common dimensions found in the literature have height ranges between 150 to 1500 µm, with a base width of 50 to 250 µm and a tip diameter of 1 to 25 µm [22]. In terms of shape, needle tips come in a variety of shapes, including triangular, cylindrical, and pentagonal [23]. The design and size of MNs have been identified as the primary characteristics to be modified for optimal performance of an MNs system. To maximize efficiency, the length of the MN can be customized to achieve the desired depth of penetration. The shape, the number of needles in an array, the height, the aspect ratio (the ratio of the base to the height of the needle), the material, and the thickness of the backing block (if needed), are all criteria that define MN design. In addition, the volume that can be collected and loaded by the array is determined by these criteria. The volume, in turn, contributes to determining the type of MN that best suits the desired application [24]. Based on applications, MNs can be categorized into various types. MNs systems have mostly been developed for biomolecular/drug delivery and microinjection [25–32]. The design of the MNs device is crucial for the efficient performance of the system, and different materials can be used in MNs fabrication [33]. The two fundamental designs that are employed to construct MNs are in-plane and out-of-plane (Figure 1A). In contrast to out-of-plane MN arrays, which rise vertically from the base, in-plane MN arrays are parallel to the top fabrication surface [34]. Typically, due to the numerous microstructures and variety of strategies for the delivery of drugs, MNs are divided into two main categories: traditional needles (solid, coated, or hollow), and emerged needles (dissolving, hydrogel-forming) [35]. In terms of materials, MNs can be divided into degradable and non-degradable materials, such as metal, silicon, ceramic and carbon for non-degradable and natural polymers for degradable ones [36,37]. Figure 1B represents the two main categories with the approaches of the six most used MNs. A more comprehensive review of these MNs structural strategies can be found elsewhere [38].

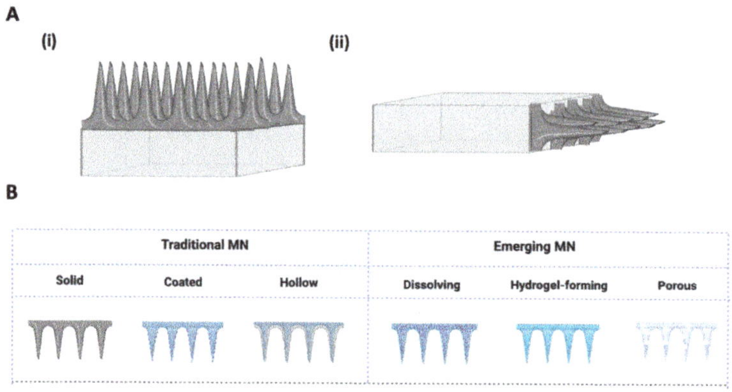


**Figure 1.** Schematic representation of MNs. (**A**) (**i**) out-of-plane and (**ii**) in-plane construction. (**B**) Traditional and emerging MNs structuring approaches according to drug delivery application.

Concerning the fabrication methods, several have been described in the literature, but the most commonly used are micro-molding, microfabrication technologies (e.g., lithography, laser, etching), additive manufacturing (i.e., 3D printing), and layer-by-layer assembly [39]. Briefly, microfabrication can also be divided into three main processes: deposition, patterning, and etching. Deposition includes film formation by physical vapor deposition or chemical vapor deposition. The patterning technique shapes the desired geometry on a film, substrate, or wafer. Lithography is a common technique used for patterning, which consists in transferring the mask into a coated photosensitive film using light to develop the exposed photoresist. Although lithography allows the production of smaller feature sizes, it is considered a more complex process that requires high-tech infrastructures and equipment [40]. Etching is a technique that involves removing the unprotected sections of the substrate with a strong caustic chemical to create a microneedle design of interest. A wet or dry etching technique can be used, but the use of chemicals are required, which can contaminate the samples [41]. Laser ablation and laser cutting are also reported to be used to fabricate metal and polymeric MNs. Laser ablation removes material from a solid surface by irradiating it with a laser beam [42]. Laser cutting uses an infra-red laser to cut metallic sheets in the shape of MNs [43]. Both techniques are simple, quick and precise, with no contaminations, but require higher power consumption. Micro-molding is used to fabricate various polymeric MNs using cutting tools to sculpt the mold. Afterwards, the polymeric material that comprises the MN is poured into the micro-mold in a liquid or semi-liquid state and then solidified to achieve the desired shape. It is a simple, low-cost, versatile process with high-resolution [44,45]. More recently, 3D printing has also emerged as a process to produce MNs with the potential to simplify the fabrication of multilayer and materials in a few steps [46].

Overall, the microfabrication techniques to produce MNs and microfluidic devices are identical. Hence, it is expected that microfluidic devices and MNs can be easily combined using those fabrication techniques and in this way to create, in a synergetic way, an advanced microfluidic device for drug screening and/or organ models monitoring [47,48]. Based on this expectation, the present systematic review aims to provide a broad vision on the state-of-the-art of MNs combined with lab and/or organ-on-a-chip, especially focusing on the MNs type, fabrication strategy, materials, and function/applications.

## 2. Materials and Methods

This work was conducted taking into account the research guidelines for systematic reviews proposed by PRISMA [49,50].

### 2.1. Data Sources and Search Strategy

The search was performed using three different databases: ScienceDirect, PubMed and Scopus, until the 1st of December 2022. The search string used was ("organoids" OR "organ-on-a-chip" OR "organ on a chip") AND ("microneedle (s)") AND ("lab-on-a-chip" OR "microfluidics" OR lab on a chip") AND ("microneedle (s)").

### 2.2. Validity Assessment

Review articles, conference papers, short communications, and non-English written articles were removed from the search results, either manually or using the filters from the database. After the elimination of duplicates, the articles were selected based on the relevance of their title in the context of this review. Further screening was performed to evaluate which paper presented the defined inclusion or exclusion criteria presented below. To avoid biases, the two first authors screened and selected the research papers separately and then compared the classifications. Disagreements or doubts regarding the classification were solved by a third author.

### 2.3. Inclusion and Exclusion Criteira

The studies included in this review followed the criteria:

- Published since 2000;
- Use of microfluidic platforms or organs-on-a-chip in combination with MNs;
- Use of microfluidic platforms or lab-on-a-chip in combination with MNs;
- MNs for media/ISF collection;
- MNs for cell injection;
- MNs for biomarkers detection.
- MNs for biofluid extraction, microneedle sensors, and analyte-capturing MNs, or combinations thereof.

The study did not present the excluded criteria.

## 3. Results

### 3.1. Data Collection Results

As previously mentioned, the authors followed the PRISMA-recommended guidance to conduct systematic reviews. Based on the title, 91 potentially relevant articles were identified from the three databases selected. In total, 80 studies were included after removing duplicates. After the evaluation of abstracts, 24 articles were dismissed due to a lack of data and different study strategies; thus, 56 full papers were analyzed. In the end, a total of 35 full-text articles were selected. Figure 2 shows the PRISMA flow chart for the selection process of studies incorporated in this systematic review.

Additionally, a metadata analysis was carried out using the Scopus database with the searched keywords "MNs + microfluidic" and "MNs + organ-on-a-chip" and "MNs + lab-on-a-chip" between 2000 (the year of the first work reported in the literature) and 2022, which shows a total sum in this period of 82 papers (67 articles and 15 reviews) (Figure 3).

Among the included studies, 30% corresponded to studies that have addressed the integration of MNs into microfluidic devices. The number of publications tended to increase over the past 20 years, where the majority of the publications were original research articles. This reflects researchers' increased interest in combining MNs with lab/organ-on-a-chip. Among the most published areas were Engineering, Material Sciences, and Physics and Astronomy, representing a total of 63.4%.

Based on the selected articles from the defined criteria, 36 works were included in this systematic revision, which had as main topic MNs applied in advanced microfluidic devices (i.e., lab/organ-on-a-chip), and subdivided into two main applications: (1) devices for extraction and biomarker detection, and (2) devices for drug delivery and microinjection, as follows in the sub-chapter.

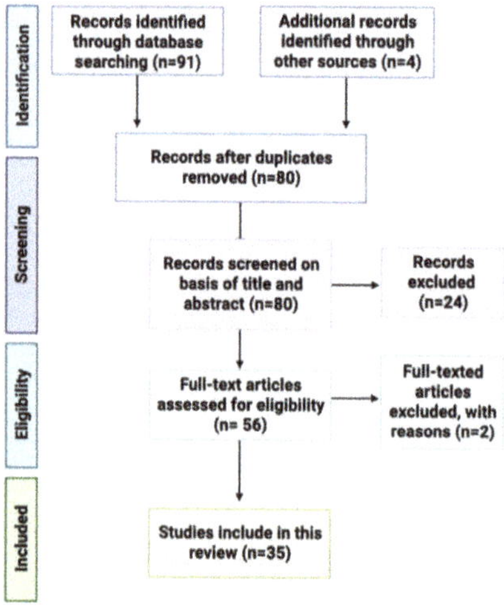


**Figure 2.** PRISMA flow diagram displaying the procedure of study selection.

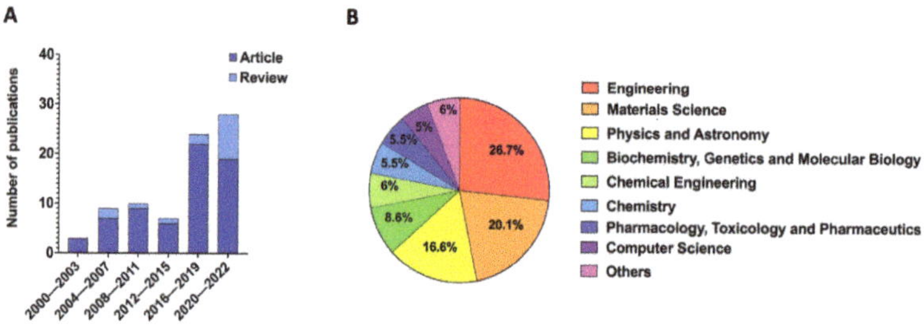


**Figure 3.** Metadata analysis of the keywords "MNs + microfluidic" and "MNs + organ-on-a-chip" and "MNs + Lab-on-a-chip" between 2000 and 2022. (**A**) Number of publications per combined years. (**B**) Documents by subject area.

### *3.2. MNs Applied in Advanced Microfluidic Devices*

An increased research effort has been focused on the use of MNs for direct or indirect sensing. This new trend has germinated naturally from former efforts of the use of MNs for OoC and LoC devices. As is possible to observe in Table 1, the majority of the applications of MNs in the microfluidic field are LoC approaches (approximately 89% of papers analyzed). Generally, an MN array is connected to a reservoir to serve as an interstitial fluid (ISF) absorption device or connected with a reservoir to serve as drug storage to release drugs.

Hollow MNs are regarded as the best choice for extract/release systems, since they provide the exact amount of drug needed at the desired location in a faster and controlled way. Therefore, hollow MNs are the most common type of MN employed in microfluidic devices, mostly made of silicon, but metals and glass are also used (Table 1). Such devices act as a conduit to access dermal biofluids for on-chip analysis in microfluidic chambers [51]. However, besides hollow MNs, the application of porous and solid MNs in microfluidic devices are also established (Table 1).

To identify the presence of a particular target analyte, microneedle-based biofluid extraction products are mainly combined with downstream analytical techniques [52]. For example, Wang et al., 2021 explored an MN patch for fast in vivo sampling and on-needle quantification of target protein biomarkers [53]. Microneedle-based in vivo sensors have been used in diagnostic systems functioning as electrodes, particularly for glucose testing [54]. To overcome the gap between extracting ISF and further analysis, some authors proposed solutions that incorporate the biosensor on the patch of porous MNs [55]. For example, Kusama et al., 2021, proposed a porous MNs patch combined with anodes and cathodes for efficient drug delivery (penetration) and analysis (extraction) [56].

Ultimately, MNs systems can provide results and detect different biomarkers in real-time, which can be used to monitor in vivo tissues, or in vitro organoids and cell cultures. The main advantage of MNs is that they can be repeatedly used to collect cellular contents without causing cell lysis. They may also promote a decrease in lateral diffusion [57].

Overall, studies show that MNs are mainly used in microfluidic applications for biomarker detection [58–68], cargo delivery [69–73], and cell microinjection [74,75]. Table 1 shows the types of MNs, materials, applications and hydrodynamic forces used in microfluidic devices. The works reviewed show that MNs are designed in two configurations, in-plane and out-of-plane (as shown in Figure 1A). An in-plane MN configuration enables the manipulation of the length and shape of MNs and the time required to produce it. It simplifies the integration into an embedded microfluidic network resulting in a device with fewer layers and steps process. Parameters, such as mechanical rigidity, can be easily tailored by varying the subtract thickness or width of MNs [76–78]. As a result, these MNs are often longer than out-of-plane MNs [79]. Out-of-plane MNs can also enhance the efficiency of drug delivery/fluid extraction by increasing the MN array density. However, achieving a higher length is more difficult because of the risk of clogging and collapsing [58,80,81].

Another interesting aspect in the design and application of MNs in microfluidic devices is the type of hydrodynamic force mechanism employed, which can be passive, such as capillary force, or active, such as by using micropumps. For instance, the detection of analytes in fluids may be facilitated by the use of capillary action in a microneedle-assisted biosensing [82]. In this case, capillary forces can propel the fluid to/from the reservoir and then to a biosensor platform. However, in some cases a micropump can be requested to supply specified volumes at higher flow rates, which in turn adds more complexity to the system [83]. Nevertheless, in many designs, capillary forces are enough and allow the liquid to flow through the MNs on its own, simplifying the manufacture and use of the device [84]. When natural hydrodynamic forces, such as capillary, are not enough, other components such as pumps, valves, and bubble traps must be combined in order to achieve the system. This, as already mentioned, can be challenging from a fabrication and integration standpoint [59]. In some revised works, planar micropumps were used because of their advantage in being simple to integrate and having the ability to change the flow operation (extraction/injection) by just flipping the valve direction. For LoC devices with in-plane MNs, this approach is further explored [60,70], although leaks between the inlet and outlet can occur.

Regarding fabrication strategies and materials, typically porous MNs are fabricated using a PDMS mold followed by a leaching method to remove the porogenic casted materials [61,62], or by using a microfabrication process to directly obtain the MNs' structure, followed by leaching [64]. The majority of solid MNs are built of metallic components or silicon, or a combination of both [65,73,85]. In the studied papers, the solid MNs were produced through micromachining processes, including the use of SU-8 photoresist. On the other hand, coated MNs are in general solid MNs that suffer a process of coating. For example, Trzebinski et al., 2012, developed a microfluidic device with enzyme-coated MNs by immersing the MNs in a solution with the desired enzyme [67]. Kang et al., 2021 used a silicon-coated MN with Cr/Au by deposition [71]. In contrast, different types of lithography are commonly used in the case of hollow MNs [63,86,87]. Deep reactive ion etching (DRIE) and sacrificial layer sharpening are two other techniques that have been extensively researched in MNs and used in the investigated microfluidic devices [70,74–78,81]. New fabrication processes, such as 3D printing, are starting to be developed as well. A comprehensive review concerning this fabrication methodology for the design of MN for biomedical application can be found elsewhere [88].

**Table 1.** Reviewed MNs-based systems concerning MN type, MN–chip connection, fabrication strategy, material, employed hydrodynamic force, function, application and microfluidic system.

| MNType | In/Out-of-Plane | MN–Chip Connection | Fabrication Strategy | Material Chip/MN | Forces | Function | Application | Microfluidic System | Reference |
|---|---|---|---|---|---|---|---|---|---|
| Porous MNs | Out-of-plane | MN integrated in the inlets of the microdevice | Microfabrication + Leach method | Polylactic acid (PLA)/PDMS | Pump | Biomarker detection | ISF collection and glucose detection | Lab-on-a-chip | [61,62] |
| Porous MNs | Out-of-plane | Integrated as MN patch | Mold + Leach method | PDMS/Ethoxylated trimethylolpropane triacrylate (ETPTA) | Capillary Action | Biomarker detection | Extraction and detection of skin interstitial fluid biomarkers | Lab-on-a-chip | [64] |
| Solid MNs | Out-of-plane | MN integrated in the inlets of the microdevice | Microfabrication (SU-8) | PDMS/SU-8 | Pressure | Drug delivery | Delivery functions for inflammation treatment | Lab-on-a-chip | [73] |
| Solid MNs | In-of-plane | MN integrated perpendicular to the microfluidic channel | Microfabrication | Oxide layer + metallic layer/Silicon | - | Biomarker Detection | Microneedle biosensor for direct label-free real-time protein detection | Lab-on-a-chip | [65] |
| Solid MNs | Out-of-plane | MN integrated perpendicular to the microfluidic channel | - | PDMS/Tungsten + parylene | Syringe pump | Cell Detection | Detection of cells in suspension | Lab-on-a-chip | [85] |
| Coated MNs | Out-of-plane | MN integrated above microfluidic channel | Microfabrication | PDMS/Silicon + Cr/AU | Capillary Forces | Delivery | Chemical delivery capability | Lab-on-a-chip | [71] |
| Coated MNs | Out-of-plane | MN integrated above chamber | Microfabrication (two-photon lithography) | PDMS/Gold + enzyme layer | Syringe pump | Biomarker detection/Biosensor | 3D microspike array-based glucose and lactate biosensor | Lab-on-a-chip | [67] |
| Coated MNs | Out-of-plane | MN integrated above microfluidic channel | SU-8 | PDMS/SU-8 resin | Syringe pump | Biomarker detection/Biosensor | Drug delivery and body fluid sampling applications | Lab-on-a-chip | [68] |
| Hollow MNs | Out-of-plane | MN integrated above microfluidic channel | Microfabrication | - | Micropump | Biomarker detection | Nonenzymatic microfluidic glucose sensor | Lab-on-a-chip | [60] |

**Table 1.** *Cont.*

| MNType | In/Out-of-Plane | MN–Chip Connection | Fabrication Strategy | Material Chip/MN | Forces | Function | Application | Microfluidic System | Reference |
|---|---|---|---|---|---|---|---|---|---|
| Hollow MNs | Out-of-plane | MN integrated in organoid chamber | Microfabrication (Photolithography) | PMMA/Silicon | Pneumatic interface | Biomarker detection | Microfluidic sampling system for tissue analytics | Organ-on-a-chip | [87] |
| Hollow MNs | Out-of-plane | MN integrated above microfluidic channel | Microfabrication | Pyrex/Silicon | Capillary action and evaporation | Biomarkerdetection | Microneedle-based glucose monitor | Lab-on-a-chip | [58] |
| Hollow MNs | Out-of-plane | MN integrated above microfluidic channel | Microfabrication/ DRIE | Aluminum + Silicon/Silicon | Capillary forces | Extraction | ISF extraction | Lab-on-a-chip | [81] |
| Hollow MNs | Out-of-plane | MN integrated above microfluidic channel | Microfabrication (two-photon lithography) | PDMS/Eshell 300 | Pump | Analysis | Sensor for on-chip potentiometric determination of $K^+$ | Lab-on-a-chip | [63] |
| Hollow MNs | Out-of-plane | MN integrated perpendicular to the microfluidic channel | Soft lithography | PDMS + SU-8/Glass | Valve actuation | Micro-injection | Single cells microinjection system | Organ-on-a-chip | [74] |
| Hollow MNs | Out-of-plane | MN integrated above microfluidic channel | Direct laser writing | PMMA/Photosensitive material | Syringe | Extraction/ delivery | A system for fluid injection and extraction | Lab-on-a-chip | [86] |
| Hollow and sharp MNs | Out-of-plane | MN integrated above microfluidic channel | Laser Ablation | Glass/SU-8 | Syringe pump | Perfusion | 3D micro perfusion system | Organ-on-a-chip | [89] |
| Hollow MNs | Out-of-plane | Integrated as MN patch | Soft lithography | PDMS/metal | Pressure | Extraction | Extraction and transport of blood | Lab-on-a-chip | [90] |
| Hollow MNs | Out-of-plane | Integrated as MN patch | Soft lithography | PDMS + paper sensor | Pressure | Biomarker detection | POCT biosensors for quantification of glucose and cholesterol in blood | Lab-on-a-chip | [66] |
| Hollow MNs | Out-of-plane | MN integrated perpendicular to the microfluidic channel | 3D printing + DRIE | PDMS/Glass | Vacuum pump | Microinjection | Microfluidic device for localized microinjection | Lab-on-a-chip | [75] |

**Table 1.** *Cont.*

| MNType | In/Out-of-Plane | MN–Chip Connection | Fabrication Strategy | Material Chip/MN | Forces | Function | Application | Microfluidic System | Reference |
|---|---|---|---|---|---|---|---|---|---|
| MN with open capillary | In-plane | Connected with microfluidic device | DRIE + photolithography | Silicon | Pressure | Insertion into skin | Extraction/delivery | Lab-on-a-chip | [76,77] |
| MN with open capillary | In-plane | Connected with microfluidic device | DRIE + photolithography | Titanium | Pressure | Insertion into skin | Extraction/delivery | Lab-on-a-chip | [78] |
| MN with open capillary | In-plane | Connected with microfluidic device | MEMS + glass cover on silicon technology | Silicon | Syring pump | Drug Infusion | System for brain drug infusion | Lab-on-a-chip/organ-on-a-chip | [72] |
| MN with open capillary | In-plane | Connected with microfluidic device | MEMS + DRIE | Silicon | Planar Micropump | Drug Delivery | Continuous on-chip micropumping for microneedle enhanced drug delivery | Lab-on-a-chip | [70] |

#### 3.2.1. Devices for Extraction and Biomarker Detection

The use of microfluidic components combined with MNs for glucose measurement has received the greatest attention [67,91]. As is possible to observe in Table 1, and as mentioned above, hollow MNs are the most developed for fluid extraction that serve for biomarker detection. In general, such devices act as a conduit to access dermal biofluids for on-chip analysis. Historically, the first LoC devices were designed with hollow MNs [58,81]. For instance, Mukerjee et al., 2004 integrated a hollow MN array with microchannels to measure glucose levels in situ. The fabrication process was a combination of DRIE and isotropic etching to produce out-of-plane hollow MNs integrated with microchannels and reservoirs. The chip was designed to draw fluid from the MN tip to microchannels by capillary forces. To achieve it, the surface tension was optimized by studied geometry, contact angle and an MN cross-section, and it was concluded that the best silicon MN profile for extracting fluid was the "snake fang". The device was able to successfully pierce the skin and extract fluid, and glucose was measured by calorimetry with the fluid in the reservoir (Figure 4A) [81]. However, the study reported that an inflammatory response was observed. Another extraction system was described by Lee et al., 2012, in which the system integrated an ultrahigh-aspect-ratio (UHA) microneedle with a novel elastic self-recovery actuator. This device successfully extracted and transported blood from a rabbit [90]. In addition, biosensors started to be combined into the microfluidic system/device with microneedles. As described by Zimmermann et al., 2003, a disposable minimally invasive self-calibrating sensor for continuous glucose monitoring was developed, consisting of hollow out-of-plane MNs to sample ISF from the epidermis that was placed in a shallow flow channel. Capillary action and evaporation drove the ISF through the MNs into the integrated glucose sensor. However, it was a prototype test, and the authors suggested that more investment was needed for the fluid to reach the biosensor. In addition, it was reported that the passing fluid gradually washed away the immobilized enzyme [58].

As a possible solution, Najmi et al., 2022, developed and simulated a nonenzymatic glucose detection device by integrating a microfluidic system and a semi-permeable membrane located at the MN base to separate the dialysis fluid from the waste fluid. In this case, an amperometric sensor was used [60]. However, some leakage was observed from outlet-to-inlet (Figure 4B).

Mansor et al., 2017, created a device for the detection of cells in suspension. The microfluidic chip consists of two MNs integrated at both sides of the channel to detect impedance measurements of passing cells through the applied electric field. The MNs can be reused, but each PDMS microchip can only be used for one cycle. Due to the low fabrication cost and more than one functionality (solution detection and cell concentration detection), this device was described as suitable for various applications, such as cancer cell detection and water contamination [85] (Figure 4C).

Miller et al., 2014, developed an ion-sensitive microfluidic chip with hollow MNs, one approach that provides an attractive platform for an on-body sensing system for monitoring potassium, which can be easily expanded to other relevant physiological markers for the next generation of point-of-care diagnostic devices. This work was the first ion-selective-electrode MN sensor integrated into a microfluidic device [63] (Figure 4D). A multi-diagnostic system including a PDMS touch-switch, a paper multisensory, and a hollow MN was described by Li et al. 2015 (Figure 4E). The cholesterol and glucose levels in rabbit blood were measured using this device [66]. The main benefit of this method is that it only requires one finger press to activate. With just one finger, enough pressure is applied to the PDMS touch-switch to enable the MN entry into the blood vessel. The deformable chamber returns to its former shape after the finger is released, creating a negative pressure that allows blood to be extracted through the hollow MN and into the sensor-chamber [66]. Sarabi et al., 2021, described an MN array integrated with a microchip for body fluid samples powered by finger press, and the process of fluid flow and its transport across the device was modeled and simulated with a finite model [92].

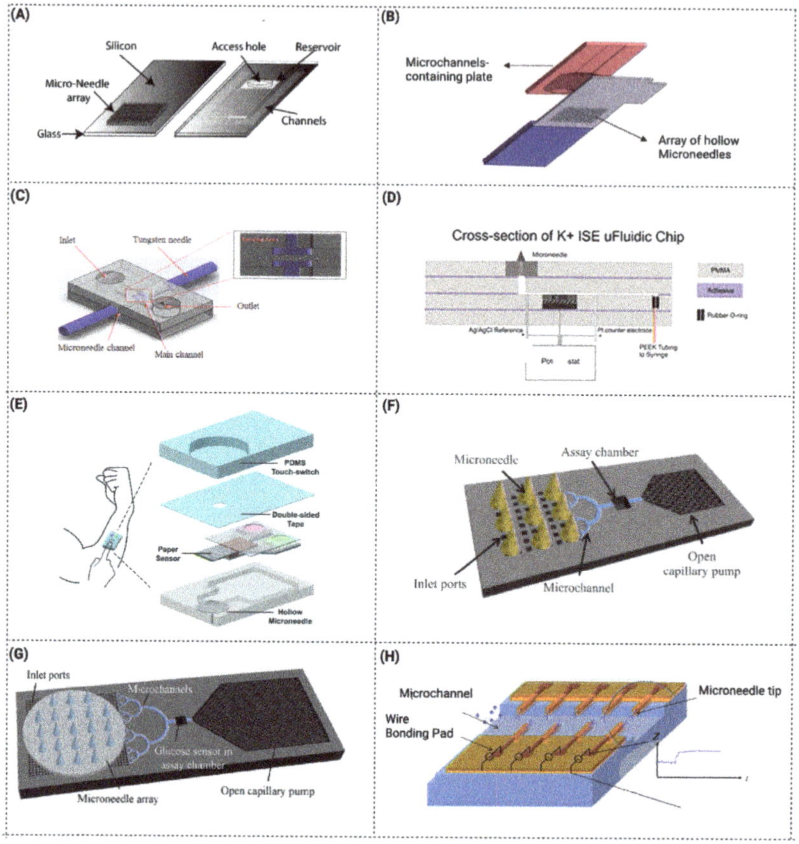


**Figure 4.** Schematic compilation of MN microfluidic devices for extraction and biomarker detection (**A**) Design of MN array. Reprinted from [81]. Copyright © 2023, with permission from Elsevier. (**B**) Integrated device for regular glucose measurement. Reprinted from [60]. Copyright © 2023, with permission from Elsevier. (**C**) 3D schematic diagram of design structure. Reprinted from [85]. Copyright © 2023, with permission from MDPI. (**D**) CorelDraw rendering of a cross-section of the $K^+$ ion-sensitive electrode microfluidic chip. Reprinted from [63]. Copyright © 2023, with permission from John Wiley and Sons, Ltd. (**E**) Schematic representation of the one-touch-activated blood multi-diagnostic system. Reprinted from [66]. Copyright © 2023, with permission from Royal Society of Chemistry. (**F**) Schematic of the proposed minimally invasive blood glucose monitoring system integrating an array of porous MNs in a microfluidic chip. Reprinted from [61]. Copyright © 2023, with permission from Springer. (**G**) Modified and improved system of 4F. Reprinted from [62] Copyright © 2023, with permission from Springer. (**H**) Schematic of an array of horizontal microneedle biosensors in the channel. Reprinted from [65]. Copyright © 2023, with permission from Elsevier.

Although hollow MNs are further explored, some devices incorporate other types of MNs, such as porous MNs. The fundamental benefit of porous MNs is that biodegradable polymers can be used, since their porous structure does not require the micromachining procedures used for hollow structures. Takeuchi et al., 2019, (Figure 4F) developed a microfluidic system with a hydrodynamically designed interface between a porous PDMS MN array and microchannels to enable a direct analysis of liquids extracted by the porous MN array [61]. A porous MN array connected to a microfluidic chip was inserted into agarose gel for evaluation of the collected fluid. This strategy demonstrated a lower flow rate than in the microchip itself, which can be due to the porous MN array increasing the hydraulic resistance of the fluidic connection from the gel to the assay chamber. More recently, a similar system was improved by an additional interface to mechanically and fluidically connect the MN array to microfluidic channels, and tested to show the potential of incorporating MNs in a microfluidic device (Figure 4G) [62]. In another study, Yi et al., 2021, developed a device with porous MNs for the extraction and detection of skin ISF. In this work, a combination of porous MNs with aptamer immobilization was developed, which created an innovative device [64]. In some devices, the detecting method is incorporated in the MN itself, as described by Esfandyarpour et al., 2013, where a solid MN biosensor (with four layers) was developed with the ability to directly measure biomolecular binding as a function of time. This strategy is described as useful for measuring reaction kinetic constants for various biomolecular species [65]. The MNs' position in this platform differs from the standard presenting horizontal MNs. The vertical construction is described to have the advantage of increasing the transducer sensitivity due to the smaller sensing area, whereas the horizontal form is preferable owing to the simplicity of production (Figure 4H). However, the use of MNs integrated in microfluidic devices can have some limitations for the extraction and detection of biomarkers. Typically, by using these MN-integrated microfluidic systems, a limited volume of sample is collected by unit of time, which can cause a limited detection of biomarkers. This can be particularly challenging for applications that require analysis of biomarkers that are presented in low concentrations, and thus, need more volume to achieve the limit of detection (LOD) in the biosensing unit. Additionally, the accuracy to detect biomarkers in these devices, strongly depends on the specificity and sensitivity of the detection method used. An example is the employment of electrochemical sensors, where their sensitivity can decrease over time due to passing fluid that can wash away the immobilized recognition molecule (antibody/aptamer), or by cleaning steps between readings. Therefore, these limitations are important parameters that should to be taken into account for this application.

#### 3.2.2. Devices for Drug Delivery and Microinjection

Microfluidic devices integrated with MNs can be used for drug delivery due to the precise control of drugs released by means of microfluidic components, such as micropumps. This strategy enhances continuous-on-chip drug delivery. Zhan et al., 2004, describe a delivery system with in-plane MNs with a microchannel and an outlet. This design allows for the decoupling of the mechanical and fluidic performance of the device (Figure 5A) [70]. For example, by using thicker substrates and/or larger shanks, needle shank stiffness can be easily raised without compromising flow rate or inlet pressure. Similarly, by employing larger substrates and more deeply etched channels, the flow rate can be enhanced without increasing inlet pressure or lowering stiffness. Based on this design, but with a different method of fabrication, Lee et al., 2015 proposed and demonstrated a MEMS MNs system for deep brain drug infusion [72].

The first flexible microneedle patch incorporating microfluidic components for on-chip loading and delivery control was produced by Xiang et al., 2015 [73]. The ease of use and cost-effectiveness of the proposed microneedle-fluidic system allow it to be a suitable and promising disposable medical device. Additionally, the device was used in the first in vivo experiment where the local inflammatory phenomena were treated by delivering diclofenac solution transdermally into tissues.

In another study, Kang et al., 2021, fabricated a flexible array base microfluidic neural interface to add a chemical delivery capability to three-dimensional electrode arrays comprising a collection of MNs (a silicon MN coated with Cr/Au) positioned perpendicular to the array base [71]. In this device, the fluid flows along the surfaces of MNs from the base, resulting in fluid delivery directly to the brain surface, but indirectly to the electrodes (Figure 5B). Thus, combining drug/chemical delivery with sensing.

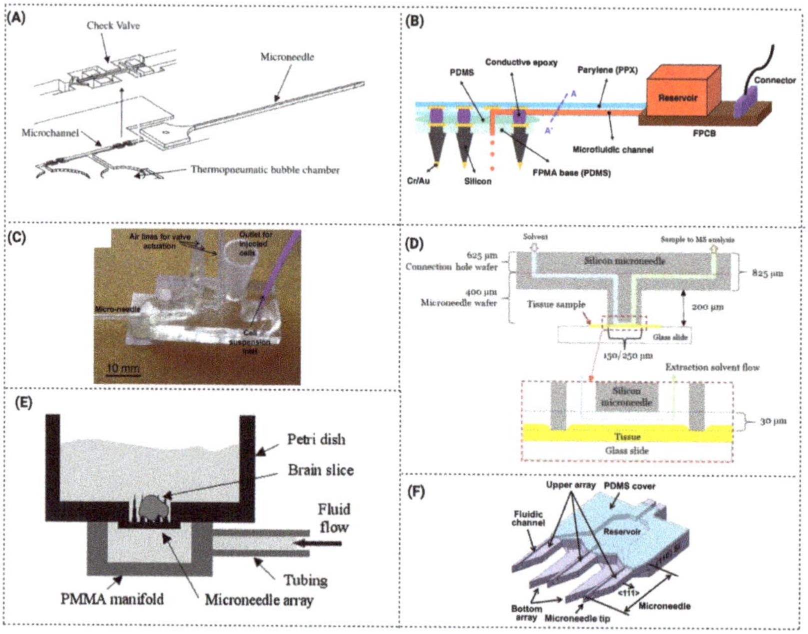


**Figure 5.** Schematic compilation of MN microfluidic devices for drug delivery and microinjection. (**A**) Schematic of an integrated micropump/microneedle device. The top shows a closeup of a planar free floating directional microvalve. Reprinted from [70]. Copyright © 2023, with permission from Springer. (**B**) The flexible penetrating microelectrode array is integrated with the microfluidic interconnection cable (μFIC). Reprinted from [71]. Copyright © 2023, with permission from Nature. (**C**) Assembled microinjection device. Reprinted from [74]. Copyright © 2023, with permission from Royal Society of Chemistry. (**D**) Silicon microneedle structure showing the solvent injection and sample aspiration during microneedle extraction. Reprinted from [87]. Copyright © 2023, with permission from American Institute of Physics. (**E**) A photomicrograph shows the microneedle array perfusing a brain slice. The microfluidic perfusion system integrates microneedle arrays in a packaged system for fluid containment. Reprinted from [89]. Copyright © 2023, with permission from Springer. (**F**) Schematic illustration of the proposed 2D in-plane microneedle chip. Reprinted from [77]. Copyright © 2023, with permission from Springer.

The first microfluidics-based microinjection system was suggested by Adamo et al., 2008, in which single cells were propelled by fluid streams and subsequently injected via MNs with the aid of flexible valve actuation (Figure 5C) [74]. In another strategy, this time based on nanoneedles, Huang et al., 2019 used a microfluidic chip and a nanoneedle array to disrupt the cell membrane, enhancing the passive transfusion of biomolecules to the cytoplasm [93]. Using microinjection-microfluidic systems allows transferring of bioactive agents to many cells in parallel, efficiently transfecting, and works in cell lines difficult to transfect. Zabihihesari et al., 2020, demonstrated the first microfluidic platform that enables immobilization and localized microinjection of a larva due to an integration of a microneedle in the device [75].

As described above, the incorporation of MNs is more developed for LoC devices than for OoC devices. Among the OoC examples is the work of Hokkanen et al., 2015, which developed an automatic microfluidic sample system for tissue analysis. In this work, a microscope and robot were used for positioning the MNs and samples for real-time biopsies (Figure 5D). The blunt-tip silicon MN chips were used to measure indicative cancer biomarkers from the tissues. This system is reported as able to be used to extract lipids from small biopsies [87].

In another OoC study, Choi et al., 2007, described a microfluidic perfusion system that integrates microneedle arrays in a packaged system for fluid containment. The hollow MNs were made with a thin body, a sharp tapered tip, and a microfluidic port along the tower's side to deliver medium to the inside of the target area (Figure 5E) [89]. The 3D perfusion design provides convective mass transport to the tissue interior for experiments on large tissue preparations over extended time periods.

In-plane MN with an open capillary was another strategy developed for LoC. Jung et al., 2015, fabricated in-plane MNs with side openings with a microchannel inside the MN that connected to a reservoir (Figure 5F) [77]. The fabricated microdevice was described to be applied for minimally invasive drug delivery or sample extraction.

Overall, these papers show the vast potential and versatility of applications for MN in microfluidic devices. However, in general, these devices are made using time-consuming fabrication processes that involve numerous steps and additional sealing layers to enhance the total thickness of the structures. The width of microchannels is frequently constrained by small openings created for successful sealing, making it difficult to reliably seal long microchannels. To overcome this fabrication constraint, Trautmann et al., 2019 described a POCT system combining femtosecond laser-generated microfluidic channels and direct laser-written MN arrays that simplify the fabrication process in only a few processing steps. This is an advantage over multiple processing methods [86]. With this method, hollow MNs of various designs were created, and a flow test using rhodamine B was performed to validate the microchip. Nevertheless, there are some other limitations that must be considered when designing MN-integrated microfluidic platforms for drug delivery and microinjection. For instance, the limited volume of drug that may be administered or injected by unit of time must be considered. This can be especially difficult for applications requiring high therapeutic dosages. In addition, many drug treatments require specific formulations and combinations of formulations, which can pose a challenge for researchers and pharmaceutical companies to adapt to MN administration. This includes using an MN-system applying soluble MNs with specific kinetic drug release. Additionally, for this application, the selected material that will act as MNs must be adequate to not react with the drug formulation. As an example, PDMS is known to capture hydrophilic molecules, which can decrease the release of available drug [94]. Considering the application of MN to be used in OoC or to act as drug delivery in a biological matrix, a challenge that may develop is the MN breaking and clogging during the insertion/extraction of MNs into the biological tissue, which can compromise the functionality of the device. Therefore, the selection and specificity of the material chosen to act as MNs and to be integrated within the microfluidic device is one of the most important parameters in the fabrication of such platforms.

## 4. Conclusions

Microfluidic devices with MNs are a relatively novel and appealing method of fluid transport that offers numerous benefits and applications. Because of the multiple possible applications in the field of biomedicine, the attention to these devices has increased significantly in recent years, as shown by the increasing number of published of lab/organ-on-a-chip systems with MNs. These combined structures are compatible with the current biotech requirements for both operation and assessment, including automated liquid management, plate shuttling, biomarker detection and delivery features. Some of the described LoC devices were tested pre-clinically, which shows the end-use applicability of them. However, systems integration and manufacturing MNs present substantial challenges (e.g., clogging effect, biocompatibility, fluid leakage, numerous fabrication steps and high costs). This inherent complexity can negatively influence the manufacture of such devices' dependability and repeatability. One of the challenges in the integration of MNs with microfluidic devices is ensuring that the MNs are precisely aligned with the fluidic channels. This is necessary to guarantee that the fluid flows smoothly through the device and the MNs are able to perform their intended function. Another challenge is ensuring that the MNs' material corresponds to the practical demands of the application that the device is being developed for, as previously outlined in this work.

Overall, the integration of MNs with microfluidic devices is a complex process that requires careful consideration of a number of factors, including design of the MNs, manufacturing techniques, possible functionalization of MN surfaces, and combination or integration with (bio)sensing and actuation systems. As researchers continue to develop new techniques to fabricate MNs-integrated microfluidic devices, the potential application for these devices is expected to expand. As a result, simple fabrication methods and new materials are being explored.

Among MNs, hollow MNs are the ones most employed in microfluidic devices, due to their capability to collect and release higher amounts of fluid. Regarding the MN material, different types of materials from metallic to non-metallic were described in the literature reviewed, which are highly dependent on their application. For instance, MNs designed to penetrate the skin or tissue must be fabricated with materials that provide enough strength and biocompatibility.

Among the microfluidic type of devices, LoC systems with MNs are being explored for extraction, biomarker detection, microinjection, and drug delivery, which can be combined for two or more of these applications in the same device. On the other hand, MN-fluidic systems for OoC/cell-culture monitoring are in the early stages of development. Nevertheless, its potentiality for cell/tissue monitoring is high, as MN structures can measure protein levels directly inside a living cell, without lyse and at real-time. For that, a thin MN can be inserted into a living cell, or in a cluster of cells (tissue), to assess its microenvironment and homeostasis. This can be used for a variety of purposes, including protein expression monitoring, homeostasis assessment, precise drug delivery, and DNA or RNA therapy. Similarly with LoC, one of the most significant advantages of OoC is the versatility of these devices for multiple applications, which has a wide scope for further development. However, the intricate structure of microfluidic devices, as well as challenges in integrating with other devices and fabrication requirements, all contribute to an untapped potential for MNs in the biomedical field. Nevertheless, work is being conducted to overcome this challenge, as shown by a recent published Patent WO/2022/180595, which presents a multiorgan-on-a-chip containing an MN-(bio)sensing platform for the validation and study of nanomaterials, drugs, or mixtures thereof, intended to be used in biomedical and/or pharmaceutic applications [95].

In addition, several researchers are focusing their efforts on developing simpler and low-cost fabrication methodologies to create powerful MN-microfluidic devices, where the integration of the different components, such as biosensing modules, are more easily achieved. One of the newest approaches is the development of microfluidic devices and biosensors using bioprinting technology, which can fabricate in a few steps. This technology, although promising, is also in its first stages. Therefore, there is plenty of room for the MN-microfluidic technology to progress, from material science and microfluidics to tissue engineering. Furthermore, a wide range of applications can be explored, not only biomedical, but also in the sea and in space.

**Author Contributions:** Conceptualization, R.O.R. and R.M.; methodology, R.M. and V.C.; validation, R.O.R., R.L. and G.M.; formal analysis, V.C.; investigation, R.M. and V.C.; data curation, R.M.; writing—original draft preparation, R.M. and V.C.; writing—review and editing, R.O.R., R.L. and G.M.; supervision, R.O.R.; project administration, R.O.R.; funding acquisition, R.O.R. All authors have read and agreed to the published version of the manuscript.

**Funding:** This work was supported by the project EXPL/EMD-EMD/0650/2021, and partially supported by the project PTDC/EEI-EEE/2846/2021, through national funds (OE), within the scope of the Scientific Research and Technological Development Projects (IC&DT) program in all scientific domains (PTDC), through the Foundation for Science and Technology, I.P. (FCT, I.P). This project also received funding from the European Union's Horizon 2020 research and innovation program under the Marie Sklodowska-Curie grant agreement No 101032481. V.C. is grateful for her Ph.D. grant from Fundação para a Ciência e Tecnologia (FCT) with reference UI/BD/151028/2021 and Fulbright Grant for Research with the support of FCT, AY2022/2023. R.O.R. thanks FCT for her contract funding provided through 2020.03975.CEECIND. The authors also acknowledge the partial financial support within the R&D Unit Project Scope: UIDB/04436/2020, UIDB/04077/2020, UIDB/00532/2020, LA/P/0045/2020.

**Institutional Review Board Statement:** Not applicable.

**Informed Consent Statement:** Not applicable.

**Data Availability Statement:** Not applicable.

**Conflicts of Interest:** The authors declare no conflict of interest.

## References

1. Patabadige, D.E.W.; Jia, S.; Sibbitts, J.; Sadeghi, J.; Sellens, K.; Culbertson, C.T. Micro Total Analysis Systems: Fundamental Advances and Applications. *Anal. Chem.* **2016**, *88*, 320–338. [CrossRef]
2. Lafleur, J.P.; Jönsson, A.; Senkbeil, S.; Kutter, J.P. Recent advances in lab-on-a-chip for biosensing applications. *Biosens. Bioelectron.* **2016**, *76*, 213–233. [CrossRef] [PubMed]
3. Mohammed, M.I.; Haswell, S.; Gibson, I. Lab-on-a-chip or Chip-in-a-lab: Challenges of Commercialization Lost in Translation. *Procedia Technol.* **2015**, *20*, 54–59. [CrossRef]
4. Jung, W.; Han, J.; Choi, J.-W.; Ahn, C.H. Point-of-care testing (POCT) diagnostic systems using microfluidic lab-on-a-chip technologies. *Microelectron. Eng.* **2015**, *132*, 46–57. [CrossRef]
5. Samper, I.C.; Gowers, S.A.N.; Booth, M.A.; Wang, C.; Watts, T.; Phairatana, T.; Vallant, N.; Sandhu, B.; Papalois, V.; Boutelle, M.G. Portable Microfluidic Biosensing System for Real-Time Analysis of Microdialysate in Transplant Kidneys. *Anal. Chem.* **2019**, *91*, 14631–14638. [CrossRef]
6. Zhang, L.; Tian, Z.; Bachman, H.; Zhang, P.; Huang, T.J. A Cell-Phone-Based Acoustofluidic Platform for Quantitative Point-of-Care Testing. *ACS Nano* **2020**, *14*, 3159–3169. [CrossRef]
7. Yan, J.; Li, Z.; Guo, J.; Liu, S.; Guo, J. Organ-on-a-chip: A new tool for in vitro research. *Biosens. Bioelectron.* **2022**, *216*, 114626. [CrossRef]
8. Ribas, J.; Pawlikowska, J.; Rouwkema, J. Microphysiological systems: Analysis of the current status, challenges and commercial future. *Microphysiol. Syst.* **2018**, *2*, 10. [CrossRef]
9. Halldorsson, S.; Lucumi, E.; Gómez-Sjöberg, R.; Fleming, R.M.T. Advantages and challenges of microfluidic cell culture in polydimethylsiloxane devices. *Biosens. Bioelectron.* **2015**, *63*, 218–231. [CrossRef]
10. Syama, S.; Mohanan, P.V. Microfluidic based human-on-a-chip: A revolutionary technology in scientific research. *Trends Food Sci. Technol.* **2021**, *110*, 711–728. [CrossRef]
11. Zheng, Y.; Ma, L.; Wu, J.; Wang, Y.; Meng, X.; Hu, P.; Liang, Q.; Xie, Y.; Luo, G. Design and fabrication of an integrated 3D dynamic multicellular liver-on-a-chip and its application in hepatotoxicity screening. *Talanta* **2022**, *241*, 123262.
12. Zhang, F.; Qu, K.-Y.; Zhou, B.; Luo, Y.; Zhu, Z.; Pan, D.-J.; Cui, C.; Zhu, Y.; Chen, M.-L.; Huang, N.-P. Design and fabrication of an integrated heart-on-a-chip platform for construction of cardiac tissue from human iPSC-derived cardiomyocytes and in situ evaluation of physiological function. *Biosens. Bioelectron.* **2021**, *179*, 113080.
13. Haring, A.P.; Sontheimer, H.; Johnson, B.N. Microphysiological Human Brain and Neural Systems-on-a-Chip: Potential Alternatives to Small Animal Models and Emerging Platforms for Drug Discovery and Personalized Medicine. *Stem Cell Rev. Rep.* **2017**, *13*, 381–406. [PubMed]
14. Nieskens, T.T.; Magnusson, O.; Persson, M.; Andersson, P.; Söderberg, M.; Sjögren, A. Development of a kidney-on-a-chip model that replicates an antisense oligonucleotide-induced kidney injury biomarker response. *Toxicol. Lett.* **2021**, *350*, S58. [CrossRef]
15. Joseph, X.; Akhil, V.; Arathi, A.; Mohanan, P.V. Comprehensive Development in Organ-On-A-Chip Technology. *J. Pharm. Sci.* **2022**, *111*, 18–31. [PubMed]
16. Rodrigues, R.O.; Sousa, P.C.; Gaspar, J.; Bañobre-López, M.; Lima, R.; Minas, G. Organ-on-a-Chip: A Preclinical Microfluidic Platform for the Progress of Nanomedicine. *Small* **2020**, *16*, 2003517.
17. Meng, X.; Zhang, Z.; Li, L. Micro/nano needles for advanced drug delivery. *Prog. Nat. Sci. Mater. Int.* **2020**, *30*, 589–596.
18. Angkawinitwong, U.; Courtenay, A.J.; Rodgers, A.M.; Larrañeta, E.; McCarthy, H.O.; Brocchini, S.; Donnelly, R.F.; Williams, G.R. A Novel Transdermal Protein Delivery Strategy via Electrohydrodynamic Coating of PLGA Microparticles onto Microneedles. *ACS Appl. Mater. Interfaces* **2020**, *12*, 12478–12488. [CrossRef]
19. Chiappini, C.; De Rosa, E.; Martinez, J.O.; Liu, X.; Steele, J.; Stevens, M.M.; Tasciotti, E. Biodegradable silicon nanoneedles delivering nucleic acids intracellularly induce localized in vivo neovascularization. *Nat. Mater* **2015**, *14*, 532–539. [PubMed]
20. Zhuang, J.; Rao, F.; Wu, D.; Huang, Y.; Xu, H.; Gao, W.; Zhang, J.; Sun, J. Study on the fabrication and characterization of tip-loaded dissolving microneedles for transdermal drug delivery. *Eur. J. Pharm. Biopharm.* **2020**, *157*, 66–73. [PubMed]
21. Bhise, N.S.; Ribas, J.; Manoharan, V.; Zhang, Y.S.; Polini, A.; Massa, S.; Dokmeci, M.R.; Khademhosseini, A. Organ-on-a-chip platforms for studying drug delivery systems. *J. Control. Release* **2014**, *190*, 82–93. [PubMed]
22. Waghule, T.; Singhvi, G.; Dubey, S.K.; Pandey, M.M.; Gupta, G.; Singh, M.; Dua, K. Microneedles: A smart approach and increasing potential for transdermal drug delivery system. *Biomed. Pharmacother.* **2019**, *109*, 1249–1258. [PubMed]

23. Chang, K.-T.; Shen, Y.-K.; Fan, F.-Y.; Lin, Y.; Kang, S.-C. Optimal design and fabrication of a microneedle arrays patch. *J. Manuf. Process.* **2020**, *54*, 274–285.
24. Sonetha, V.; Majumdar, S.; Shah, S. Step-wise micro-fabrication techniques of microneedle arrays with applications in transdermal drug delivery—A review. *J. Drug Deliv. Sci. Technol.* **2022**, *68*, 103119.
25. Matsumoto, D.; Rao Sathuluri, R.; Kato, Y.; Silberberg, Y.R.; Kawamura, R.; Iwata, F.; Kobayashi, T.; Nakamura, C. Oscillating high-aspect-ratio monolithic silicon nanoneedle array enables efficient delivery of functional bio-macromolecules into living cells. *Sci. Rep.* **2015**, *5*, 15325. [PubMed]
26. Kaur, R.; Arora, S.; Goswami, M. Advancement in microneedles as minimally invasive delivery system for pharmaceutical and biomedical application: A review. *Mater. TodayProc.* **2022**. [CrossRef]
27. Yang, L.; Yang, Y.; Chen, H.; Mei, L.; Zeng, X. Polymeric microneedle-mediated sustained release systems: Design strategies and promising applications for drug delivery. *Asian J. Pharm. Sci.* **2022**, *17*, 70–86.
28. McAlister, E.; Kirkby, M.; Donnelly, R.F. 6—Microneedles for drug delivery and monitoring. In *Microfluidic Devices for Biomedical Applications*, 2nd ed.; Li, X. (James), Zhou, Y., Eds.; Woodhead Publishing Series in Biomaterials; Woodhead Publishing: Sawston, UK, 2021; pp. 225–260. ISBN 978-0-12-819971-8.
29. Nguyen, N.-T.; Shaegh, S.A.M.; Kashaninejad, N.; Phan, D.-T. Design, fabrication and characterization of drug delivery systems based on lab-on-a-chip technology. *Adv. Drug Deliv. Rev.* **2013**, *65*, 1403–1419.
30. Sanjay, S.T.; Zhou, W.; Dou, M.; Tavakoli, H.; Ma, L.; Xu, F.; Li, X. Recent advances of controlled drug delivery using microfluidic platforms. *Adv. Drug Deliv. Rev.* **2018**, *128*, 3–28.
31. Sawon, M.A.; Samad, M.F. Design and optimization of a microneedle with skin insertion analysis for transdermal drug delivery applications. *J. Drug Deliv. Sci. Technol.* **2021**, *63*, 102477.
32. Chow, Y.T.; Chen, S.; Liu, C.; Liu, C.; Li, L.; Kong, C.W.M.; Cheng, S.H.; Li, R.A.; Sun, D. A High-Throughput Automated Microinjection System for Human Cells With Small Size. *IEEE/ASME Trans. Mechatron.* **2016**, *21*, 838–850.
33. Naveen, N.R.; Goudanavar, P.S.; Ramesh, B.; Kumar, G.K. Prospection of fabrication techniques and material selection of microneedles for transdermal drug delivery: An update on clinical trials. *Mater. Today Proc.* **2022**, *69*, 187–192.
34. Bhadale, R.S.; Londhe, V.Y. A systematic review of carbohydrate-based microneedles: Current status and future prospects. *J. Mater. Sci. Mater. Med.* **2021**, *32*, 89. [PubMed]
35. Meng, F.; Hasan, A.; Mahdi Nejadi Babadaei, M.; Hashemi Kani, P.; Jouya Talaei, A.; Sharifi, M.; Cai, T.; Falahati, M.; Cai, Y. Polymeric-based microneedle arrays as potential platforms in the development of drugs delivery systems. *J. Adv. Res.* **2020**, *26*, 137–147. [PubMed]
36. Singh, J.; Rathi, A.; Rawat, M.; Gupta, M. Graphene: From synthesis to engineering to biosensor applications. *Front. Mater. Sci.* **2018**, *12*, 1–20.
37. Nagarkar, R.; Singh, M.; Nguyen, H.X.; Jonnalagadda, S. A review of recent advances in microneedle technology for transdermal drug delivery. *J. Drug Deliv. Sci. Technol.* **2020**, *59*, 101923.
38. Aldawood, F.K.; Andar, A.; Desai, S. A Comprehensive Review of Microneedles: Types, Materials, Processes, Characterizations and Applications. *Polymers* **2021**, *13*, 2815.
39. Tarbox, T.N.; Watts, A.B.; Cui, Z.; Williams, R.O. An update on coating/manufacturing techniques of microneedles. *Drug Deliv. Transl. Res.* **2018**, *8*, 1828–1843.
40. Takahashi, H.; Jung Heo, Y.; Arakawa, N.; Kan, T.; Matsumoto, K.; Kawano, R.; Shimoyama, I. Scalable fabrication of microneedle arrays via spatially controlled UV exposure. *Microsyst. Nanoeng.* **2016**, *2*, 16049.
41. Jung, P.G.; Lee, T.W.; Oh, D.J.; Hwang, S.J.; Jung, I.; Lee, S.; Ko, J. Nickel Microneedles Fabricated by Sequential Copper and Nickel Electroless Plating and Copper Chemical Wet Etching. *Sens. Mater.* **2008**, *20*, 45–53.
42. Wang, Q.L.; Zhu, D.D.; Liu, X.B.; Chen, B.Z.; Guo, X.D. Microneedles with Controlled Bubble Sizes and Drug Distributions for Efficient Transdermal Drug Delivery. *Sci. Rep.* **2016**, *6*, 38755. [PubMed]
43. Aoyagi, S.; Izumi, H.; Isono, Y.; Fukuda, M.; Ogawa, H. Laser fabrication of high aspect ratio thin holes on biodegradable polymer and its application to a microneedle. *Sens. Actuators A Phys.* **2007**, *139*, 293–302. [CrossRef]
44. Kim, J.D.; Kim, M.; Yang, H.; Lee, K.; Jung, H. Droplet-born air blowing: Novel dissolving microneedle fabrication. *J. Control. Release* **2013**, *170*, 430–436. [PubMed]
45. Faraji Rad, Z.; Prewett, P.D.; Davies, G.J. Rapid prototyping and customizable microneedle design: Ultra-sharp microneedle fabrication using two-photon polymerization and low-cost micromolding techniques. *Manuf. Lett.* **2021**, *30*, 39–43.
46. Pere, C.P.P.; Economidou, S.N.; Lall, G.; Ziraud, C.; Boateng, J.S.; Alexander, B.D.; Lamprou, D.A.; Douroumis, D. 3D printed microneedles for insulin skin delivery. *Int. J. Pharm.* **2018**, *544*, 425–432. [PubMed]
47. Häfeli, U.O.; Mokhtari, A.; Liepmann, D.; Stoeber, B. In vivo evaluation of a microneedle-based miniature syringe for intradermal drug delivery. *Biomed. Microdevices* **2009**, *11*, 943–950.
48. Valdés-Ramírez, G.; Windmiller, J.R.; Claussen, J.C.; Martinez, A.G.; Kuralay, F.; Zhou, M.; Zhou, N.; Polsky, R.; Miller, P.R.; Narayan, R.; et al. Multiplexed and switchable release of distinct fluids from microneedle platforms via conducting polymer nanoactuators for potential drug delivery. *Sens. Actuators B Chem.* **2012**, *161*, 1018–1024.
49. Liberati, A.; Altman, D.G.; Tetzlaff, J.; Mulrow, C.; Gøtzsche, P.C.; Ioannidis, J.P.A.; Clarke, M.; Devereaux, P.J.; Kleijnen, J.; Moher, D. The PRISMA Statement for Reporting Systematic Reviews and Meta-Analyses of Studies That Evaluate Health Care Interventions: Explanation and Elaboration. *PLoS Med.* **2009**, *6*, e1000100.

50. Moher, D.; Liberati, A.; Tetzlaff, J.; Altman, D.G. Preferred reporting items for systematic reviews and meta-analyses: The PRISMA statement. *BMJ* **2009**, *339*, b2535. [CrossRef]
51. Ventrelli, L.; Marsilio Strambini, L.; Barillaro, G. Microneedles for Transdermal Biosensing: Current Picture and Future Direction. *Adv. Healthc. Mater.* **2015**, *4*, 2606–2640.
52. Li, C.G.; Lee, C.Y.; Lee, K.; Jung, H. An optimized hollow microneedle for minimally invasive blood extraction. *Biomed. Microdevices* **2013**, *15*, 17–25. [PubMed]
53. Wang, Z.; Luan, J.; Seth, A.; Liu, L.; You, M.; Gupta, P.; Rathi, P.; Wang, Y.; Cao, S.; Jiang, Q.; et al. Microneedle patch for the ultrasensitive quantification of protein biomarkers in interstitial fluid. *Nat. Biomed. Eng.* **2021**, *5*, 64–76. [PubMed]
54. Takeuchi, K.; Kim, B. Functionalized microneedles for continuous glucose monitoring. *Nano Converg.* **2018**, *5*, 28.
55. Dardano, P.; Rea, I.; De Stefano, L. Microneedles-based electrochemical sensors: New tools for advanced biosensing. *Curr. Opin. Electrochem.* **2019**, *17*, 121–127.
56. Kusama, S.; Sato, K.; Matsui, Y.; Kimura, N.; Abe, H.; Yoshida, S.; Nishizawa, M. Transdermal electroosmotic flow generated by a porous microneedle array patch. *Nat. Commun.* **2021**, *12*, 658.
57. Azizgolshani, H.; Coppeta, J.R.; Vedula, E.M.; Marr, E.E.; Cain, B.P.; Luu, R.J.; Lech, M.P.; Kann, S.H.; Mulhern, T.J.; Tandon, V.; et al. High-throughput organ-on-chip platform with integrated programmable fluid flow and real-time sensing for complex tissue models in drug development workflows. *Lab Chip* **2021**, *21*, 1454–1474. [PubMed]
58. Zimmermann, S.; Fienbork, D.; Stoeber, B.; Flounders, A.W.; Liepmann, D. A microneedle-based glucose monitor: Fabricated on a wafer-level using in-device enzyme immobilization. In Proceedings of the TRANSDUCERS '03, 12th International Conference on Solid-State Sensors, Actuators and Microsystems, Digest of Technical Papers (Cat. No.03TH8664), Boston, MA, USA, 8–12 June 2003; Volume 1, pp. 99–102.
59. Najmi, A.; Saidi, M.S.; Shahrokhian, S.; Hosseini, H.; Kazemzadeh Hannani, S. Fabrication of a microdialysis-based nonenzymatic microfluidic sensor for regular glucose measurement. *Sens. Actuators B Chem.* **2021**, *333*, 129569.
60. Najmi, A.; Saidi, M.S.; Kazemzadeh Hannani, S. Design of the micropump and mass-transfer compartment of a microfluidic system for regular nonenzymatic glucose measurement. *Biotechnol. Rep.* **2022**, *34*, e00723.
61. Takeuchi, K.; Takama, N.; Kim, B.; Sharma, K.; Paul, O.; Ruther, P. Microfluidic chip to interface porous microneedles for ISF collection. *Biomed. Microdevices* **2019**, *21*, 28.
62. Takeuchi, K.; Takama, N.; Sharma, K.; Paul, O.; Ruther, P.; Suga, T.; Kim, B. Microfluidic chip connected to porous microneedle array for continuous ISF sampling. *Drug Deliv. Transl. Res.* **2022**, *12*, 435–443. [CrossRef]
63. Miller, P.R.; Xiao, X.; Brener, I.; Burckel, D.B.; Narayan, R.; Polsky, R. Microneedle-Based Transdermal Sensor for On-Chip Potentiometric Determination of $K^+$. *Adv. Healthc. Mater.* **2014**, *3*, 876–881. [PubMed]
64. Yi, K.; Wang, Y.; Shi, K.; Chi, J.; Lyu, J.; Zhao, Y. Aptamer-decorated porous microneedles arrays for extraction and detection of skin interstitial fluid biomarkers. *Biosens. Bioelectron.* **2021**, *190*, 113404. [PubMed]
65. Esfandyarpour, R.; Esfandyarpour, H.; Javanmard, M.; Harris, J.S.; Davis, R.W. Microneedle biosensor: A method for direct label-free real time protein detection. *Sens. Actuators B Chem.* **2013**, *177*, 848–855. [PubMed]
66. Li, C.G.; Joung, H.-A.; Noh, H.; Song, M.-B.; Kim, M.-G.; Jung, H. One-touch-activated blood multidiagnostic system using a minimally invasive hollow microneedle integrated with a paper-based sensor. *Lab Chip* **2015**, *15*, 3286–3292. [PubMed]
67. Trzebinski, J.; Sharma, S.; Radomska-Botelho Moniz, A.; Michelakis, K.; Zhang, Y.; Cass, A.E.G. Microfluidic device to investigate factors affecting performance in biosensors designed for transdermal applications. *Lab Chip* **2012**, *12*, 348–352.
68. Kim, K.; Lee, J.-B. High aspect ratio tapered hollow metallic microneedle arrays with microfluidic interconnector. *Microsyst. Technol.* **2006**, *13*, 231–235.
69. Singh, R.R.T.; Tekko, I.; McAvoy, K.; McMillan, H.; Jones, D.; Donnelly, R.F. Minimally invasive microneedles for ocular drug delivery. *Expert Opin. Drug Deliv.* **2017**, *14*, 525–537.
70. Zahn, J.D.; Deshmukh, A.; Pisano, A.P.; Liepmann, D. Continuous On-Chip Micropumping for Microneedle Enhanced Drug Delivery. *Biomed. Microdevices* **2004**, *6*, 183–190. [CrossRef]
71. Kang, Y.N.; Chou, N.; Jang, J.-W.; Choe, H.K.; Kim, S. A 3D flexible neural interface based on a microfluidic interconnection cable capable of chemical delivery. *Microsyst. Nanoeng.* **2021**, *7*, 66.
72. Lee, H.J.; Son, Y.; Kim, D.; Kim, Y.K.; Choi, N.; Yoon, E.-S.; Cho, I.-J. A new thin silicon microneedle with an embedded microchannel for deep brain drug infusion. *Sens. Actuators B Chem.* **2015**, *209*, 413–422.
73. Xiang, Z.; Wang, H.; Pastorin, G.; Lee, C. Development of a Flexible and Disposable Microneedle-Fluidic-System With Finger-Driven Drug Loading and Delivery Functions for Inflammation Treatment. *J. Microelectromech. Syst.* **2015**, *24*, 565–574. [CrossRef]
74. Adamo, A.; Jensen, K.F. Microfluidic based single cell microinjection. *Lab Chip* **2008**, *8*, 1258. [CrossRef] [PubMed]
75. Zabihihesari, A.; Hilliker, A.J.; Rezai, P. Localized microinjection of intact *Drosophila melanogaster* larva to investigate the effect of serotonin on heart rate. *Lab Chip* **2020**, *20*, 343–355. [CrossRef] [PubMed]
76. Li, Y.; Zhang, H.; Yang, R.; Tazrin, F.; Zhu, C.; Kaddoura, M.; Blondeel, E.J.M.; Cui, B. In-plane silicon microneedles with open capillary microfluidic networks by deep reactive ion etching and sacrificial layer based sharpening. *Sens. Actuators A Phys.* **2019**, *292*, 149–157. [CrossRef]
77. Jung, M.; Jeong, D.; Yun, S.-S.; Lee, J.-H. Fabrication of a 2-D in-plane micro needle array integrated with microfluidic components using crystalline wet etching of (110) silicon. *Microsyst. Technol.* **2016**, *22*, 2287–2294. [CrossRef]

78. Parker, E.R.; Rao, M.P.; Turner, K.L.; Meinhart, C.D.; MacDonald, N.C. Bulk Micromachined Titanium Microneedles. *J. Microelectromech. Syst.* **2007**, *16*, 289–295. [CrossRef]
79. Griss, P.; Stemme, G. Side-opened out-of-plane microneedles for microfluidic transdermal liquid transfer. *J. Microelectromech. Syst.* **2003**, *12*, 296–301. [CrossRef]
80. Zhu, J.; Cao, Y.; Wang, H.; Li, Y.; Chen, X.; Chen, D. Fabricating process of hollow out-of-plane Ni microneedle arrays and properties of the integrated microfluidic device. *J. Micro/Nanolith. MEMS MOEMS* **2013**, *12*, 033019. [CrossRef]
81. Mukerjee, E.V.; Collins, S.D.; Isseroff, R.R.; Smith, R.L. Microneedle array for transdermal biological fluid extraction and in situ analysis. *Sens. Actuators A Phys.* **2004**, *114*, 267–275. [CrossRef]
82. Dixon, R.V.; Skaria, E.; Lau, W.M.; Manning, P.; Birch-Machin, M.A.; Moghimi, S.M.; Ng, K.W. Microneedle-based devices for point-of-care infectious disease diagnostics. *Acta Pharm. Sin. B* **2021**, *11*, 2344–2361. [CrossRef]
83. Ashraf, M.W.; Tayyaba, S.; Afzulpurkar, N. Micro Electromechanical Systems (MEMS) Based Microfluidic Devices for Biomedical Applications. *IJMS* **2011**, *12*, 3648–3704. [CrossRef]
84. Gao, B.; Guo, M.; Lyu, K.; Chu, T.; He, B. Intelligent Silk Fibroin Based Microneedle Dressing (i-SMD). *Adv. Funct. Mater.* **2021**, *31*, 2006839. [CrossRef]
85. Mansor, M.; Takeuchi, M.; Nakajima, M.; Hasegawa, Y.; Ahmad, M. Electrical Impedance Spectroscopy for Detection of Cells in Suspensions Using Microfluidic Device with Integrated Microneedles. *Appl. Sci.* **2017**, *7*, 170. [CrossRef]
86. Trautmann, A.; Roth, G.-L.; Nujiqi, B.; Walther, T.; Hellmann, R. Towards a versatile point-of-care system combining femtosecond laser generated microfluidic channels and direct laser written microneedle arrays. *Microsyst. Nanoeng.* **2019**, *5*, 6. [CrossRef]
87. Hokkanen, A.; Stuns, I.; Schmid, P.; Kokkonen, A.; Gao, F.; Steinecker, A.; Budczies, J.; Heimala, P.; Hakalahti, L. Microfluidic sampling system for tissue analytics. *Biomicrofluidics* **2015**, *9*, 054109. [CrossRef]
88. Dabbagh, S.R.; Sarabi, M.R.; Rahbarghazi, R.; Sokullu, E.; Yetisen, A.K.; Tasoglu, S. 3D-printed microneedles in biomedical applications. *iScience* **2021**, *24*, 102012. [CrossRef] [PubMed]
89. Choi, Y.; McClain, M.A.; LaPlaca, M.C.; Frazier, A.B.; Allen, M.G. Three dimensional MEMS microfluidic perfusion system for thick brain slice cultures. *Biomed. Microdevices* **2007**, *9*, 7–13. [CrossRef] [PubMed]
90. Li, C.G.; Lee, K.; Lee, C.Y.; Dangol, M.; Jung, H. A Minimally Invasive Blood-Extraction System: Elastic Self-Recovery Actuator Integrated with an Ultrahigh- Aspect-Ratio Microneedle. *Adv. Mater.* **2012**, *24*, 4583–4586. [CrossRef]
91. Ju, J.; Li, L.; Regmi, S.; Zhang, X.; Tang, S. Microneedle-Based Glucose Sensor Platform: From Vitro to Wearable Point-of-Care Testing Systems. *Biosensors* **2022**, *12*, 606. [CrossRef]
92. Sarabi, M.R.; Ahmadpour, A.; Yetisen, A.K.; Tasoglu, S. Finger-Actuated Microneedle Array for Sampling Body Fluids. *Appl. Sci.* **2021**, *11*, 5329. [CrossRef]
93. Huang, D.; Zhao, D.; Li, J.; Wu, Y.; Du, L.; Xia, X.-H.; Li, X.; Deng, Y.; Li, Z.; Huang, Y. Continuous Vector-free Gene Transfer with a Novel Microfluidic Chip and Nanoneedle Array. *CDD* **2018**, *16*, 164–170. [CrossRef] [PubMed]
94. Wang, J.D.; Douville, N.J.; Takayama, S.; ElSayed, M. Quantitative Analysis of Molecular Absorption into PDMS Microfluidic Channels. *Ann. Biomed. Eng.* **2012**, *40*, 1862–1873. [CrossRef] [PubMed]
95. Minas, H.; Maria, G.; Rodrigues, R.O.; de Sousa, T.; Jorge, P.; De Lima, M.M.; Alberto, R.; De Sousa, S.; Catarina, P.; Cabanas, C.; et al. WO2022180595—Multiorgan-on-Chip Device with Integrated Microbiosensors, Methods and Uses Thereof. WO/2022/180595. Available online: https://patentscope.wipo.int/search/en/detail.jsf?docId=WO2022180595&_cid=P20-L7J87M-45311-1 (accessed on 10 January 2023).

*pharmaceutics*

MDPI

*Article*

# Promotion of Hair Regrowth by Transdermal Dissolvable Microneedles Loaded with Rapamycin and Epigallocatechin Gallate Nanoparticles

**Yali Lin [1,2], Ruomei Shao [1], Tong Xiao [1,3] and Shuqing Sun [1,*]**

1 Institute of Biopharmaceutical and Health Engineering, Shenzhen International Graduate School, Tsinghua University, Shenzhen 518055, China; lin-yl19@mails.tsinghua.edu.cn (Y.L.); shruomei@aliyun.com (R.S.); xiaot21@mails.tsinghua.edu.cn (T.X.)
2 Department of Biomedical Engineering, Tsinghua University, Beijing 100084, China
3 Department of Chemical Engineering, Tsinghua University, Beijing 100084, China
* Correspondence: sun.shuqing@sz.tsinghua.edu.cn; Tel.: +86-755-2603-6026

**Abstract:** Interest in transdermal delivery methods for stimulating hair regrowth has been increasing recently. The microneedle approach can break the barrier of the stratum corneum through puncture ability and improve drug delivery efficiency. Herein, we report a dissolvable microneedle device for the co-delivery of rapamycin and epigallocatechin gallate nanoparticles that can significantly promote hair regeneration. Compared with the mice without any treatment, our strategy can facilitate hair growth within 7 days. Higher hair shaft growth rate and hair follicle density with inconspicuous inflammation were exhibited in C57BL/6 mice, elucidating its potential for clinical application.

**Keywords:** hair regrowth; microneedles; nanoparticles; rapamycin

## 1. Introduction

Hair loss, a common and distressing symptom, has become a condition that plagues billions of people worldwide [1,2]. Currently, topical minoxidil [3], oral finasteride [4], and hair follicle transplantation [5] are common clinical treatments but still face challenges such as uncontrolled adverse effects, high cost, poor compliance of patients, and time commitment [6,7]. Although other pharmacological treatments, such as valproic acid [8], Ru58841 [9], etc., as well as phytochemicals from botanicals [10], were demonstrated to promote hair growth, most drug formulations are prepared for topical administration [11]. However, because of the protective barrier of the stratum corneum, the percutaneous absorption of drugs is hindered, resulting in low percutaneous permeability and poor treatment compliance [12,13]. Therefore, effective treatments are urgently needed.

Transdermal delivery systems are required for successful therapeutic application beyond conventional venous injections and oral or topical administration [14–17]. Microneedles (MNs) with three-dimensional microstructures with microscale lengths (usually less than 1000 μm) are a potential direction, which can overcome the complex and dynamic barriers of the stratum corneum, control the delivery dose, and improve the efficiency and accuracy of drugs [16,18]. In recent years, microneedle drug delivery systems therapy for alopecia disease has received extensive attention and fueled the hair loss therapy research field [19–22]. However, individual differences have led to an ever-increasing need for precise hair growth.

In this study, a dissolvable microneedle device to deliver nanoparticles (NPs) was designed (Figure 1). Polyvinylpyrrolidone (PVP), with good biocompatibility, mechanical properties, and water-soluble properties, served as a microneedle structure [23]. When the microneedle penetrated into the skin, it dissolved rapidly and released nanoparticles, enabling controlled and sustained release of drug nanoparticles into the skin. Rapamycin

(RAPA) and epigallocatechin gallate (EGCG) were selected as target drugs. Rapamycin, an autophagy-activating small molecule, can induce the transition of the hair cycle from the telogen to anagen phase, thereby promoting hair regrowth [24,25]. The nanoparticles were formed by polylactic–glycolic acid copolymer (PLGA) with encapsulation of rapamycin (RAPA-PLGA NPs), which helps to improve the sustained-release effect and prolong the incubation period of rapamycin [26]. In addition, EGCG has antioxidation and anagen activation effects [27]. Keratin (KE) is the main component of hair [28]. Crosslinking keratin with EGCG to form nanoparticles (EGCG-KE NPs) can not only provide nutrition for hair but also benefit the proliferation of hair follicle cells. From a series of in vitro and in vivo experiments, we demonstrated that the RAPA-PLGA and EGCG-KE NP-loaded MN device (DMN) can promote hair regeneration within as few as 7 days.

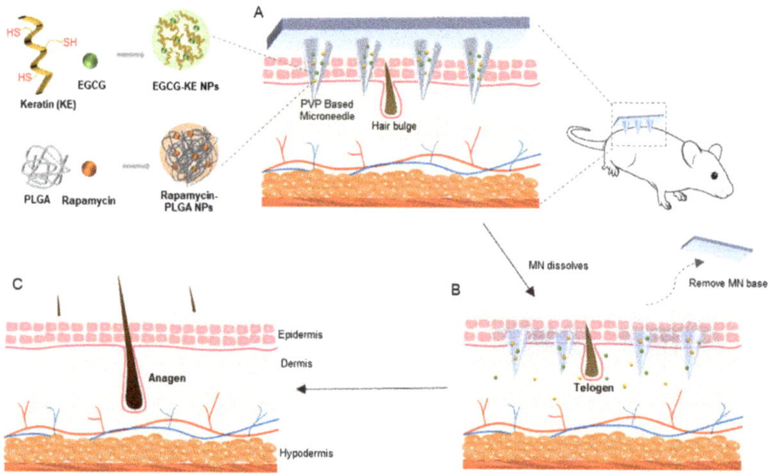


**Figure 1.** Schematic of the microneedle device for hair regrowth. (**A**) Our DMN (PVP-based microneedle loaded with RAPA-PLGA and EGCG-KE NPs) penetrate the skin. (**B**) The microneedles dissolve rapidly and release nanoparticles and drug transport into the hair follicle niche. (**C**) Drugs can activate the healthy hair cycle, accelerate the transition of hair follicles from telogen to anagen, and promote hair regrowth.

## 2. Materials and Methods

### 2.1. Materials and Animals

Poly(lactic-co-glycolic acid) (PLGA, 50/50), rapamycin (RAPA, 98%), Keratin(KE) solution (5 mg/mL, Aladdin, Shanghai, China), epigallocatechin gallate (EGCG, 95%, Aladdin, Shanghai), polyvinyl pyrrolidone (PVP, Mw 400,000), acetone, dithiothreitol (DTT), polyethylene-polypropylene glycol (F68), polydimethylsiloxane (PDMS, Dow Corning Sylgard 184), formaldehyde, C57BL/6 mice (6 weeks old, Guangdong Medical Laboratory Animal Center). All mouse experiments were approved by the Animal Care Committee of Tsinghua University.

### 2.2. Preparation of Nanoparticles

RAPA-PLGA NPs: 10 mg of PLGA and 1 mg of rapamycin were dissolved in 1 mL of acetone solution. PLGA solution was added dropwise to 10 mL of 0.1% F68 solution with stirring at room temperature overnight. After centrifugation at 10,000 r/min for 20 min, the collected nanoparticles were dispersed in pure water and stored at 4 °C.

EGCG-KE NPs: 10 mL of keratin solution (1 mg/mL) was reduced by 20 μg of DTT for 4 h, and then 40 mL of EGCG solution (5 mg/mL) was added. Then, 100 μL of 37% formaldehyde solution was added dropwise into the mixture with stirring at room temperature for 12 h. After centrifugation at 10,000 r/min for 20 min, the collected nanoparticles were dispersed in pure water and stored at 4 °C.

*2.3. Fabrication of DMN*

A 10 × 10 array microneedle (a round base diameter of 320 μm, a height of 680 μm in each microneedle, 600 μm of tip–tip spacing) anode model was prepared by Suzhou Machinery (China). Then, the PDMS cathode mold was prepared by the template method. PVP solution (1 g/mL) mixed with the drug (RAPA-PLGA NPs and/or EGCG-KE NPs) was added to the PDMS microneedle mold and then vacuumed for 2 min. The excess PVP solution was removed using a spin coater. Then, 13% PVA/sucrose solution was added as the MN substrate. The whole model was placed in a desiccator for 2 days until completely dry. The microneedle patch was peeled off from the PDMS model and stored in a desiccator.

An example of how to prepare a MN patch with 1 μg of RAPA is shown. Next, 1 g of PVP was mixed with 1 mL of RAPA-PLGA NPs solution (containing 1 mg RAPA encapsulated in NPs). Then, the microneedle wells (2 μL/MN patch) were filled with PVP solution (0.5 mg/mL RAPA) by vacuum. The excess PVP solution was removed by a spin coater to ensure wells contained only drugs. Thus, the microneedle wells contained 1 μg (2 μL × 0.5 mg/mL) of RAPA. Different dosage amounts of model drugs in MN were controlled in the same way.

*2.4. Characterizations of NPs and DMN*

Ultraviolet spectroscopy (UV): the aqueous solution of the samples (nanoparticles, KE, rapamycin, EGCG) was measured by an ultraviolet spectrophotometer in the wavelength range of 200–400 nm.

Dynamic light scattering (DLS): the nanoparticles were ultrasonically dispersed in pure water, and their size and zeta potential were obtained using a Malvern Mastersizer 3000 analyzer.

Scanning electron microscopy (SEM): the lyophilized nanoparticle powder or MN was placed in a silicon wafer. The surface of the sample was sprayed with gold, and the morphology of the nanoparticles was observed under a scanning electron microscope (5 kV).

Mechanical strength test: the microneedle was pressed by the top sensor at a speed of 0.1 mm/min until destroyed, and the force-displacement data were recorded by an electromechanical universal testing machine.

In vitro drug release study: a vertical Franz diffusion was used for the PLGA nanoparticle release study. The upper diffusion pool was added to the nanoparticle dispersion, and the lower pool was filled with 0.1% F68 PBS solution (pH = 7.4). A filter membrane (0.2 μm) was located between the diffusion pool and the supply pool. The Franz diffusion cell was stirred at 37 °C. One milliliter of solution from the supply pool at the setting time was used to detect the concentration of rapamycin by UV.

*2.5. Animals Experiments*

Rapamycin MN: following anesthesia by 1.25% tribromoethanol, dorsal skin hair (an area of approximately 2 cm × 2 cm) was shaved using an electric hair clipper and hair removal cream. Six-week-old C57BL/6 mice with MN administration were treated on the first and seventh day. The microneedle was pressed into the dorsal skin with the thumb for 30 s, followed by fixation with medical tape paste and the microneedle base was peeled off after 2 h. In rapamycin MN groups, dosage from low to high (0.001 μg, 0.01 μg, 0.1 μg, 1 μg, 10 μg rapamycin/MN patch) was applied to the treatment area. In the topical dosing groups, 30 μL of rapamycin lecithin gel (low dose to high dose: 0.2 μM, 2 μM, 20 μM) was applied to the treatment area (2 cm × 2 cm) every other day. The shaved untreated mice served as controls.

DMN: following anesthesia by 1.25% tribromoethanol, the dorsal skin hair (an area of approximately 2 cm × 2 cm) was shaved by using an electric hair clipper and hair removal cream. Six-week-old C57BL/6 mice with MN administration were treated on the first and seventh day. The microneedle was pressed into the dorsal skin with the thumb for 30 s, followed by fixation with medical tape paste, and the microneedle base was then peeled off after 2 h. In the topical dosing group, 30 μL of rapamycin lecithin gel (2 μM) or 20 μL of 2% EGCG ethanol solution was applied on the treatment area (2 cm × 2 cm) every other day. The shaved untreated mice served as controls.

### 2.6. Histology and Immunofluorescent

At the time point, mice were sacrificed, and skin samples were collected from the back. Samples were fixed with 4% paraformaldehyde solution for 24 h and then dehydrated and embedded in wax using an automatic tissue dehydrator. After sectioning, the samples were subjected to hematoxylin and eosin (H&E) staining. H&E staining images were collected by optical microscopy.

For immunofluorescence, the sample slices were immersed in 0.01 M Tris-EDTA solution for antigen retrieval and then blocked in 5% goat serum. The samples were incubated with primary antibody-targeting (CD3, CD68; 1:100; Bioscience) working solution for 12 h at 4 °C, and then washed with PBS three times. For secondary antibody incubation, the sections were stained with FITC- and rhodamine-conjugated secondary antibodies, and counterstained with DAPI. The fluorescent images were collected by fluorescence microscopy.

### 2.7. Western Blotting

Skin tissue samples from the shaved dorsal area were lysed with lysis buffer for protein extraction. Next, equal amounts of protein were separated on SDS–PAGE gels by electrophoresis (100 V, 120 min) and transferred to nitrocellulose membranes (300 mA, 40 min). The protein membrane was rinsed and blocked with BSA solution at room temperature for 60 min. Next, the membrane was incubated with primary antibodies (β-catenin, LC3, P62, AKT, p-AKT) at 4 °C overnight and then incubated with HRP-labeled secondary antibody for 1 h at room temperature.

### 2.8. Statistical Analysis

All experiments were independently repeated at least 3 times ($n \geq 3$). The results are presented as the mean ± standard deviation. Data analysis was processed by SPSS and GraphPad software. A probability value ($p < 0.05$) by $t$-test was considered significant (* $p < 0.05$, ** $p < 0.01$, *** $p < 0.001$).

## 3. Results and Discussion

### 3.1. Characterization of MNs and Nanoparticles

The microneedles were prepared using a two-step template method (Figure 2A). First, PVP-based microneedles were prepared, and then PVA/sucrose was covered as a flexible substrate. The finished microneedle patch was a 10 × 10 microneedle array on a 1 cm × 1 cm base. Scanning electron microscopy (Figure 2B,C) and laser confocal microscopy (Figure 2D) showed that the DMN was smooth and uniform, maintaining a good conical shape and sharp needle tip. The base diameter of each microneedle was 320 μm, and the height was 680 μm. Since the epidermal layer of skin is the main barrier for transdermal drug delivery, studies discovered that a force of at least 0.1 N/needle is required to penetrate the skin [29]. According to the mechanical strength test, the force–displacement curve of the microneedle showed linear continuity, indicating that the PVP microneedles have good mechanical properties and are not easy to destroy during the compression process (Figure 2E). When half of the needle length (300 μm) was compressed, the mechanical strength of a single microneedle was 300 mN. This demonstrated that the microneedle can satisfy the mechanical conditions for penetrating the skin.

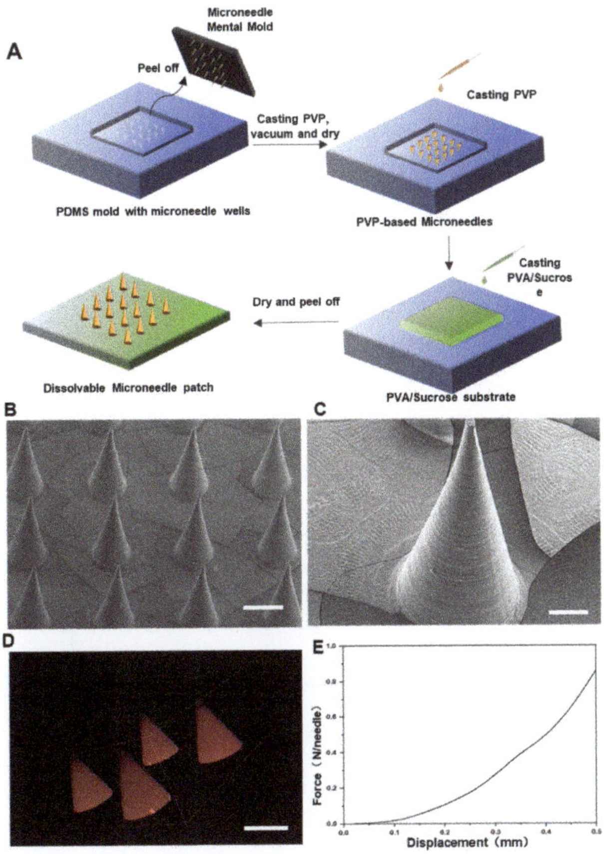


**Figure 2.** Characterization of MNs. (**A**) Preparation scheme of a drug NP-loaded MN. (**B**) SEM images of MNs. Scale bar: 300 μm. (**C**) SEM images of MNs. Scale bar: 100 μm. (**D**) Laser confocal microscopy image of MNs. Scale bar: 300 μm. (**E**) Mechanical strength of MNs and photograph after compression.

In this study, EGCG and RAPA were used as drugs to activate hair follicle regeneration. Rapamycin nanoparticles were prepared using the emulsification and volatilization method (oil-in-water O/W method) to form microemulsions dispersed in water, which is a common synthetic method for biodegradable polymer nanoparticles. Hydrophobic rapamycin was encapsulated in the PLGA polymer. In contrast, EGCG nanoparticles were formed by chemical cross-linking with keratin, and the formation mechanism was the polycondensation reaction of methyl of KE and the thiol groups (-SH) of EGCG [30]. To characterize the physicochemical properties of the nanoparticles, scanning electron microscopy showed that both NPs were spherical, with good dispersibility and good singleness (Figure 3A,B). DSL illustrated that the average diameters of PLGA nanoparticles (Figure 3E) and EGCG nanoparticles (Figure 3F) were 150 nm and 100 nm, respectively. Notably, the UV absorption peaks of rapamycin and EGCG were 280 nm and 275 nm, respectively. The synthesized nanoparticles (Figure 3C,D) also had the same absorption peak, indicating that the optical properties of the drugs were not affected during the nanoparticle formation process. In addition, the loading capacity is an important index to evaluate the quality of nanoparticles. The loading capacities of RAPA and EGCG NPs were 82% and 76%, respectively. The in vitro drug release curve (37 °C, pH = 7.4) demonstrated the sustained-release effect of PLGA NPs, with a slow release of 70% RAPA in 13 days (Figure 3G).

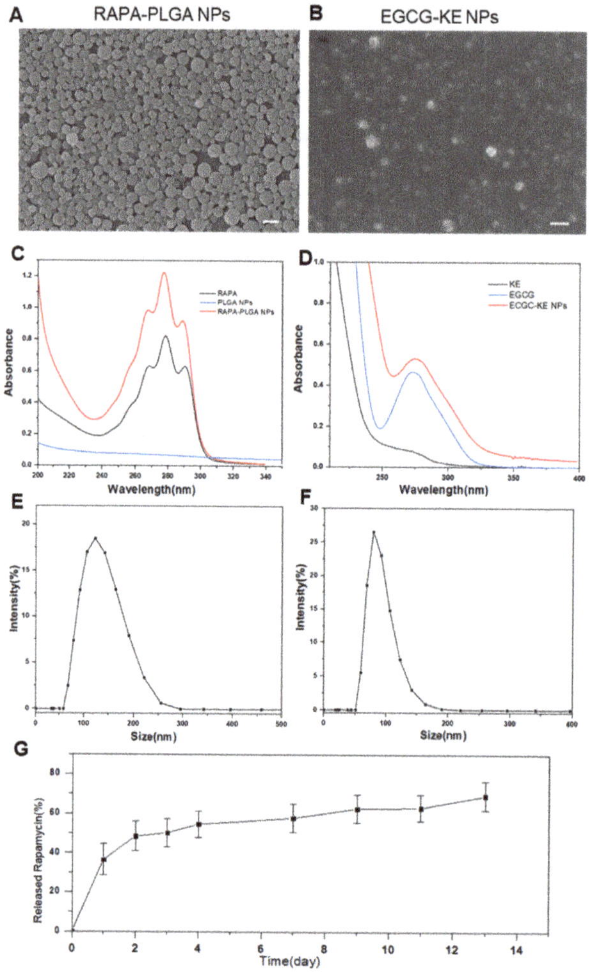


**Figure 3.** Characterization of NPs. SEM image of PLGA-RAPA NPs (**A**) and EGCG-KE NPs (**B**). Scale bar: 200 nm. UV–vis of PLGA-RAPA NPs (**C**) and EGCG-KE NPs (**D**). Particle size distribution with a photograph of PLGA-RAPA NPs (**E**) and EGCG-KE NPs (**F**) in water. (**G**) In vitro release test of RAPA-PLGA NPs ($n = 3$, mean $\pm$ SD).

## 3.2. Transcutaneous Permeation Analyses

To evaluate the transcutaneous permeation and biocompatibility of microneedles, a series of in vitro and in vivo experiments was performed. When the microneedle pierced the mouse dorsal skin for 30 s followed by 5 min of waiting, H&E staining demonstrated that the microneedle created a microchannel, confirming the transdermal function of the microneedles (Figure 4A). The deepest penetration depth could reach around 480 μm. The average insertion depth of MN was around 400~450 μm because of skin natural elasticity. Since the skin thickness on mice was 300~700 μm through the hair cycle, the depth of pore formation made it easy and acceptable for drugs to deliver into hair follicles [31]. At the same time, the MN base could be peeled off the skin after 2 h, leaving the microneedles dissolved in the skin. To verify the solubility of the microneedles, Figure 3B illustrates that the dissolution degree of PVP microneedles pierced into porcine cadaver skin was higher with a longer residence time. The microneedles were completely dissolved in 60 s, proving the high solubility of PVP microneedles. In clinical safety experiments, after microneedles were pierced into mice, microneedle patterns appeared in the dorsal skin and the treated skin recovered within 60 min (Figure 4C). To further verify the cause of inflammation, we evaluated the biosafety of the DMN group, the PVP microneedle group, and the control group by immunofluorescence staining. CD68 is a marker for macrophages, and CD3 is a marker for T cells. Figure 3D illustrates that CD68 and CD3 were not significantly expressed in all groups and indicated no inflammatory reaction, proving the biocompatibility of DMN.

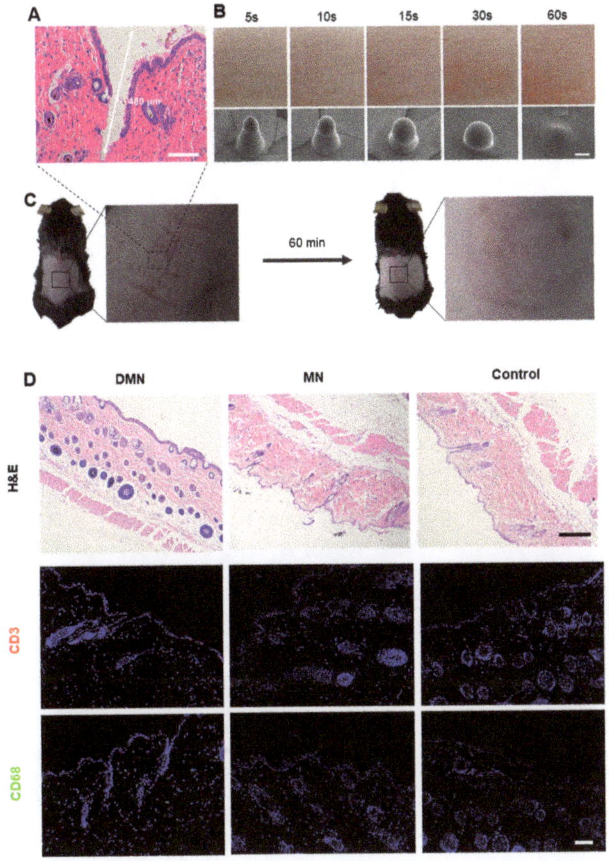


**Figure 4.** In vitro and in vivo administration of MNs. (**A**) H&E staining image of the mouse dorsal skin after MN penetration. Scale bar: 100 μm. (**B**) Photographs of porcine cadaver skin and SEM images of MNs after penetration at different time points. Scale bar: 100 μm. (**C**) Photographs of mice after penetration and at 60 min postinsertion with removal of MNs. (**D**) H&E and immunofluorescence staining of treated mouse skin at day 10. CD3 (marker of lymphocyte infiltration) is shown in red, CD68 (marker of macrophages) is shown in green, and cell nuclei (DAPI) are shown in blue. Scale bar: 50 μm.

### 3.3. Hair Regrowth Evaluation

C57BL/6J mice with obvious hair cycling are known to enter a prolonged telogen phase by six weeks of age [32]. Thus, hair-shaved mice were commonly used as animal models for hair regrowth evaluation to induce the transformation of the hair cycle. In our study, rapamycin dosage can affect the process of hair regeneration. Therefore, we first determined the dosage of rapamycin nanoparticles loaded in microneedles. Forty-two-day C57BL/6 mice were divided into nine groups (mice number: $n = 5$/group): five microneedle administration groups from low dose to high dose, three topical administration groups with different dosages, and a control group without any treatment. Figure 5A shows representative images of mice during the treatments, and Figure 5B illustrates the hair loss therapy in each group. Hair regrowth was observed on day 10 after shaving when the dosage of rapamycin was 0.01 μg~1 μg/DMN. The longest hair shaft length was obtained in mice treated with 0.1 μg of rapamycin (Figure 5C). In contrast, the control group without treatment showed almost no hair growth. Western blotting (Figure 5D) confirmed that rapamycin could induce autophagy. β-Catenin is a marker of hair follicle cycle activation, while p62 and LC3 are autophagy marker proteins that regulate hair follicle morphogenesis. Figure 5D demonstrates that the protein expression levels of β-catenin, p62 and LC3 with low-dose rapamycin were much higher, which further illustrated that low-dose rapamycin can effectively promote hair regeneration.

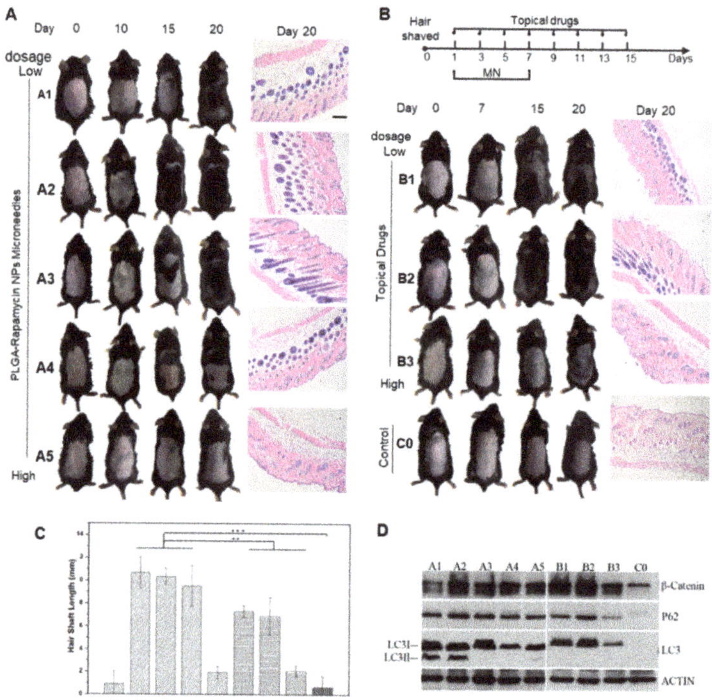


**Figure 5.** In vivo hair regrowth study by treatments with different dosages of rapamycin. (**A**) Schematic illustration of the hair loss treatments. (**B**) Physical and H&E staining images (scale bar: 100 μm) of mice treated with RAPA-PLGA NP-loaded MNs and topical RAPA. The untreated mice served as a control. (**C**) Hair shaft analysis chart of new hair grown on treated mouse dorsal skin ($n = 3$, mean ± SD). (**D**) Western blotting assay of the expression level of proteins related to hair follicle growth activation (β-Catenin) and autophagy (p62 and LC3). A probability value ($p < 0.05$) by $t$-test was considered significant (** $p < 0.01$, *** $p < 0.001$).

Compared with topical administration, a reduced dosage of drugs is used via the MN delivery strategy. Our DMN patch was loaded with 0.1 μg of rapamycin and 4 μg of EGCG. To evaluate the therapeutic effect, mice were divided into six groups, and photographs of hair growth states at each time point are shown in Figure 6A. A faster hair growth rate was observed in the rapamycin administration groups (H1, H2, H4), while a higher hair follicle density was shown in the EGCG administration groups (H1, H3, H5) (Figure 6B,C). H&E staining of longitudinal and transverse sections of mouse skin was conducted to reveal hair regeneration behavior (Figure 6E). In general, compared with other groups, DMN for the codelivery of RAPA and EGCG generated the best therapeutic effect on hair regeneration. Hair in the DMN region was significantly the longest and densest. Western blotting further indicated higher expression levels of β-catenin (hair follicle regulatory protein) and p-AKT (a marker of hair follicle cells for proliferation and anti-aging) via DMN dorsal skin to activate hair follicles to enter a new hair cycle (Figure 6D).

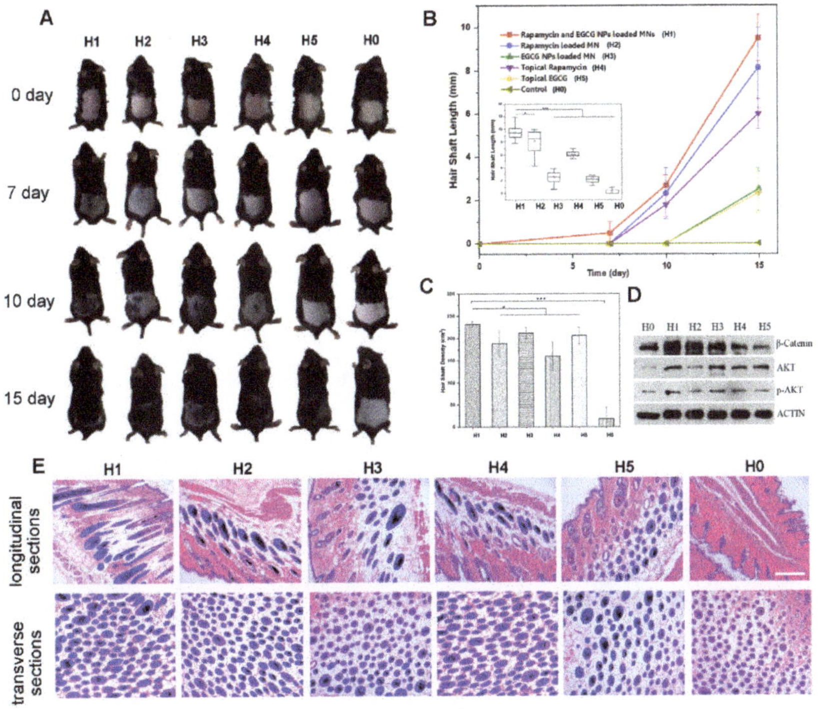


**Figure 6.** In vivo study of DMN for hair regrowth. (**A**) Physical images of mice treated with RAPA-PLGA and EGCG-KE NP-loaded MNs (H1), RAPA-PLGA-loaded MNs (H2), EGCG-KE NP-loaded MNs (H3), topical RAPA (H4), and topical EGCG (H5). Untreated mice (H0) served as a control. (**B**) Hair shaft analysis chart of new hair grown on treated mouse dorsal skin as a function of treatment time and day 15 ($n$ = 3, mean ± SD). (**C**) Hair follicle density analysis chart of new hair grown on treated dorsal skin at day 15 ($n$ = 3, mean ± SD). (**D**) Western blotting assay of the expression level of proteins related to hair follicle growth activation (β-Catenin, p-AKT). (**E**) H&E staining images of longitudinal sections (top) and transverse sections (bottom) of mouse dorsal skin (scale bar: 100 μm). A probability value ($p < 0.05$) by $t$-test was considered significant (* $p < 0.05$, *** $p < 0.001$).

## 4. Conclusions

In summary, a dissolvable PVP-based microneedle patch was prepared for the codelivery of RAPA and EGCG nanoparticles. Microneedles were constructed with high mechanical properties to break the barrier of the stratum corneum via punctuation and then dissolve rapidly, transporting RAPA and EGCG nanoparticles to the hair follicle niche. In vivo experiments demonstrated that the DMN can significantly improve hair regrowth with biocompatibility. Our findings indicate that it is expected to be utilized as a potential candidate to address hair loss in a minimally invasive manner.

**Author Contributions:** Conceptualization, S.S.; methodology, Y.L.; formal analysis, Y.L.; investigation, Y.L, T.X. and R.S.; data curation, Y.L.; writing—original draft preparation, Y.L.; writing—review and editing, S.S.; project administration, Y.L. All authors have read and agreed to the published version of the manuscript.

**Funding:** This research was funded by the National Natural Science Foundation of China (Grant No. 21874082) and Fundamental Research Program of Shenzhen (Committee of Scientific and Technological Innovation of Shenzhen) (JCYJ20170413104646428 and JCYJ20170307153548350).

**Institutional Review Board Statement:** The study was conducted according to the guidelines of the Declaration of Helsinki and approved by the Ethics Committee of Tsinghua University Shenzhen International Graduate school (Approval No. 202154, 20 July 2021).

**Acknowledgments:** We acknowledge the support of Tsinghua University.

**Conflicts of Interest:** The authors declare no conflict of interest.

## References

1. Lolli, F.; Pallotti, F.; Rossi, A.; Fortuna, M.C.; Caro, G.; Lenzi, A.; Sansone, A.; Lombardo, F. Androgenetic alopecia: A review. *Endocrine* **2017**, *57*, 9–17. [CrossRef] [PubMed]
2. Pratt, C.H.; King, L.E.; Messenger, A.G., Jr.; Christiano, A.M.; Sundberg, J.P. Alopecia areata. *Nat. Rev. Dis. Primers* **2017**, *3*, 17011. [CrossRef] [PubMed]
3. Goren, A.; Naccarato, T. Minoxidil in the treatment of androgenetic alopecia. *Dermatol. Ther.* **2018**, *31*, e12686. [CrossRef] [PubMed]
4. Gupta, A.K.; Carviel, J.; MacLeod, M.A.; Shear, N. Assessing finasteride-associated sexual dysfunction using the FAERS database. *J. Eur. Acad. Dermatol. Venereol.* **2017**, *31*, 1069–1075. [CrossRef]
5. Mohammadi, P.; Youssef, K.K.; Abbasalizadeh, S.; Baharvand, H.; Aghdami, N. Human Hair Reconstruction: Close, But Yet So Far. *Stem Cells Dev.* **2016**, *25*, 1767–1779. [CrossRef]
6. Traish, A.M. Health Risks Associated with Long-Term Finasteride and Dutasteride Use: It's Time to Sound the Alarm. *World J. Mens Health* **2020**, *38*, 323–337. [CrossRef]
7. Goren, A.; Castano, J.A.; McCoy, J.; Bermudez, F.; Lotti, T. Novel enzymatic assay predicts minoxidil response in the treatment of androgenetic alopecia. *Dermatol. Ther.* **2014**, *27*, 171–173. [CrossRef]
8. Jo, S.J.; Shin, H.; Park, Y.W.; Paik, S.H.; Park, W.S.; Jeong, Y.S.; Shin, H.J.; Kwon, O. Topical valproic acid increases the hair count in male patients with androgenetic alopecia: A randomized, comparative, clinical feasibility study using phototrichogram analysis. *J. Dermatol.* **2014**, *41*, 285–291. [CrossRef]
9. Sawaya, M.E.; Roth, W.I.; Hevia, O.; Flowers, F.P. Significance of Ru58841 as a Therapeutic Agent Effecting Androgen Receptor Molecular-Interactions in Human Hair-Follicles. *J. Investig. Dermatol.* **1995**, *104*, 606.
10. Daniels, G.; Akram, S.; Westgate, G.E.; Tamburic, S. Can plant-derived phytochemicals provide symptom relief for hair loss? A critical review. *Int. J. Cosmet. Sci.* **2019**, *41*, 332–345. [CrossRef]
11. Ashique, S.; Sandhu, N.K.; Haque, S.N.; Koley, K. A Systemic Review on Topical Marketed Formulations, Natural Products, and Oral Supplements to Prevent Androgenic Alopecia: A Review. *Nat. Prod. Bioprospect.* **2020**, *10*, 345–365. [CrossRef] [PubMed]
12. Kumar, R.; Philip, A. Modified Transdermal technologies: Breaking the barriers of drug permeation via the skin. *Trop. J. Pharm. Res.* **2007**, *6*, 633–644. [CrossRef]
13. Moser, K.; Kriwet, K.; Naik, A.; Kalia, Y.N.; Guy, R.H. Passive skin penetration enhancement and its quantification in vitro. *Eur. J. Pharm. Biopharm.* **2001**, *52*, 103–112. [CrossRef]
14. Wokovich, A.M.; Prodduturi, S.; Doub, W.H.; Hussain, A.S.; Buhse, L.F. Transdermal drug delivery system (TDDS) adhesion as a critical safety, efficacy and quality attribute. *Eur. J. Pharm. Biopharm.* **2006**, *64*, 1–8. [CrossRef]
15. Vogt, A.; Wischke, C.; Neffe, A.T.; Ma, N.; Alexiev, U.; Lendlein, A. Nanocarriers for drug delivery into and through the skin—Do existing technologies match clinical challenges? *J. Control. Release* **2016**, *242*, 3–15. [CrossRef]
16. Quinn, H.L.; Kearney, M.C.; Courtenay, A.J.; McCrudden, M.T.C.; Donnelly, R.F. The role of microneedles for drug and vaccine delivery. *Expert Opin. Drug Deliv.* **2014**, *11*, 1769–1780. [CrossRef]
17. Singh, S.; Singh, J. Transdermal Drug-Delivery by Passive Diffusion and Iontophoresis—A Review. *Med. Res. Rev.* **1993**, *13*, 569–621. [CrossRef]
18. Donnelly, R.; Douroumis, D. Microneedles for drug and vaccine delivery and patient monitoring. *Drug Deliv. Transl. Res.* **2015**, *5*, 311–312. [CrossRef]
19. Lahiji, S.F.; Seo, S.H.; Kim, S.; Dangol, M.; Shim, J.; Li, C.G.; Ma, Y.; Lee, C.; Kang, G.; Yang, H.; et al. Transcutaneous implantation of valproic acid-encapsulated dissolving microneedles induces hair regrowth. *Biomaterials* **2018**, *167*, 69–79. [CrossRef]
20. Fang, J.H.; Liu, C.H.; Hsu, R.S.; Chen, Y.Y.; Chiang, W.H.; Wang, H.M.D.; Hu, S.H. Transdermal Composite Microneedle Composed of Mesoporous Iron Oxide Nanoraspberry and PVA for Androgenetic Alopecia Treatment. *Polymers* **2020**, *12*, 1392. [CrossRef]

21. Yang, G.; Chen, Q.; Wen, D.; Chen, Z.W.; Wang, J.Q.; Chen, G.J.; Wang, Z.J.; Zhang, X.D.; Zhang, Y.Q.; Hu, Q.Y.; et al. A Therapeutic Microneedle Patch Made from Hair-Derived Keratin for Promoting Hair Regrowth. *ACS Nano* **2019**, *13*, 4354–4360. [CrossRef] [PubMed]
22. Hong, C.; Zhang, G.; Zhang, W.; Liu, J.; Zhang, J.; Chen, Y.; Peng, H.; Cheng, Y.; Ding, X.; Xin, H.; et al. Hair grows hair: Dual-effective hair regrowth through a hair enhanced dissolvable microneedle patch cooperated with the pure yellow light irradiation. *Appl. Mater. Today* **2021**, *25*, 101188. [CrossRef]
23. Broekhuizen, C.A.; de Boer, L.; Schipper, K.; Jones, C.D.; Quadir, S.; Feldman, R.G.; Vandenbroucke-Grauls, C.M.; Zaat, S.A. The influence of antibodies on Staphylococcus epidermidis adherence to polyvinylpyrrolidone-coated silicone elastomer in experimental biomaterial-associated infection in mice. *Biomaterials* **2009**, *30*, 6444–6450. [CrossRef] [PubMed]
24. Yoshihara, N.; Ueno, T.; Takagi, A.; Trejo, J.A.O.; Haruna, K.; Suga, Y.; Komatsu, M.; Tanaka, K.; Ikeda, S. The significant role of autophagy in the granular layer in normal skin differentiation and hair growth. *Arch. Dermatol. Res.* **2015**, *307*, 159–169. [CrossRef] [PubMed]
25. Chai, M.; Jiang, M.; Vergnes, L.; Fu, X.; de Barros, S.C.; Doan, N.B.; Huang, W.; Chu, J.; Jiao, J.; Herschman, H.; et al. Stimulation of Hair Growth by Small Molecules that Activate Autophagy. *Cell Rep.* **2019**, *27*, 3413–3421.e3. [CrossRef] [PubMed]
26. Astete, C.E.; Sabliov, C.M. Synthesis and characterization of PLGA nanoparticles. *J. Biomater. Sci. Polym. Ed.* **2006**, *17*, 247–289. [CrossRef]
27. Kwon, O.S.; Han, J.H.; Yoo, H.G.; Chung, J.H.; Cho, K.H.; Eun, H.C.; Kim, K.H. Human hair growth enhancement in vitro by green tea epigallocatechin-3-gallate (EGCG). *Phytomedicine* **2007**, *14*, 551–555. [CrossRef]
28. Hill, P.; Brantley, H.; Van Dyke, M. Some properties of keratin biomaterials: Kerateines. *Biomaterials* **2010**, *31*, 585–593. [CrossRef]
29. Lee, J.W.; Park, J.H.; Prausnitz, M.R. Dissolving microneedles for transdermal drug delivery. *Biomaterials* **2008**, *29*, 2113–2124. [CrossRef]
30. Yi, Z.; Cui, X.; Chen, G.; Chen, X.; Jiang, X.; Li, X. Biocompatible, Antioxidant Nanoparticles Prepared from Natural Renewable Tea Polyphenols and Human Hair Keratins for Cell Protection and Anti-inflammation. *ACS Biomater. Sci. Eng.* **2021**, *7*, 1046–1057. [CrossRef]
31. Hansen, L.S.; Coggle, J.E.; Wells, J.; Charles, M.W. The influence of the hair cycle on the thickness of mouse skin. *Anat. Rec.* **1984**, *210*, 569–573. [CrossRef] [PubMed]
32. Müller-Röver, S.; Handjiski, B.; van der Veen, C.; Eichmüller, S.; Foitzik, K.; McKay, I.A.; Stenn, K.S.; Paus, R. A comprehensive guide for the accurate classification of murine hair follicles in distinct hair cycle stages. *J. Investig. Dermatol.* **2001**, *117*, 3–15. [CrossRef] [PubMed]

pharmaceutics

MDPI

Article

# A Novel Approach for Skin Regeneration by a Potent Bioactive Placental-Loaded Microneedle Patch: Comparative Study of Deer, Goat, and Porcine Placentas

Kritsanaporn Tansathien [1], Phuvamin Suriyaamporn [1], Tanasait Ngawhirunpat [1], Praneet Opanasopit [1] and Worranan Rangsimawong [2,*]

[1] Pharmaceutical Development of Green Innovations Group (PDGIG), Faculty of Pharmacy, Silpakorn University, Nakhon Pathom 73000, Thailand; isomeroff@gmail.com (K.T.); puvamin.su.55@ubu.ac.th (P.S.); ngawhirunpat_t@su.ac.th (T.N.); opanasopit_p@su.ac.th (P.O.)

[2] Division of Pharmaceutical Chemistry and Technology, Faculty of Pharmaceutical Sciences, Ubon Ratchathani University, Ubon Ratchathani 34190, Thailand

* Correspondence: worranan.r@ubu.ac.th; Tel.: +66-(045)-353605; Fax: +66-(045)-353626

**Abstract:** The aims of this study were to investigate the skin regeneration potential of bioactive placenta (deer placenta (DP), goat placenta (GP), and porcine placenta (PP)) and fabricate bioactive extract-loaded dissolving microneedles (DMNs) as a dermal delivery approach. The placentas were water-extracted, and the active compounds were evaluated. Bioactivity studies were performed in dermal fibroblasts and keratinocytes. DMNs were fabricated to deliver the potent bioactive placenta extract into the skin. All placental extracts expressed high amounts of protein, growth factors (EGF, FGF, IGF-1 and TGF-β1), and amino acids. These extracts were not toxic to the skin cells, while the proliferation of fibroblast cells significantly increased in a time-dependent manner. GP extract that exhibited the maximum proliferation, migration, and regeneration effect on fibroblast cells was loaded into DMN patch. The suitable physical properties of DMNs led to increased skin permeation and deposition of bioactive macromolecules. Moreover, GP extract-loaded DMNs showed minimal invasiveness to the skin and were safe for application to human skin. In conclusion, placental extracts act as potent bioactive compounds for skin cells, and the highest bioactive potential of GP-loaded DMNs might be a novel approach to regenerate the skin.

**Keywords:** deer placenta; goat placenta; porcine placenta; bioactive extract; skin regeneration; dissolving microneedles

## 1. Introduction

The placenta is an organ containing many active molecules, such as hormones, proteins, lipids, nucleic acids, glycosaminoglycans, amino acids, vitamins, and minerals, which are required for life sustenance and proliferation of the fetus [1]. Placental therapy has been used to stimulate the recovery of disease and tissue regeneration since the early 1900s, in which various clinical applications have exhibited a range of remarkable therapeutic attributes encompassing antioxidant, antimicrobial, anti-inflammation, pain reliever, hair growth stimulation, health improvement, cellular proliferation, tissue regeneration, and wound healing properties [2]. In many countries (e.g., Japan, Korea, and China), porcine placenta (PP) extract containing water-soluble active compounds have been used as a non-prescription drug for analeptic medicine, healthy foods, and cosmetics [3]. Previous studies have shown that peptides from goat placenta (GP) extract and human placenta have numerous bioactivities, such as antioxidant and anti-inflammatory activities [4–6]. Deer placenta (DP) also contains some bioactive compounds, such as glycoproteins and alpha-fetoprotein [7]. However, no comparative scientific data of DP, GP, and PP on skin regeneration have yet been reported.

For the healing and repair mechanisms in the skin, growth factors consist of a large group of secreted proteins that are important in regulating and stimulating the growth, proliferation, migration, and differentiation of cells [8]. Placental extracts are rich in growth factors, such as insulin-like growth factor-1 (IGF-1), epidermal growth factor (EGF), fibroblast growth factor (FGF), transforming growth factor-β1 (TGF-β1), vascular endothelial growth factor, granulocyte-colony stimulating factor, granulocyte-macrophage colony stimulating factor, hepatocyte growth factor, and platelet-derived growth factor, referring to physiological effects ranging from immunomodulation, anti-inflammation, wound healing, cellular proliferation, and regeneration [2]. Many exogenous growth factors have been reported as a potential regenerative medicine to replace or repair damaged cells, tissues, and organs [9]. Amino acids are also found in the placentas, including alanine, aspartic acid, arginine, histidine, leucine, lysine, phenylalanine, proline, tyrosine, tryptophan, and valine, which stimulate fibroblast and collagen production and decrease skin pigmentation [2].

The rejuvenating and revitalizing effect of the placenta on the skin have been applied either via mesotherapy or topically along with cosmeceutical aesthetic procedure. Mesotherapy, generally known as "biorejuvenation" or "biorevitalization", is a technique used to regenerate the skin by using transdermal injection of a multivitamin solution and natural plant extracts to repair the signs of skin aging [10]. However, hypodermic injection is painful, generates dangerous medical wastes, and poses the risk of disease transmission by needle reuse. Self-administered transdermal systems show the improvement of patient compliance and are generally inexpensive [11]. Microneedles can be used to overcome the limitations of conventional approaches. The micron-sized needles arranged on a small patch can deliver hydrophilic macromolecular compounds bypassing the layer of stratum corneum and entering into the skin. This technique provides a fast onset of action, the best patient compliance, self-administration, and improvement of permeability and efficacy. Additionally, dissolving microneedles (DMNs) are fabricated with biodegradable polymers to encapsulate many drugs into the polymer. After inserting these microneedles into the skin, efficient drug delivery without skin irritation has been reported [12]. Therefore, DMNs should be used to deliver bioactive macromolecules into the skin.

The aims of this study were to investigate the skin regeneration potential of bioactive placentals and fabricate a bioactive extract loaded into DMNs as a dermal delivery device. DP, GP, and PP were water-extracted by probe sonication, and the protein, growth factor, and amino acid contents were evaluated. Bioactivity studies were performed for skin cells, such as human dermal fibroblasts (NHFs) and human immortalized keratinocytes (HaCaTs), evaluating the cytotoxicity, cell proliferation and migration, and skin regeneration after UVB-induced skin damage. Subsequently, DMNs were fabricated to deliver bioactive placental extract into the skin. The in vitro skin permeation was determined using Franz-type diffusion cells. Confocal laser scanning microscopy (CLSM) visualized the deposition of macromolecular proteins in the skin. Skin histology was observed after applying the formulation. Moreover, in vivo study was also performed with human volunteers.

## 2. Materials and Methods

### 2.1. Materials

Fresh DP, GP, and PP were gifts from Image Focus Holding Co., Ltd., Bangkok, Thailand, and Payayen Dairy Co., Ltd., Nakhon Ratchasima, Thailand, and CCF Energy Supplement Co., Ltd., Ratchaburi, Thailand, respectively. NHFs and HaCaT cells were obtained from the American-Type Culture Collection (ATCC), Rockville, MD, USA. Dulbecco's modified Eagle's medium (DMEM), fetal bovine serum (FBS), trypsin–ethylenediaminetetraacetic acid (EDTA), L-glutamine (Glutamax$^{TM}$), nonessential amino acids, and penicillin–streptomycin were purchased from Gibco BRL, Rockville, MD, USA. The 3-(4,5-dimethyl-2-thiazolyl)-2,5-diphenyl-2H-tetrazolium bromide (MTT) and polydimethylacrylamide (PDMA) were purchased from Sigma, Aldrich, St. Louis, MO, USA. Hyaluronic acid was obtained from the P.C. drug center, Bangkok, Thailand. All other chemical agents were of analytical grade.

### 2.2. Extraction of DP, GP and PP

Fresh DP, GP, and PP were stored in tight containers for freezer storage (−20 °C) before processing. These materials were placed at room temperature for thawing of frozen materials. The extraction method was performed by the sonication method [13]. Then, DP, GP, or PP was mashed with phosphate-buffered saline (PBS), pH 7.4 (1:1), and then weighed 1 g to soak with 20 mL of distilled water. A probe sonicator (Vibra-Cell™, High-Intensity Ultrasonic Processor VCX500, Sonics & Materials, Inc., Newtown, CT, USA) with a frequency of 20 kHz at 20% amplitude was applied for 30 min in an ice bath. Centrifugation was performed at 4000 rpm for 15 min to collect the supernatants. Freeze-drying process was done at −49 °C for 3 days using a freeze dryer (FreeZone 2.5, Labconco, UK) to obtain the dry powder. After that, the extracts were weighed and determined the percentage of yield as Equation (1).

$$\%\text{Yield} = \frac{\text{Weight of extract}}{\text{Weight of fresh placenta used}} \times 100 \quad (1)$$

### 2.3. Determination of Protein, Growth Factors and Amino Acids

The soluble protein compositions were determined by SDS-polyacrylamide gel electrophoresis (SDS–PAGE) on a 12% gel. The soluble proteins were dissolved in sterile water (100 mg/mL). The samples were mixed with 2-mercaptoethanol (1:4) to reduce the disulfide bonds and irreversibly denature the proteins. These samples were run at 100 mV for 2 h, and then the gel was stained with a silver staining kit (ProteoSilver™ Silver Stain Kit, Sigma–Aldrich, St. Louis, MO, USA) according to the manufacturer's protocol.

The total protein content was measured using a bicinchoninic acid (BCA) protein assay kit (Novagen®, EMD Millipore Corp., Taunton, MA, USA) using bovine serum protein (BSA) as a standard. Growth factors, such as EGF, FGF, IGF-1, and TGF-β1, were analyzed by the enzyme-linked immunosorbent assay (ELISA kits; Abcam, Cambridge, MA, USA) following the manufacturer's protocol. The amino acid content was determined by an amino acid analyzer (Hitachi L8900, Hitachi High Technologies Corporation, Tokyo, Japan).

### 2.4. Cytotoxicity Study of Skin Cells

NHF and HaCaT cells were cultured in DMEM supplemented with 10% FBS, 1% penicillin–streptomycin, 1% Glutamax®, and 1% nonessential amino acids and incubated under a humidified atmosphere (5% $CO_2$, 95% air, 37 °C) until they reached 70–80% confluence. NHFs ($10^4$ cells/well) or HaCaTs ($5 \times 10^3$ cells/well) were seeded into 96-well plates and incubated until cell confluence was achieved. Each extract was diluted to obtain various concentrations (0–5000 μg/mL). After removing the cell medium from the cell plates and washing with PBS, pH 7.4, each concentration of diluted extract was added and incubated for 24 h. The cell viability was measured by the MTT assay [14], in which the diluted extracts were removed, and the cells were washed with PBS, pH 7.4. Medium containing MTT (0.5 mg/mL) was added to the plate and incubated for 3 h. Subsequently, the medium was removed, and 100 μL of DMSO was added to each well to dissolve the formazan crystals that had formed in living cells. Subsequently, the absorbance was analyzed by a microplate reader (VICTOR Nivo™ Multimode Plate Reader, PerkinElmer, Pontyclun, UK) at 550 nm. The percentage of cell viability was calculated using Equation (2).

$$\%\ \text{Cell viability} = \frac{\text{Absorbance of treated cells}}{\text{Absorbance of untreated cells}} \times 100 \quad (2)$$

### 2.5. Determination of Cell Proliferation and Migration

NHFs ($5 \times 10^3$ cells/well) were seeded into a 96-well plate and incubated overnight. Each extract was diluted to obtain various concentrations (0–2000 μg/mL). The old medium was removed, followed by washing with PBS, pH 7.4, and each concentration was added to the cells for 24–72 h. Cell proliferation was determined by the MTT assay, after which the percent cell proliferation was calculated using the same equation as the percent cell viability [14].

For cell migration, an in vitro scratch assay was used to evaluate skin cells [15]. NHF cells ($2 \times 10^5$ cells/well) were cultured in 6-well plates and incubated until 70–80% cell confluency. Marking lines were performed as a straight line using a 200-μL pipette tip, and then the medium was removed. The extracts (1000 and 2000 μg/mL) were added to NHF cells. The negative control was serum-free DMEM (DMEM supplemented with 1% penicillin/streptomycin), and the positive control was EGF standard solution (200 pg/mL). Images were acquired using an inverted microscope (Nikon® T-DH, Nikon, Tokyo, Japan) after 0, 24, and 48 h of incubation time. The gap of marked lines in the cell plate was measured.

### *2.6. Measurement of Skin Regeneration after UVB-Induced Skin Damage*

NHF cells at $8 \times 10^3$ cells/mL were seeded into a 96-well plate and incubated at 37 °C and 5% $CO_2$/95% humidity. After washing the cells with PBS, pH 7.4, 100 μL of PBS was added. Subsequently, the plate was immediately exposed to UVB rays for 20 min, and then the PBS was removed. Various concentrations of the placental extracts (GP, DP, or PP) were used to treat the cells for 24 h. The percent cell viability was measured by the MTT assay and calculated as Equation (2).

### *2.7. Fabrication and Characterization of DMNs Loading Placenta Extract*

Hyaluronic acid (10% *w*/*w*) and PDMA (0.5% *w*/*w*) were used as the main biodegradable polymers for the fabrication of DMNs. Placenta extract or bovine serum albumin-fluorescein isothiocyanate conjugate (BSA-FITC) was mixed with aqueous blends containing biodegradable polymers. All DMNs were fabricated using the micro-molding technique [16]. The formulation was weighted onto laser-engineered silicone micromold templates. The tips of the needle cavities were filled by centrifugation of the microneedle molds at 4000 rpm and 25 °C for 20 min. Microneedle arrays were dried at room temperature for 48 h and then removed from the molds to evaluate the physical properties in terms of appearance, mechanical strength, protein content in DMN patch, and dissolution time.

The physical appearance of microneedles was imaged under a Dino-Lite Edge/5MP digital microscope, AM7915 series (Dino-Lite, Hsinchu, Taiwan), in which the height, width, and interspace of microneedle arrays were measured using dino-capture 2.0 software. For mechanical strength, a texture analyzer (TA. XT plus, Stable Micro Systems, Godalming, UK) with the probe (P/25P) in compression mode was performed at 4.0–20.0 N for 30 s. The percent height change was calculated from Equation (3).

$$\%\text{Height change} = \frac{\text{Height before tested–Height after tested}}{\text{Height before tested}} \times 100 \quad (3)$$

For protein content, DMN patch loading placenta extract was dissolved in PBS pH 7.4 and analyzed protein content as described above. To evaluate the dissolution time of the DMNs in the full thickness of neonatal porcine skin, the skin was stretched on dustless tissue paper and saturated with PBS. DMN patch was pressed into skin with a strength of 10 N of dumble for 2 min. Next, the MNs applied to porcine skin were incubated at 37 °C for different time periods. After withdrawing DMN patch from the skin, the decreased height of DMNs was determined using a Dino-Lite digital microscope.

### *2.8. In Vitro Skin Permeation Study*

Abdominal porcine skins were collected from intrapartum stillborn animals from a local farm in Sisaket Province, Thailand. The subcutaneous layer was carefully removed with medical scissors. The skin was 600–700 μm-thick and was kept at −20 °C and thawed in PBS, pH 7.4, at 25 °C before use.

Generally, endogenous proteins and peptides in the skin can interfere with the determined amount of exogenous proteins and growth factors' permeation into the skin. In this study, BSA-FITC was used as a model macromolecular protein. The skin permeation of macromolecular protein was performed by vertical Franz-type diffusion cells [17]. Approximately 12 mL of PBS, pH 7.4 was added into a receptor compartment and continuously stirred using a magnetic stirrer. The temperature was maintained at 32 °C. The DMN patch was pressed on the skin (2.01 $cm^2$ of skin area) with 10 N of dumble for 2 min. A total of 0.5 mL of receiver medium was collected at 1, 2, 4, 6, and 8 h for fluorescence analysis by a microplate reader at an excitation wavelength of 485 nm and an emission wavelength of 535 nm. The receiver compartment was filled with the same volume of PBS to maintain a constant volume. Each sample was analyzed in triplicate.

Fick's law of diffusion was used as a mathematical model to calculate the parameters of skin permeation. The cumulative permeation amount ($\mu g/cm^2$) against time (h) was plotted, and steady-state flux was measured from the slope of the linear portion in each formulation. The permeability coefficient ($K_p$) was the ratio of flux and the donor concentration of the formulation.

### 2.9. CLSM Study

In this study, green fluorescent BSA-FITC was used as a model macromolecular protein [17]. After 8 h of in vitro skin permeation, the treated skins were washed with PBS to remove excess formulation. The fluorescent compound that permeated throughout skin was immersed in sufficient methyl salicylate. The top layer and permeation depth of skin were visualized under a confocal laser scanning microscope (CLSM; an inverted Zeiss LSM 800 microscope, Carl Zeiss, Jena, Germany) equipped with diode lasers (405, 488, and 561 nm). Confocal images were observed at a 10× objective lens. The fluorescence intensities were evaluated at the middle horizontal line of each image using ZEISS ZEN software. The mean fluorescence intensity was plotted against the skin depth.

### 2.10. Skin Histology

The skin was treated with the DMN formulation for 24 h. The skin sample was fixed in 10% formaldehyde solution for 8 h, dehydrated with ethanol, embedded in paraffin wax, and cut vertically along the surface. The cross-sectioned skin was marked with hematoxylin and eosin (H&E) and observed under light microscopy.

### 2.11. In Vivo Human Skin Study

The study involved 15 healthy human volunteers (between 20 and 35 years old) who agreed to participate in a clinical trial. This study was approved by an Investigational Review Board (Human Studies Ethics Committee, Faculty of Pharmacy, Silpakorn University; COE 65.0223-032). Two different points in the forearm were marked, and DMN patches were applied by pressing the thumb on the patch for 30 s. Subsequently, each DMN patch was covered with waterproof tape (OPSITE◊ Post-Op, Smith&nephew, Hull, UK) for 24 h. The DermaLab® series (SkinLab Combo; Cortex technology, Hadsund, Denmark) was used to evaluate the skin (transepidermal water loss (TEWL), hydration and erythema).

The TEWL data are presented as the Δ value compared with the baseline (untreated skin). The percent change in skin hydration was calculated (%hydration; Equation (4)). Moreover, the effect of formulations on erythema (vascularity) was determined by generating the value of the percent erythema as shown in Equation (5).

$$\% \text{ Hydration} = \frac{\text{Ht} - \text{H}}{\text{H}} \times 100 \tag{4}$$

where Ht is the hydration value of treated skin, and H is the hydration value of untreated skin;

$$\% \text{ Erythema} = \frac{\text{Et} - \text{E}}{\text{E}} \times 100 \tag{5}$$

where Et is the erythema value of treated skin, and E is the erythema value of untreated skin [17].

*2.12. Data Analysis*

All data were presented as the mean ± standard deviation (S.D.). Statistically significant difference was analyzed by one-way ANOVA, followed by Tukey's post-hoc test. In case of in vivo human study, the Wilcoxon signed rank test was determined. The significance level was set at $p < 0.05$.

## 3. Results and Discussion

*3.1. Physicochemical Properties of DP, GP and PP Extracts*

As shown in Figure 1, extraction of DP, GP, and PP provided a brownish-red fibrous texture, in which the percent extraction yields of all extracts ranged from 2.17 to 2. 77. The SDS–PAGE profiles of water-soluble proteins from crude extracts were compared with protein markers (molecular weights ranging from 250 kDa to 10 kDa), in which the bands at 66 kDa, 37 kDa, 24 kDa, 20 kDa, and ~10 kDa were similar to the molecular weights of albumin, glyceraldehyde-3-phosphate dehydrogenase, trypsinogen, trypsin inhibitor, and polypeptide, respectively. All extracts clearly showed bands of high-molecular-weight proteins of albumin and polypeptides (i.e., growth factor); thus, the total protein and growth factors (EGF, FGF, IGF-1, and TGF-β1) showed that the GP extract had higher protein and growth factor contents than the DP and PP extracts (Table 1).

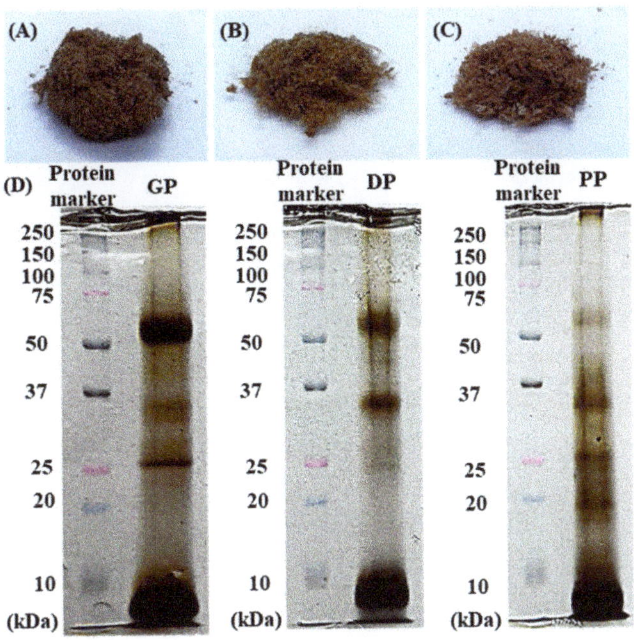


**Figure 1.** Appearance of GP extract (**A**), DP extract (**B**), and PP extract (**C**) and proteins from the placental extract analyzed by electrophoresis on a 12% SDS–PAGE gel (**D**).

**Table 1.** The protein and growth factor contents in GP, DP, and PP extract.

| Compounds | Contents (per 1 g of Extract) | | |
|---|---|---|---|
| | GP Extract | DP Extract | PP Extract |
| **Protein** | 705.51 ± 4.70 mg/g | 198.34 ± 3.26 mg/g | 151.44 ± 3.65 mg/g |
| **Growth factors** | | | |
| EGF | 171.18 ± 8.65 pg/g | 39.02 ± 2.92 pg/g | 5.79 ± 2.47 pg/g |
| FGF | 401.79 ± 24.07 ng/g | 448.99 ± 4.29 ng/g | 65.34 ± 6.56 ng/g |
| IGF-1 | 155.58 ± 27.82 ng/g | 23.07 ± 3.19 ng/g | 40.38 ± 6.00 ng/g |
| TGF-β1 | 56.52 ± 15.61 pg/g | 14.21 ± 0.58 pg/g | 55.20 ± 1.21 pg/g |

Each data represents mean ± S.D. ($n$ = 3).

For the amino acid content, as presented in Table 2, the DP extract was found to contain 14 amino acids in the following order: lysine > alanine > tyrosine > threonine > isoleucine > aspartic acid > glutamic acid > asparagine > valine > serine > leucine > glycine > arginine > histidine. The PP extract had 12 amino acids as follows: cysteine > lysine > valine > glutamic acid > leucine > threonine > phenylalanine > tyrosine > isoleucine > methionine > serine > histidine. The GP extract had nine amino acids as follows: aspartic acid > lysine > methionine > tyrosine > glutamic acid > isoleucine > phenylalanine > arginine > histidine. Although various types of amino acids were found in DP extract, the total amino acid content in GP was higher than that in DP and PP extracts. Aspartic acid was higher content than other amino acids and found predominantly in GP extract. Recently, aspartic acid has been reported as an active ingredient with potential to repair the sign of skin aging and improve the skin condition by stimulating proteins of the dermal extracellular matrix (ECM) [18]. Treatment with amino acids contribute to the collagen and elastin synthesis, leading to increase proteins in fibroblasts. Moreover, the mixture of various amino acids (glycine, proline, lysine, leucine, valine, and alanine) with hyaluronic acid was reported to increased ECM genes in cultured human fibroblasts [19]. Therefore, various types of amino acids in DP extract may also affect the proteins in fibroblasts.

**Table 2.** Type and content of amino acids in GP, DP, and PP extract.

| Compounds | Contents (per 1 g of Extract) | | |
|---|---|---|---|
| | GP Extract | DP Extract | PP Extract |
| Alanine | ND | 2841.08 μg/g | ND |
| Arginine | 0.23 μg/g | 34.94 μg/g | ND |
| Asparagine | ND | 1126.98 μg/g | ND |
| Aspartic acid | 23,842.50 μg/g | 1449.57 μg/g | ND |
| Cysteine | ND | ND | 124.72 μg/g |
| Glutamic acid | 15.45 μg/g | 1356.54 μg/g | 48.73 μg/g |
| Glycine | ND | 340.07 μg/g | ND |
| Histidine | 0.08 μg/g | 0.38 μg/g | 1.04 μg/g |
| Isoleucine | 6.16 μg/g | 1608.14 μg/g | 16.29 μg/g |
| Leucine | ND | 598.14 μg/g | 45.15 μg/g |
| Lysine | 47.69 μg/g | 3062.68 μg/g | 74.00 μg/g |
| Methionine | 40.14 μg/g | ND | 12.24 μg/g |
| Phenylalanine | 3.14 μg/g | ND | 26.63 μg/g |
| Serine | ND | 627.39 μg/g | 11.35 μg/g |
| Threonine | ND | 1757.01 μg/g | 38.64 μg/g |
| Tyrosine | 21.82 μg/g | 1860.82 μg/g | 16.96 μg/g |
| Valine | ND | 1027.41 μg/g | 51.43 μg/g |

ND indicated Not Detected.

### 3.2. *Cytotoxicity of Placental Extracts on Skin Cells*

As shown in Figure 2, none of the placental extracts (GP, DP, and PP) were toxic to fibroblast skin cells at concentrations of 1–2000 μg/mL and significantly exhibited the highest percent NHF cell viability at a concentration of 2000 μg/mL. However, at a concentration of all placental extracts greater than 2000 μg/mL, NHF cell viability was decreased, especially in the PP extract, which decreased the percent cell viability to less than 100%. This result indicated that these placental extracts at concentrations over 2000 μg/mL were toxic to fibroblast cells. For keratinocytes, these extracts at concentrations of 1–5000 μg/mL were not toxic to HaCaT cells and slightly increased the percent cell viability of HaCaTs at concentrations of 1000–2000 μg/mL. These results indicated that at concentrations lower than 2000 μg/mL, the extracts showed no toxicity on either skin cell line and might induce fibroblast proliferation.

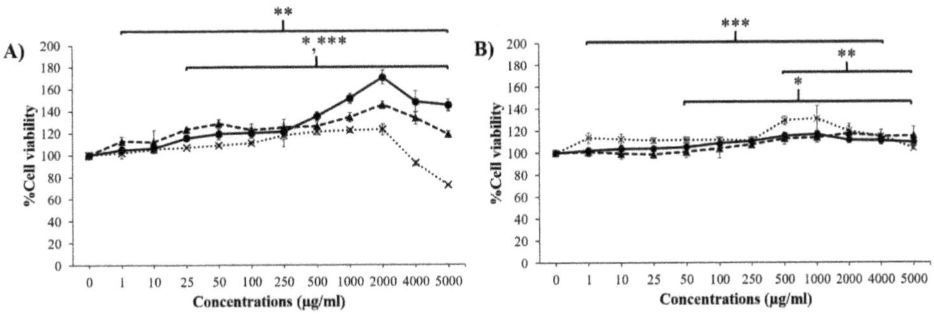


**Figure 2.** Percentages of cell viability of NHFs (**A**) and HaCaTs (**B**) after treatment with various concentrations of GP extract (—●—), DP extract (-▲--), and PP extract (···✕···). Data are presented as the mean ± S.D. ($n = 3$). *, **, and *** indicate that the GP extract, DP extract, and PP extract were significantly different from the control group (untreated cells), respectively ($p < 0.05$).

### 3.3. Effect of Placental Extracts on Cell Proliferation and Migration

To evaluate the skin-regenerating activity of placental extracts, the effect on NHF cell proliferation was measured. As shown in Figure 3, all placental extracts significantly enhanced cell growth in a concentration- and time-dependent manner ($p < 0.05$). GP and DP extracts at concentrations of 100–2000 μg/mL significantly promoted cell proliferation at 48 h and 72 h when compared to untreated cells, in which the maximum proliferation effect was found at 2000 μg/mL GP and DP extracts. While the PP extract significantly proliferated NHFs at concentrations between 50 and 2000 μg/mL after 72 h of treatment, the highest percent cell proliferation was found with 500 μg/mL PP extract. The results indicated that stimulation of fibroblast proliferation with the GP and DP extracts had a greater effect than that of PP extract.

For the cell migration study shown in Figure 4, treatment with placental extracts significantly accelerated gap area closure compared with a negative control ($p < 0.05$). After treatment with all placental extracts (1000 μg/mL and 2000 μg/mL) for 48 h, the gap areas were completely closed when compared to a negative control (56.17 ± 8.56%). After treatment with placental extracts for 24 h, the width of the scratch area was closed in the following order: GP 2000 μg/mL (88.85 ± 3.42%), GP 1000 μg/mL (87.86 ± 2.46%), EGF (87.81 ± 1.92%), PP 2000 μg/mL (85.65 ± 2.23%), DP 1000 μg/mL (81.14 ± 4.50%), DP 2000 μg/mL (78.75 ± 9.81%), PP 1000 μg/mL (60.04 ± 0.80%), negative control (44.34 ± 8.52%), which indicated that the placental extracts increased human dermal fibroblast migration, and the GP extract provided higher bioactivity on dermal fibroblasts than the other extracts.

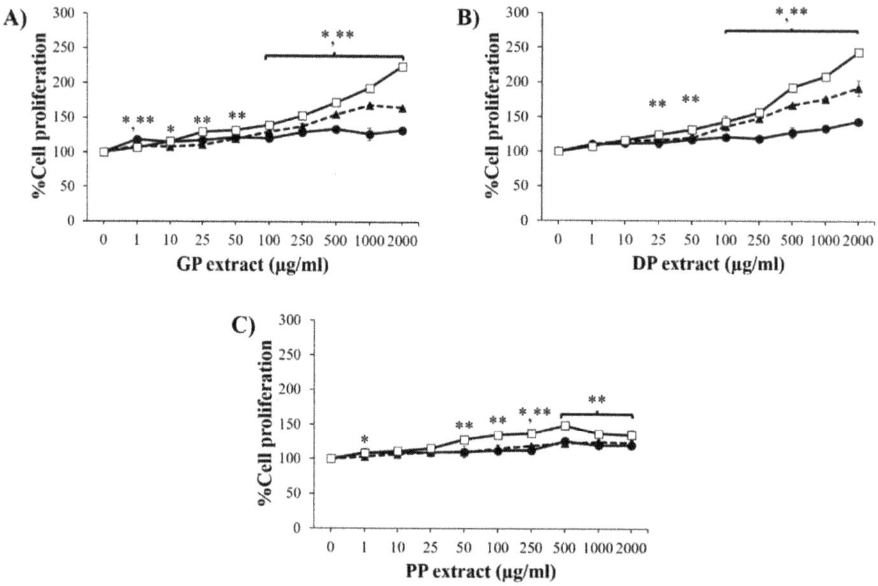


**Figure 3.** Percent cell proliferation of NHFs after treatment with various concentrations of GP extract (**A**), DP extract (**B**), and PP extract (**C**). Data are presented as the mean ± S.D. ($n = 3$). * and ** indicate that the percent cell proliferation at 48 h (-▲-) and 72 h (-□-) were significantly different from the untreated cells at 24 h (-●-) ($p < 0.05$).

Placental tissue is an excellent resource for total protein and growth factors, such as EGF, fibroblast growth factor basic (bFGF), and TGF-β1 [20]. These proteins, growth factors, or cytokines have key roles in dermal or epidermal rejuvenation by inducing proliferation, migration, and extracellular matrix synthesis [21]. Growth factors play an important role in signaling pathways to control cell regeneration and repair. FGF can induce fibroblast skin cell proliferation by accumulating collagen and stimulating angiogenesis [22]. The TGF-β family regulates migration, differentiation, and proliferation. In particular, TGF-β is involved in the proliferative stage, and TGF-β1 is one of three prototypic TGF-β isoforms associated with tissue repair that mediates fibroblast collagen production [23]. EGF also regulates intracellular biochemical pathways such as cell division, cell growth, and cell survival [24]. In this study, all the extracts were found to contain proteins and growth factors (e.g., EGF, IGF-1, TGF-β1, and FGF) as the bioactive compounds to regenerate the skin cells. Therefore, GP extract had the higher protein and growth factor contents, resulting in better bioactivity on dermal fibroblasts than other extracts. Moreover, GP extract containing the highest amino acids that affects the proteins in fibroblasts also resulted in high bioactivity on dermal fibroblasts.

### 3.4. *Skin Regeneration after UVB-Induced Skin Damage*

As shown in Figure 5, human dermal fibroblasts were exposed to UVB rays for 20 min, leading to significantly reduced cell viability of 60–70% ($p < 0.05$). After treatment with the placental extracts (GP, DP, and PP), the damaged skins significantly improved the regeneration effect compared to the UVB-irradiated group ($p < 0.05$). The highest cell regeneration was found in the GP extract (2000 μg/mL).

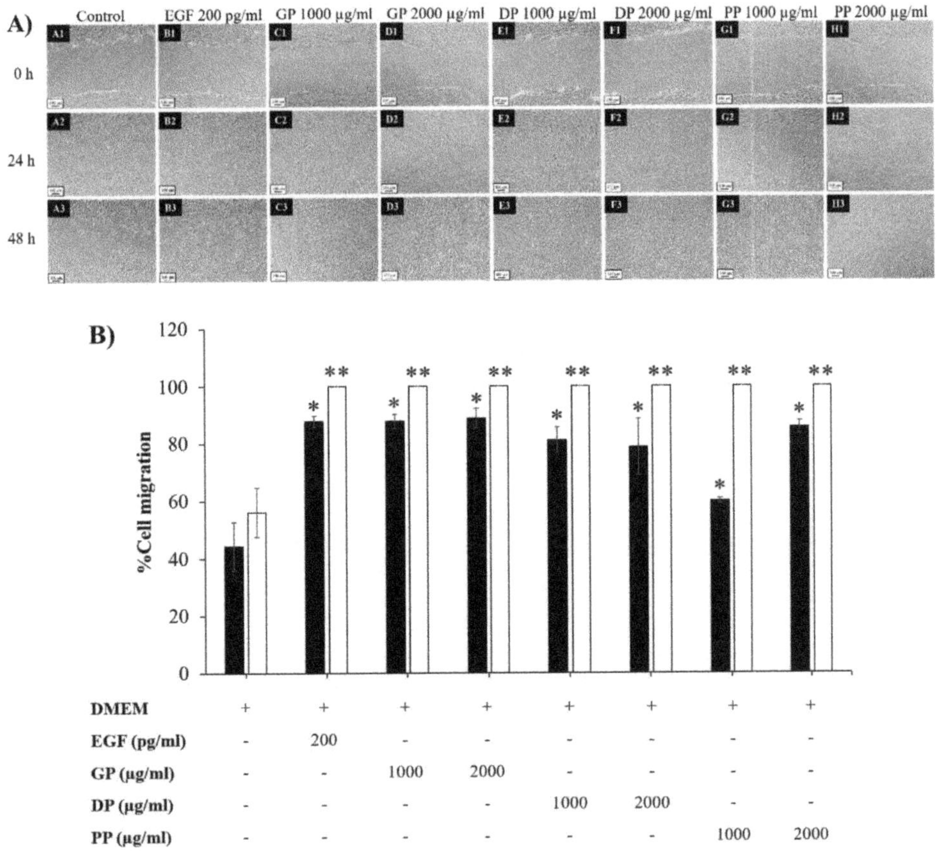


**Figure 4.** (**A**) Images of NHF cell migration after treatment with 1000 and 2000 µg/mL placental extracts (GP, DP, and PP) compared with a negative control group (untreated cells) and a positive control group (EGF 200 pg/mL) for 0, 24, and 48 h (4× objective lens) and (**B**) width of the scratch area of placental extract (GP, DP, and PP)-treated cells, negative control (untreated cells), and positive control (EGF 200 pg/mL) at 24 h (■), and 48 h (□). * and ** present a significant difference compared with the negative control at 24 and 48 h, respectively ($p < 0.05$).

In aged skin, the proliferation, metabolic activity, and functions of skin fibroblasts are impaired, resulting in abnormalities in the synthesis of structural substances such as collagen, elastin, and hyaluronic acid [22]. Growth factors and cytokines such as EGF, vascular endothelial growth factor (VEGF), and TGF-β have been reported to be involved in collagen biosynthesis and to promote skin rejuvenation [25]. In addition, human skin fibroblasts are the primary cells in the dermal layer and are associated with UVB-induced photoaging in the upper layer of these cells. In a previous report, UVB-irradiated human skin fibroblasts significantly decreased the expression of IGF-1, TGF-β1, and EGF [26]. In the previous experiments, these extracts containing some growth factors such as EGF, IGF-1, TGF-β 1, and FGF affected the skin cell proliferation and migration. After the skin cells were damaged by UVB rays, these active ingredients of placental extracts repaired the damaged dermal cells. Consequently, placental extracts (GP, DP, and PP) were useful for skin regenerative activities because they proliferated human dermal fibroblasts by increasing cell regeneration, leading to the induction of fibroblast migration, the upregulation of pro-collagen I, and the repair of UVB irradiation-damaged skin. Moreover, the results showed that GP extract had a stronger bioactive effect on skin cells than DP and PP, resulting from total protein, growth factors, and total amino acids content as the bioactive substances were predominantly found in GP extract. Therefore, GP extract was selected as a bioactive placental extract for delivery into the skin using the microneedling technique.

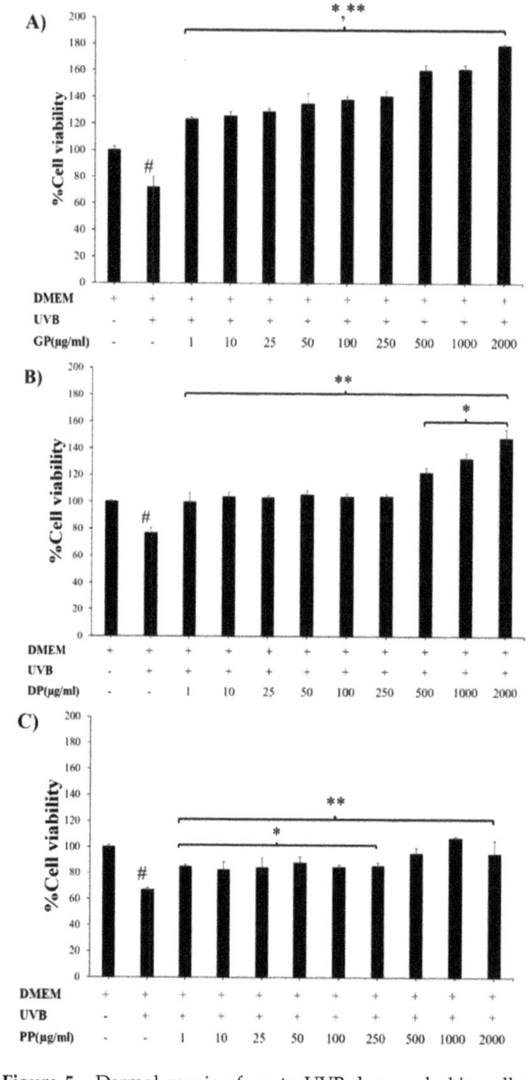


**Figure 5.** Dermal repair of acute UVB-damaged skin cells by placental extracts GP (**A**), DP (**B**), and PP (**C**) at various concentrations (1–2000 µg/mL) on NHFs treated with UVB ray ($n = 3$). * and ** represent significant differences compared with nontreated UVB and treated UVB ($p < 0.05$), respectively. # denotes a significant difference compared with nontreated UVB ($p < 0.05$).

### *3.5. DMN Loading of Bioactive Macromolecular Compounds*

As shown in Figure 6, the physical appearance of hyaluronic acid and PDMA microneedles under the digital microscope displayed sharp conical-shaped microneedle tips (11 × 11 needle arrays) with a height of 557.75 ± 2.11 µm, base width of 299.93 ± 2.31 µm, and interneedle spacing of 600.90 ± 2.22 µm. The percentage of height reduction of DMNs increased progressively with increases in the applied force from 4.0 to 20.0 N. At the average applied force for polymeric microneedles on the skin by human thumbs (20 N), DMNs showed the highest percent height reduction; however, none of the needles were brittle. These MNs deformed when applied to a stainless-steel plate, which is important from a patient safety perspective [27].

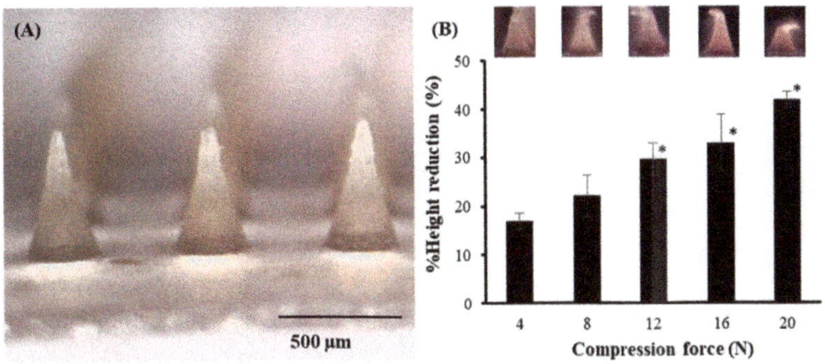


**Figure 6.** (**A**) Appearance of GP extract loaded DMN arrays and (**B**) the percent height reduction of DMNs after the application of the different compression forces. The data represents the mean ± S.D. ($n$ = 3). * represent significant differences from compression force at 4 N ($p < 0.05$).

Protein content in the DMN patch was 461.52 ± 79.43 µg per patch. Moreover, the dissolution of DMNs in the skin exhibited height reductions of 45.47 ± 4.478% and 77.28 ± 0.57% after the application for 2 h and 4 h, respectively, in which the complete dissolution of DMNs was found at an insertion time of 6 h. These results presented an appropriate system of DMNs to deliver bioactive compounds into and throughout the skin.

### 3.6. Skin Permeation and Deposition of Macromolecular Protein-Loaded DMNs

As shown in Figure 7, the cumulative amount of BSA-FITC-loaded DMNs through the skin was higher than that in solution form at every time interval. The flux of DMNs and solution was 0.1745 ± 0.12 µg/cm$^2$/h ($R^2$ = 0.7521) and 0.0610 ± 0.01 µg/cm$^2$/h ($R^2$ = 0.9381), respectively, while $K_p$ was 1.75 × $10^{-6}$ cm/h and 0.31 × $10^{-6}$ cm/h, respectively. This result indicated that DMNs increased the permeability of macromolecular protein through the skin for a 5.65-fold enhancement from solution.

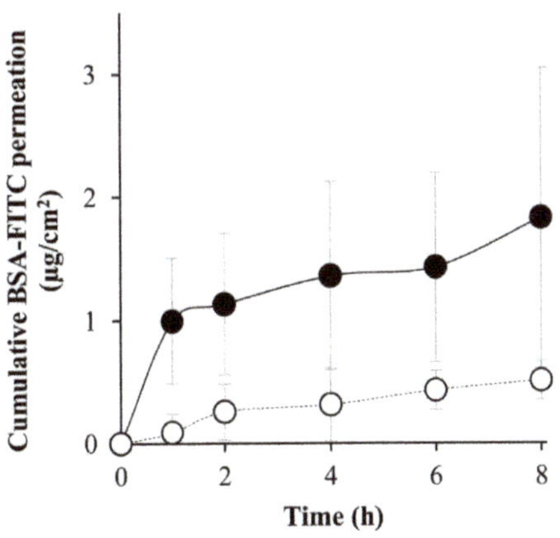


**Figure 7.** Cumulative BSA-FITC permeation-time profiles of DMNs (•) and BSA-FITC solution (○). The data represents the mean ± S.D. ($n$ = 3).

CLSM visualized the skin permeation pathway and evaluated the permeation depth of BSA-FITC-loaded DMNs (Figure 8). The X-Y serial images of skin treated with DMNs exhibited the green fluorescent BSA-FITC between 0 μm and 260 μm skin depth. The spatial distribution of BSA-FITC-loaded DMNs showed the shape of these needle arrays in the skin. For the BSA-FITC intensity, the skin treated with DMNs presented the maximum fluorescence intensity at a depth of 105 μm with a deeper skin permeation depth (260 μm) of green fluorescent BSA-FITC than the skin treated with solution (100 μm). This result indicated greater and deeper deposition in skin of macromolecular protein from DMNs than that from solution.

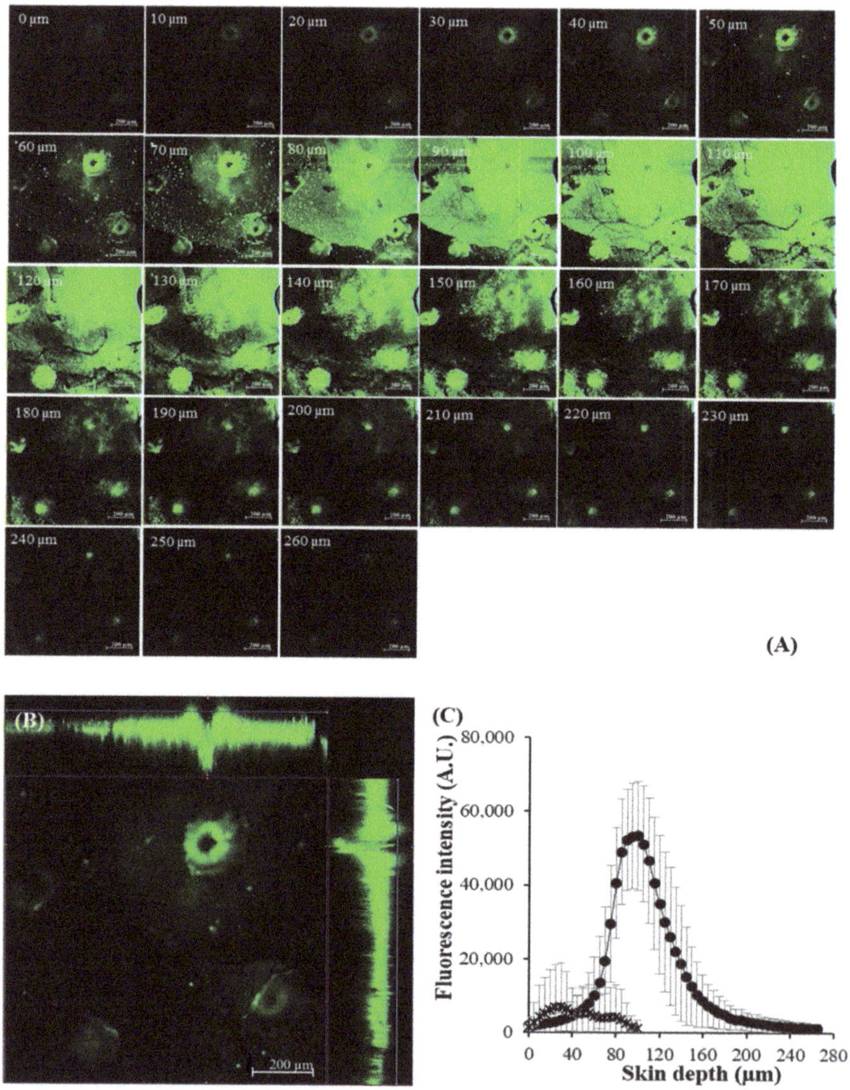


**Figure 8.** CLSM images of skins treated with DMN loading BSA-FITC for 8 h: (**A**) The X-Y serial images, (**B**) spatial distribution (X−Y, X−Z, and Y−Z planes) image, and (**C**) fluorescence intensity profile at difference skin depths (10 × objective lens).

Bioactive macromolecular proteins and growth factors are hydrophilic compounds and have a limited ability to passively penetrate skin. The outermost layer of skin, the stratum corneum barrier, is a lipophilic layer and allows only small, potent, and moderately lipophilic molecules to partition across it passively into the deeper skin layers [28]. The study showed that DMN patch enhanced the delivery of macromolecular proteins into and through the skin. DMN fabricated from hyaluronic acid can be used to encapsulate peptides and proteins, and the DMN morphology exhibited an acceptable height range for the delivery of drugs into skin with minimal invasion. The DMNs were sufficiently sharp and strong for passage through the layer of stratum corneum, for which the thicknesses of stratum corneum layer, viable epidermis, and dermis are approximately 10–20 μm, 50–100 μm, and 1–2 mm, respectively [29]. After DMN insertion into the skin, possible routes to transport protein and growth factors through the skin was created as micropores into the epidermis layer by using a minimally invasive technique, bypassing the tightly packed stratum corneum barrier and improving the ability to deliver macromolecular protein into the skin [28]. However, DMNs could not be inserted passing through the whole dermal layers completely because of the deformation and elasticity of the skin during the process of penetration [30,31]. Approximately 46% of the needle length was used to create a micropore in the skin, suggesting that the macromolecular proteins remained in the epidermal and dermal layers. Therefore, DMNs exhibited a potential delivery system for biomacromolecules into the active site of action, presenting a suitable dermal delivery system for bioactive placental extracts.

### 3.7. Skin Histology

As presented in Figure 9, the histological images of porcine skin treated with GP extract in solution and the DMN patch indicated a normal appearance of the skin structure, in which the stratum corneum, viable epidermal, and dermal layers remained unchanged. However, DMN provided a minimally invasive approach for the stratum corneum barriers (~130 μm insertion depth), suggesting that GP extract-loaded DMNs were successfully inserted into the epidermal and dermal layers and did not damage the deep skin layer.

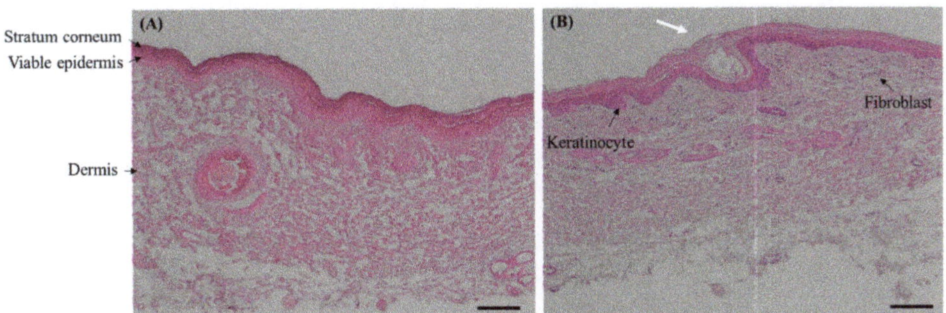


**Figure 9.** Histology of the skin treated with GP extract in solution (**A**) and DMN patch (**B**) at 24 h (H&E stain, magnification: ×10). The microneedle hole (white arrow) is ~130 μm, reaching the superficial skin.

In the staining method, the hematoxylin component in the skin stains nuclei of fibroblast cells, rough endoplasmic reticulum, ribosomes, collagen, keratohyalin granules, and elastic fibers as a blue or purple color [32], while the eosin stains cell eosinophilic structures, normally composed of intracellular or extracellular protein (e.g., cytoplasm and connective tissue fibers) as varying shades of pink, orange, and red color [33]. The skin treated with GP extract in the DMN patch showed the blue dots of hematoxylin staining more than the skin treated with GP solution, which the position of blue dots in the skin image suggested that the morphology of fibroblasts and keratinocytes [34]. Therefore,

DMNs that can deliver bioactive compounds from GP extract into the skin exhibited the growth of dermal fibroblast and keratinocyte.

### 3.8. Human Study

After 24 h of DMN application in human volunteers, all subjects were measured for skin changes in TEWL, erythema, and hydration, as presented in Figure 10. No unwanted symptom was observed by visual appearance. TEWL was used to evaluate the puncturing properties at the injection sites of the skin surface, and an increase in TEWL was observed in all DMN arrays with/without GP extract, indicating that the DMN arrays caused disruption of the skin by successfully puncturing the skin and creating permeation pathways [35]. Based on the skin hydration results, almost all skin treated with DMN patches showed an increase in percent skin hydration change, demonstrating a high moisture content of the skin [36]. The erythema value was used to determine the reaction to irritant and allergy. Increasing erythema after applying the DMN patch for 24 h indicated that compression during the application might cause skin redness. Although skin irritation and disruption caused by microneedle arrays were observed, no pain and edema or severe redness of skin was found.

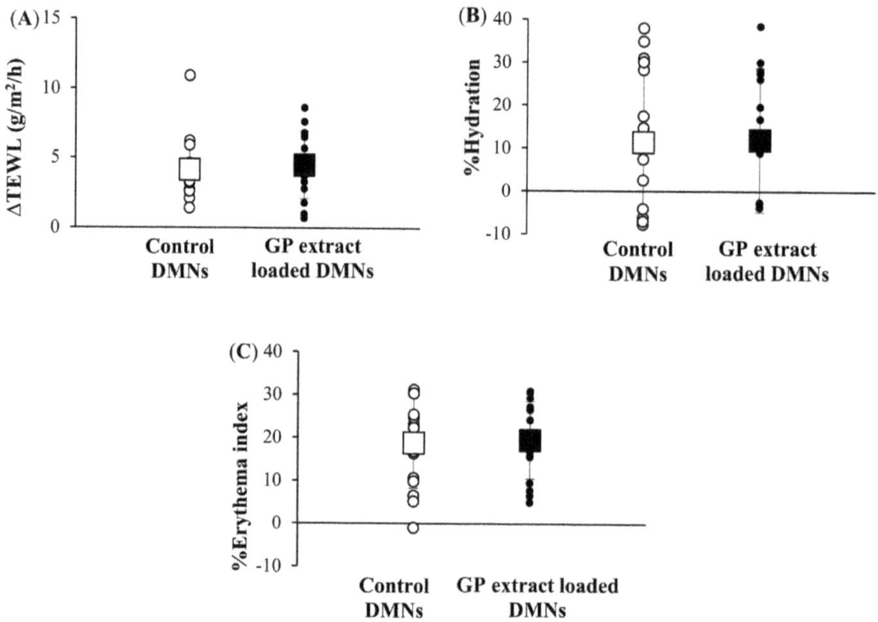


**Figure 10.** (**A**) ΔTEWL, (**B**) the percent hydration, and (**C**) the percent erythema index after control DMN patch and GP extract loaded DMN patch applied onto the skin of healthy volunteers. The data represents the mean ± S.D. ($n$ = 15).

In this study, the GP extract-loaded DMN patch showed no significant difference from the control DMN patch (no GP extract loaded) after 24 h in the human study, indicating that it served as a suitable dermal delivery device for bioactive macromolecules without altering the microneedle insertion properties. Skin irritation after application of microneedle arrays fabricated from hyaluronic acid was slight and transient, and small transdermal pathways created by these DMNs were also rapidly recovered. These results indicated that the DMN patch fabricated from hyaluronic acid was quite safe [35].

Microneedles have been reported as a potent drug delivery system by passing through the stratum corneum permeability barrier, which these needles are also easy to produce and allow the self-administration of drugs without causing pain or bleeding. Low invasiveness of microneedles is important to increase the opportunity for application in population-specific and personalized therapies, especially in pediatrics [37]. Moreover, the development of a minimally invasive needle-sensor to monitor $O_2$ levels in the brain using acupuncture needles have been shown that a small tool with minimally invasive has an ability to monitor real-time $O_2$ in vivo complex environments with minimizing pain, discomfort, and injury to the patient [38]. In addition, DMNs can be used to deliver immunologically active peptides to the epidermal and intradermal space, which these microneedles array containing 33 × 33 needles with 200 to 125 μm-diameter and 600 μm-height can release the peptides in physiological condition at therapeutic dose [39]. Therefore, DMN patch in this study could be a very useful and effective approach to improve the dermal delivery of bioactive macromolecules, especially potent bioactive placental extracts, without serious damage to the skin.

## 4. Conclusions

Three types of animal placentas (deer, goat, and porcine) were water-extracted and exhibited high protein, growth factor (EGF, FGF, IGF-1, and TGF-β1) and amino acid contents. These placental extracts were not toxic to skin cells at concentrations lower than 2000 μg/mL, while the proliferation of fibroblast cells significantly increased in a time-dependent manner. GP extracts exhibited the maximum proliferation, migration, and regeneration effect on fibroblast cells, suggesting that the GP extract had a stronger bioactive effect on skin cells compared with the other extracts. To overcome the limitation of the skin barrier, DMN patches were successfully fabricated to deliver bioactive macromolecular compounds into and through the skin. Moreover, GP extract-loaded DMNs showed successful skin insertion with minimal skin invasion, supporting their safety for application to human skin. In conclusion, placental extracts act as potent bioactive compounds for skin cells, and the highest bioactive potential of GP-loaded DMNs might play an important role in skin regeneration.

**Author Contributions:** Investigation: K.T., P.S., P.O. and W.R.; supervision: P.O., T.N. and W.R., writing—original draft preparation: K.T. and W.R.; writing—review and editing: P.O. and W.R. All authors have read and agreed to the published version of the manuscript.

**Funding:** This research was funded by the National Research Council of Thailand (NRCT; Grant No. N42A650224 and N42A650551), the Golden Jubilee Ph.D. Program (Grant No. PHD/0192/2561), and the Program Management Unit for Competitiveness (PMUC; Grant No. C10F640021).

**Institutional Review Board Statement:** The study was conducted in accordance with the Declaration of Helsinki and approved by the Institutional Review Board (Human Studies Ethics Committee) of Faculty of Pharmacy, Silpakorn University (protocol code: COE 65.0223-032 and date of approval: 23 February 2022) for studies involving humans.

**Informed Consent Statement:** Not applicable.

**Data Availability Statement:** Not applicable.

**Acknowledgments:** The authors would like to thank the National Research Council of Thailand (NRCT; Grant No. N42A650224 and N42A650551), the Golden Jubilee Ph.D. Program (Grant No. PHD/0192/2561), the Program Management Unit for Competitiveness (PMUC; Grant No. C10F640021), and faculty of pharmaceutical sciences, Ubon Ratchathani University for their financial support and facility support. We would like to thank image focus holding Co., Ltd. for the fresh DP, Phaya Yen Daily Co., Ltd. for the fresh GP, and CCF energy supplement Co., Ltd. for the fresh PP.

**Conflicts of Interest:** The authors declare no conflict of interest.

## References


1. Lee, K.; Choi, W.; Yum, K.; Song, S.; Ock, S.; Park, S.; Kim, M. Efficacy and Safety of Human Placental Extract Solution on Fatigue: A Double-Blind, Randomized, Placebo-Controlled Study. *Evid. Based Complement. Alternat. Med.* **2012**, *2012*, 130875. [CrossRef] [PubMed]
2. Pan, S.Y.; Chan, M.K.S.; Wong, M.B.F.; Klokol, D.; Chernykh, V. Placental therapy: An insight to their biological and therapeutic properties. *J. Med. Ther.* **2017**, *1*, 1–6. [CrossRef]
3. Tebakari, M.; Daigo, Y.; Ishikawa, H.; Nakamura, M.; Kawashima, J.; Takano, F. Anti-inflammatory Effect of the Water-Soluble Portion of Porcine Placental Extract in Lipopolysaccharide-Stimulated RAW264.7 Murine Macrophage Cells. *Biol. Pharm. Bull.* **2018**, *41*, 1251–1256. [CrossRef] [PubMed]
4. Chakraborty, P.D.; Bhattacharyya, D. Isolation of fibronectin type III like peptide from human placental extract used as wound healer. *J. Chromatogr. B* **2005**, *818*, 67–73. [CrossRef]
5. Park, S.Y.; Phark, S.; Lee, M.; Lim, J.Y.; Sul, D. Anti-oxidative and anti-inflammatory activities of placental extracts in benzo a pyrene-exposed rats. *Placenta* **2010**, *31*, 873–879. [CrossRef]
6. Teng, D.; Fang, Y.; Song, X.; Gao, Y. Optimization of enzymatic hydrolysis parameters for antioxidant capacity of peptide from goat placenta. *Food Bioprod. Process.* **2011**, *89*, 202–208. [CrossRef]
7. Bériot, M.; Tchimbou, A.F.; Barbato, O.; Beckers, J.F.; de Sousa, N.M. Identification of pregnancy-associated glycoproteins and alpha-fetoprotein in fallow deer (*Dama dama*) placenta. *Acta Vet. Scand.* **2014**, *56*, 4. [CrossRef]
8. Barrientos, S.; Stojadinovic, O.; Golinko, M.S.; Brem, H.; Tomic-Canic, M. Growth factors and cytokines in wound healing. *Wound Repair. Regen.* **2008**, *16*, 585–601. [CrossRef]
9. Mao, A.S.; Mooney, D.J. Regenerative medicine: Current therapies and future directions. *Proc. Natl. Acad. Sci. USA* **2015**, *112*, 14452–14459. [CrossRef]
10. El-Domyati, M.; El-Ammawi, T.S.; Moawad, O.; El-Fakahany, H.; Medhat, W.; Mahoney, M.G.; Uitto, J. Efficacy of mesotherapy in facial rejuvenation: A histological and immunohistochemical evaluation. *Int. J. Dermatol.* **2012**, *51*, 913–919. [CrossRef]
11. Prausnitz, M.R.; Langer, R. Transdermal drug delivery. *Nat. Biotechnol.* **2008**, *26*, 1261–1268. [CrossRef] [PubMed]
12. Waghule, T.; Singhvi, G.; Dubey, S.K.; Pandey, M.M.; Gupta, G.; Singh, M.; Dua, K. Microneedles: A smart approach and increasing potential for transdermal drug delivery system. *Biomed. Pharmacother.* **2019**, *109*, 1249–1258. [CrossRef] [PubMed]
13. Tansathien, K.; Suriyaamporn, P.; Charoenputtakhun, P.; Ngawhirunpat, T.; Opanasopit, P.; Rangsimawong, W. Development of Sponge Microspicule Cream as a Transdermal Delivery System for Protein and Growth Factors from Deer Antler Velvet Extract. *Biol. Pharm. Bull.* **2019**, *42*, 1207–1215. [CrossRef] [PubMed]
14. Tolosa, L.; Donato, M.T.; Gómez-Lechón, M.J. General Cytotoxicity Assessment by Means of the MTT Assay. In *Protocols in In Vitro Hepatocyte Research*; Vinken, M., Rogiers, V., Eds.; Springer: New York, NY, USA, 2015; pp. 333–348.
15. Kansom, T.; Sajomsang, W.; Saeeng, R.; Charoensuksai, P.; Opanasopit, P.; Tonglairoum, P. Apoptosis Induction and Antimigratory Activity of Andrographolide Analog (3A.1)-Incorporated Self-Assembled Nanoparticles in Cancer Cells. *AAPS PharmSciTech* **2018**, *19*, 3123–3133. [CrossRef] [PubMed]
16. Suriyaamporn, P.; Opanasopit, P.; Ngawhirunpat, T.; Rangsimawong, W. Computer-aided rational design for optimally Gantrez® S-97 and hyaluronic acid-based dissolving microneedles as a potential ocular delivery system. *J. Drug Deliv. Sci. Technol.* **2021**, *61*, 102319. [CrossRef]
17. Tansathien, K.; Chareanputtakhun, P.; Ngawhirunpat, T.; Opanasopit, P.; Rangsimawong, W. Hair growth promoting effect of bioactive extract from deer antler velvet-loaded niosomes and microspicules serum. *Int. J. Pharm.* **2021**, *597*, 120352. [CrossRef]
18. Mavon, A. Acetyl aspartic acid, a novel active ingredient, demonstrates potential to improve signs of skin ageing: From consumer need to clinical proof. *Int. J. Cosmet. Sci.* **2015**, *37*, 1–2. [CrossRef]
19. Chung, K.W.; Song, S.H.; Kim, M. Synergistic effect of copper and amino acid mixtures on the production of extracellular matrix proteins in skin fibroblasts. *Mol. Biol. Rep.* **2021**, *48*, 3277–3284. [CrossRef]
20. Russo, A.; Bonci, P.; Bonci, P. The effects of different preservation processes on the total protein and growth factor content in a new biological product developed from human amniotic membrane. *Cell Tissue Bank.* **2012**, *13*, 353–361. [CrossRef]
21. Anitua, E.; Pino, A.; Orive, G. Plasma rich in growth factors promotes dermal fibroblast proliferation, migration and biosynthetic activity. *J. Wound Care* **2016**, *25*, 680–687. [CrossRef]
22. De Araújo, R.; Lôbo, M.; Trindade, K.; Silva, D.F.; Pereira, N. Fibroblast Growth Factors: A Controlling Mechanism of Skin Aging. *Skin Pharmacol. Physiol.* **2019**, *32*, 275–282. [CrossRef] [PubMed]
23. Gilbert, R.W.D.; Vickaryous, M.K.; Viloria-Petit, A.M. Signalling by Transforming Growth Factor Beta Isoforms in Wound Healing and Tissue Regeneration. *Int. J. Dev. Biol.* **2016**, *4*, 21. [CrossRef] [PubMed]
24. Esquirol Caussa, J.; Herrero Vila, E. Epidermal growth factor, innovation and safety. *Med. Clin.* **2015**, *145*, 305–312. [CrossRef]
25. Aldag, C.; Nogueira Teixeira, D.; Leventhal, P.S. Skin rejuvenation using cosmetic products containing growth factors, cytokines, and matrikines: A review of the literature. *Clin. Cosmet. Investig. Dermatol.* **2016**, *9*, 411–419. [CrossRef] [PubMed]
26. Qin, F.; Huang, J.; Zhang, W.; Zhang, M.; Li, Z.; Si, L.; Long, X.; Wang, X. The Paracrine Effect of Adipose-Derived Stem Cells Orchestrates Competition between Different Damaged Dermal Fibroblasts to Repair UVB-Induced Skin Aging. *Stem Cells Int.* **2020**, *2020*, 8878370. [CrossRef]

27. Donnelly, R.F.; McCrudden, M.T.C.; Zaid Alkilani, A.; Larrañeta, E.; McAlister, E.; Courtenay, A.J.; Kearney, M.-C.; Singh, T.R.R.; McCarthy, H.O.; Kett, V.L.; et al. Hydrogel-Forming Microneedles Prepared from "Super Swelling" Polymers Combined with Lyophilised Wafers for Transdermal Drug Delivery. *PLoS ONE* **2014**, *9*, e111547. [CrossRef]
28. Kalluri, H.; Banga, A.K. Transdermal delivery of proteins. *AAPS PharmSciTech* **2011**, *12*, 431–441. [CrossRef]
29. Andrews, S.N.; Jeong, E.; Prausnitz, M.R. Transdermal delivery of molecules is limited by full epidermis, not just stratum corneum. *Pharm. Res.* **2013**, *30*, 1099–1109. [CrossRef]
30. Chen, M.C.; Ling, M.H.; Kusuma, S.J. Poly-γ-glutamic Acid Microneedles with a Supporting Structure Design as a Potential Tool for Transdermal Delivery of Insulin. *Acta Biomater.* **2015**, *24*, 106–116. [CrossRef]
31. Liu, S.; Wu, D.; Quan, Y.S.; Kamiyama, F.; Kusamori, K.; Katsumi, H.; Sakane, T.; Yamamoto, A. Improvement of Transdermal Delivery of Exendin-4 Using Novel Tip-Loaded Microneedle Arrays Fabricated from Hyaluronic Acid. *Mol. Pharm.* **2016**, *13*, 272–279. [CrossRef]
32. Chan, J.K. The wonderful colors of the hematoxylin-eosin stain in diagnostic surgical pathology. *Int. J. Surg. Pathol.* **2014**, *22*, 12–32. [CrossRef] [PubMed]
33. Bancroft, J.D.; Layton, C. *The hematoxylins and eosin. Bancroft's Theory and Practice of Histological Techniques*, 7th ed.; Suvarna, S.K., Layton, C., Bancroft, J.D., Eds.; Churchill Livingstone: London, UK, 2013; Volume 10, pp. 173–186.
34. Kim, E.; Rebecca, V.W.; Fedorenko, I.V.; Messina, J.L.; Mathew, R.A.; Maria-Engler, S.S.; Basanta, D.; Smalley, K.S.; Anderson, A.R. Senescent fibroblasts can drive melanoma initiation and progression. *arXiv* **2013**, arXiv:1304.1054.
35. Liu, S.; Jin, M.N.; Quan, Y.S.; Kamiyama, F.; Kusamori, K.; Katsumi, H.; Sakane, T.; Yamamoto, A. Transdermal delivery of relatively high molecular weight drugs using novel self-dissolving microneedle arrays fabricated from hyaluronic acid and their characteristics and safety after application to the skin. *Eur. J. Pharm. Biopharm.* **2014**, *86*, 267–276. [CrossRef] [PubMed]
36. Hua, W.; Fan, L.M.; Dai, R.; Luan, M.; Xie, H.; Li, A.Q.; Li, L. Comparison of two series of non-invasive instruments used for the skin physiological properties measurements: The DermaLab® from cortex technology vs. the series of detectors from courage & khazaka. *Skin Res. Technol.* **2017**, *23*, 70–78. [CrossRef]
37. Pires, L.R.; Vinayakumar, K.B.; Turos, M.; Miguel, V.; Gaspar, J. A Perspective on Microneedle-Based Drug Delivery and Diagnostics in Paediatrics. *J. Pers. Med.* **2019**, *9*, 49. [CrossRef]
38. Vieira, D.; McEachern, F.; Filippelli, R.; Dimentberg, E.; Harvey, E.J.; Merle, G. Microelectrochemical Smart Needle for Real Time Minimally Invasive Oximetry. *Biosensors* **2020**, *10*, 157. [CrossRef]
39. Pires, L.R.; Amado, I.R.; Gaspar, J. Dissolving microneedles for the delivery of peptides—Towards tolerance-inducing vaccines. *Int. J. Pharm.* **2020**, *586*, 119590. [CrossRef]

*pharmaceutics*

*Article*

# Demonstrating Biological Fate of Nanoparticle-Loaded Dissolving Microneedles with Aggregation-Caused Quenching Probes: Influence of Application Sites

**Yanping Fu [1], Chaonan Shi [1], Xiaodie Li [1], Ting Wen [2], Qiaoli Wu [3], Antian Zhang [1], Ping Hu [1], Chuanbin Wu [1], Xin Pan [2], Zhengwei Huang [1,*] and Guilan Quan [1,*]**

1 College of Pharmacy, Jinan University, Guangzhou 510632, China
2 School of Pharmaceutical Sciences, Sun Yat-sen University, Guangzhou 510006, China
3 The Fourth Affiliated Hospital of Guangzhou Medical University, Guangzhou 511300, China
* Correspondence: huangzhengw@jnu.edu.cn (Z.H.); quanguilan@jnu.edu.cn (G.Q.)

**Abstract:** Integrating dissolving microneedles (DMNs) and nanocarriers (NC) holds great potential in transdermal drug delivery because it can simultaneously overcome the stratum corneum barrier and achieve efficient and controlled drug delivery. However, different skin sites with different thicknesses and compositions can affect the transdermal diffusion of NC-loaded DMNs. There are few reports on the biological fate (especially transdermal diffusion) of NC-loaded DMNs, and inaccurate bioimaging information of intact NC limits the accurate understanding of the in vivo fate of NC-loaded DMNs. The aggregation-caused quenching (ACQ) probes P4 emitted intense fluorescence signals in intact NC while quenched after the degradation of NC, had been demonstrated the feasibility of label intact NC. In this study, P4 was loaded in solid lipid nanoparticles (SLNs), and further encapsulated into DMNs, to track the transdermal diffusion of SLNs delivered at different skin sites. The results showed that SLNs had excellent stability after being loaded into DMNs with no significant changes in morphology and fluorescence properties. The in vivo live and ex vivo imaging showed that the transdermal diffusion rate of NC-loaded DMNs was positively correlated with skin thickness, with the order ear > abdomen > back. In conclusion, this study confirmed the site-dependency of transdermal diffusion in NC-loaded DMNs.

**Keywords:** dissolving microneedles; solid lipid nanoparticles; in vivo fate; transdermal drug delivery; aggregation-caused quenching

## 1. Introduction

Transdermal drug delivery (TDD) is an administration route through the skin to achieve local or systemic therapeutic purposes [1]. It can avoid the metabolism of drugs by gastrointestinal digestive enzymes and overcome the first-pass effect of the liver [2,3]. However, the hindrance of the cutaneous stratum corneum reduces the efficiency of TDD, limiting its use in current clinical practice [4]. To overcome the stratum corneum barrier and improve the transdermal penetration of drugs, various advanced strategies (such as ultrasound, light, heat, and electroporation) have been developed [5]. These approaches, however, have still shown limited efficiency for the transdermal delivery of macromolecular drugs [6].

In recent years, microneedles (MNs) have drawn widespread attention as a novel physical permeation promotion technique. MNs consists of hundreds of tiny micron-sized needle tips attached to a base in an array pattern that can break through the stratum corneum barrier to produce multiple mechanical pores. Thus, MNs can significantly improve the efficiency of transdermal drug delivery [7]. As an intensively studied category of MNs, dissolving microneedles (DMNs) are mainly prepared by water-soluble polymers, and the drugs are distributed in the matrix of the needle tip. The needle tip can dissolve by absorbing tissue fluid after piercing the skin, and the encapsulated drugs are released [8]. DMNs have been widely explored in TDD based on the significant advantages of simple preparation methods, high drug delivery efficiency, and satisfactory patient compliance [9–12].

Nevertheless, there are still some challenges for monotonic DMNs. Firstly, the hydrophilic material of DMNs severely limits the encapsulation of hydrophobic drugs, while most available drugs in the pipeline are hydrophobic. Secondly, without release management designs, monotonic DMNs cannot achieve precise and controlled drug release [13,14]. Within decades, research based on nanocarriers (NC) in drug delivery has gained wide attention [15]. Various types of NC, such as liposomes [16], solid lipid nanoparticles (SLNs) [17], metal-organic frameworks [18], and magnetic nanoparticles [19], have shown excellent therapeutic effects. NC are capable of loading insoluble drugs and improving bioavailability in vivo [20]. In addition, the modulation of the physicochemical properties of NC enables controlled drug release in a spatiotemporal manner [21]. Therefore, the combination of NC and DMNs can simultaneously overcome the stratum corneum barrier and achieve efficient and controlled drug delivery, producing a synergistic effect.

However, to date, most studies based on NC-loaded DMNs have refrained from preclinical investigation, and it is rare to identify NC-loaded DMNs that have been introduced into the clinic or market. This is mainly attributed to the fact that little is known about the biological fate of NC-loaded DMNs.

Previously, our group preliminarily explored the effect of the length of DMNs on the in vivo fate of NC in both the temporal and spatial dimensions [22]. Noticeably, without a consensus on the standard operating procedure or clinical practice of MNs administration, the application sites of NC-loaded DMNs can be diverse, and NC will be exposed to different biological environments. Differences in skin structures and compositions at different sites [23] may affect the transdermal diffusion rate of NC-loaded DMNs. Therefore, the fate of NC-loaded DMNs depends on the encountered in vivo biological environment [24]. When studying the biological fate of NC, specific physiological conditions must be taken into account. Unfortunately, there are few reports on how different skin sites affect the biological fate of NC-loaded DMNs, which has limited their clinical translation. Even worse, in previous studies, the lack of effective tools and strategies for reliably identifying intact NC has resulted in inaccurate bioimaging information. One of the key issues in the study on the in vivo fate of NC-loaded DMNs is the integrity of NC, which is a prerequisite for improved drug targeting and local retention [25]. Thus, it is impossible to grasp a comprehensive and accurate understanding of the in vivo fate of NC-loaded DMNs.

To demonstrate the biological fate of NC-loaded DMNs administrated via different skin sites, a platform for in vivo comprehensive identification and real-time, precise monitoring of intact NC is essential. Recently, environmentally responsive fluorescent probes have been used to study the in vivo fate of NC [26–30]. The aggregation-caused quenching (ACQ) probes are environment-responsive fluorescent probes with strong hydrophobicity [31]. When ACQ probes are embedded in intact NC, they emit a fluorescent signal. When probes are released as the NC degrade, they tend to aggregate and quench spontaneously due to the ACQ effect [31,32]. Therefore, ACQ probes can identify intact NC.

In this study, we chose SLNs as model NC and further prepared them into NC-loaded DMNs, whose biological fate was scrutinized. Due to the simple production process, high biocompatibility, and excellent drug-loading ability, SLNs are promising for clinical translation [33]. In addition, SLNs are lipid-based NC with a core-shell structure: a hydrophilic surfactant shell and a hydrophobic lipid core, which is capable of effective loading of hydrophobic ACQ probes. Importantly, a series of studies have been conducted on SLNs-loaded DMNs, which showed good compatibility of SLNs with DMNs [22,28,34]. As shown in Figure 1, we first loaded ACQ probes (code P4) into SLNs (P4 SLNs), which were further encapsulated into DMNs (P4 SLNs@DMNs). Then, P4 SLNs@DMNs were applied to the skin of the ear, back, and abdomen in rats, respectively. Subsequently, the biological fate of P4 SLNs@DMNs administrated via different skin sites was monitored by in vivo and ex vivo fluorescence bioimaging. This study is expected to clarify the relationship between the administration site and the in vivo fate of NC-loaded DMNs and provide a theoretical basis for their clinical application.

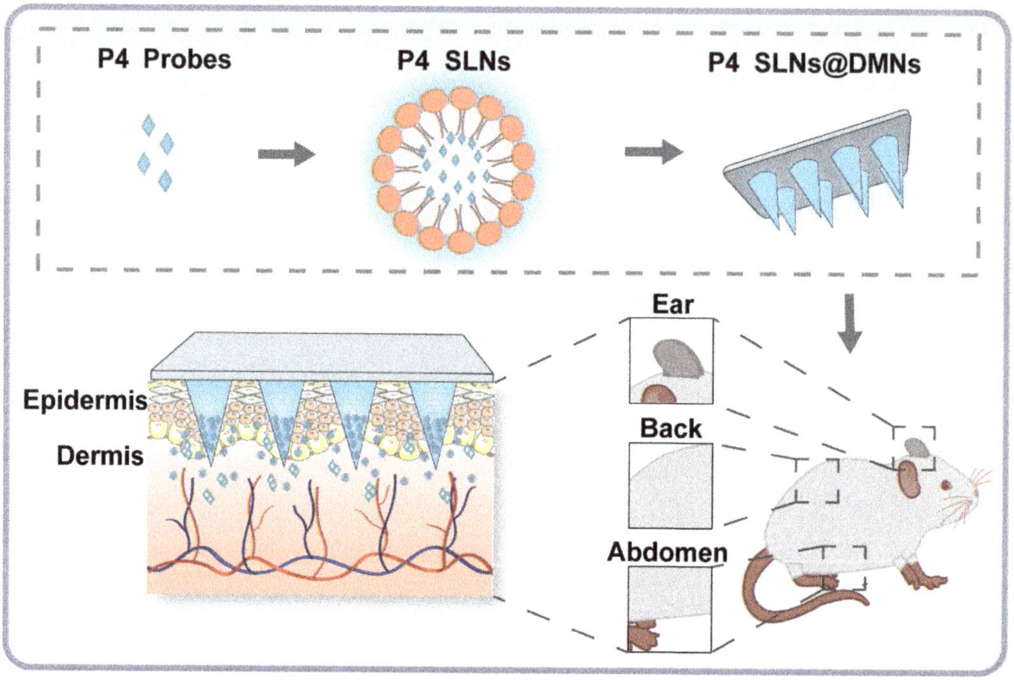


**Figure 1.** Schematic illustration of the research framework: Impact of different skin sites on in vivo fate of P4 SLNs@DMNs.

## 2. Materials and Methods

### *2.1. Materials*

The P4 probes were donated by Prof. Wei Wu's group from Fudan University (Shanghai, China). Gelatin, Tween 80 (T80), and Cetyl Palmitate (CP) were purchased from Aladdin Industrial, Inc. (Shanghai, China). Dichloromethane was acquired from Damao Chemical Reagent Factory (Tianjin, China). Polydimethylsiloxane (PDMS, Sylgard 184 Silicone Elastomer Kit) was obtained from Dow Corning Ltd. (Midland, MI, USA). Sodium hyaluronic acid (HA) (MW < 10 kDa) was supplied by Bloomage Freda Biopharm Co., Ltd. (Jinan, China). Polyvinyl pyrrolidone (PVP K90) was kindly provided by MBCHEM Ltd. (Monmouth Junction, NJ, USA).

### *2.2. Animals*

SD male rats (180–220 g) were supplied by Guangdong Medical Laboratory Animal Center (Guangzhou, China). During the experiment, rats were housed under standard conditions of 12-h light/dark cycles and with free access to food and water. All experiments were approved by the Laboratory Animals Ethics Committee of Sun Yat-sen University (Guangzhou, China). (Approval No. SYSU-IACUC-2022-001225).

### *2.3. Synthesis of P4 SLNs*

According to the previous study [22], P4 SLNs were prepared through an ultrasound approach. Briefly, 315 mg of CP was heated at 70 °C as the oil phase. At the same temperature, 210 mg of Tween 80 was mixed with 10.5 mL of ultrapure water, acting as the water phase. When CP was completely melted, 1 mL of P4 dichloromethane solution (40.4 μg/mL) was pipetted into the oil phase and stirred for 20 min to evaporate dichloromethane. Subsequently, the water phase was slowly added to the oil phase and stirred continuously at 70 °C for 45 min to form the primary emulsion. Then, the crude emulsion was sonicated for 6 min in an ice bath using an Ultrasonic Cell Disrupter (BI-LON-650Y, BILON Co., Ltd., Shanghai, China). P4 SLNs were ultimately produced after 45 min of churning in an ice bath.

### 2.4. Characterization of P4 SLNs

On days 0, 1, 3, 5, 7, and 10 following preparation, the mean particle size, polydispersity index (PDI), and zeta potential of P4 SLNs were examined using Malvern Zetasizer (Nano ZS90, Malvern Instruments Ltd., Worcestershire, UK). The samples were adequately diluted by 121 folds with ultrapure water before measurement. The fluorescence intensity change of P4 SLNs was measured using a fluorescence spectrometer (Fluoromax-4, HORIBA Ltd., Kyoto, Japan) at days 0, 1, 3, 5, 7, and 10 after preparation. The excitation/emission wavelengths of P4 were 620/660 nm, and the slit width was 4 nm. The stability of P4 SLNs was evaluated over ten days during the storage period. Transmission electron microscopy (TEM, JEM-1400Flash, JEOL Ltd., Tokyo, Japan) was used to observe the morphology of P4 SLNs. The samples were stained with phosphotungstic acid (1% *w*/*v*).

### 2.5. ACQ Property Verification of P4

#### 2.5.1. Water-Quenching Sensitivity

To verify the ACQ properties of the P4 probes, fluorescence emission spectra of P4 in water-acetonitrile co-solvent with 10–100% (*v*/*v*) water content were recorded by fluorescence spectrometer.

#### 2.5.2. Fluorescence Quenching in Biological Matrices

P4 SLNs were mixed with a 7-fold volume of phosphate-buffered saline, and homogenate of rat back, abdomen, and ear skin, respectively. The systems were incubated at 37 °C with a gas bath oscillator (TH2-82BA, Runhua Co., Ltd., Xinghua, China). At predetermined time intervals (2, 4, 6, 8, and 24 h), the fluorescence intensity was recorded by fluorescence spectrometer.

### 2.6. Fabrication and Characterization of P4 SLNs@DMNs

#### 2.6.1. Fabrication

The three-step centrifugation method, as described previously [34], was used to prepare P4 SLNs@DMNs. The female mold exhibited a hole depth of 800 μm, and it was filled with P4 SLNs suspension before being centrifuged at 4000× *g* rpm for 5 min at 4 °C and removing the excess P4 SLNs suspension. The female mold was centrifuged for 1 h under the same conditions and dried in a dryer for an additional night at room temperature. This process was carried out three times to increase the loading effectiveness of P4 SLNs in microneedles. Next, HA solution (400 mg/mL) was filled into the female mold under centrifugation at 4000× *g* rpm for 5 min at 4 °C. After removing the excess HA solution, 250 μL of PVP K90 solution (310 mg/mL) was poured, and centrifuged under the same condition to form the base part. Finally, the female mold was dried for 24 h at room temperature in a dryer, and then the P4 SLNs@DMNs were gently peeled off.

#### 2.6.2. Characterization

The distribution of P4 SLNs in DMNs was observed by confocal laser scanning microscopy (CLSM, LSM800, Carl Zeiss, Oberkochen, Germany). To evaluate the in vitro skin insertion ability, P4 SLNs@DMNs were pressed onto the excised back, abdomen, and ear skin obtained from SD rats for 2 min. After the DMNs were removed, the insertion sites were stained with 1% trypan blue and then imaged with a camera. Subsequently, the skin sites inserted by DMNs were fixed in 4% paraformaldehyde, embedded in paraffin, and then stained by hematoxylin and eosin (H&E). To simulate P4 SLNs@DMNs dissolution in vitro, the DMNs were inserted into the gelatin block with 35% water (*w/w*), and the morphology of DMNs after 10 min in the gelatin block was observed with a biomicroscope (BX53, OLYMPUS, Tokyo, Japan), and 3D fluorescence images were captured by CLSM. To evaluate the stability of P4 SLNs encapsulated into DMNs over ten days at storage period, P4 SLNs@DMNs were dissolved by ultrapure water at day ten after preparation and were observed by TEM. The fluorescence intensity change of dissolved P4 SLNs@DMNs dispersions was measured using a fluorescence spectrometer at days 0, 1, 3, 5, 7, and 10 after preparation. Triplicate measurements were performed for each sample.

### 2.7. In Vivo Live Imaging

Before the experiment, hair from the back, abdomen, and ear of SD rats was shaved off to avoid autofluorescence during imaging. After P4 SLNs@DMNs were inserted into the back, abdomen, and ear skin of rats, fluorescence was recorded using in vivo imaging system (IVIS, Lumina Series III, PerkinElmer, Waltham, Massachusetts, America) at predetermined time points (0.5, 2, 4, 8, 12, and 24 h) under excitation/emission wavelengths of 640/710 nm. Fluorescence signals were quantified by region of interest (ROI) analysis and normalized for comparison. Pharmacokinetic analysis was then performed to calculate half-life ($T_{1/2}$) and area under the curve ($AUC_{0\text{–}t}$). The rats were imaged under anesthesia with isoflurane.

### 2.8. Ex Vivo Imaging

The diffusion behavior of P4 SLNs delivered via different skin sites by DMNs was determined by CLSM. After P4 SLNs@DMNs were inserted into the skin of the back, abdomen, and ear of rats for 4 h, the skin of rats in different site administration groups was collected. The collected skin was then analyzed by 3D reconstruction using CLSM at a magnification of 20×. In addition, three rats were sacrificed in each group at 4, 12, and 24 h post-administration, and the major organs, such as the heart, liver, kidney, spleen, and lungs were collected and imaged by the IVIS system.

### 2.9. Statistical Analysis

All data are expressed as the mean ± standard deviation (SD) from multiple independent experiments, and statistical analysis was performed using one-way analysis of variance (ANOVA) via GraphPad Prism (version 8.02, GraphPad Software LLC., San Diego, CA, USA). The $p$-value < 0.05 was considered to be statistically significant.

## 3. Results

### 3.1. Preparation and Characterization of P4 SLNs

P4 SLNs were fabricated through an ultrasound method. The average hydrodynamic diameter of P4 SLNs was approximately 154 nm (Figure 2A). TEM image further demonstrated uniform particle size and spherical shape of P4 SLNs (Figure 2A). During the 10-day storage period, the particle size of P4 SLNs remained essentially unchanged, around about 150 nm, and the PDI was below 0.2 (Figure 2B). The color of the P4 SLNs solution did not change, and no aggregation and sedimentation of nanoparticles were observed (Figure 2C). In addition, the zeta potential and fluorescence intensity of P4 SLNs did not change significantly within ten days (Figure 2D,E). These results indicated the excellent compatibility of P4 probes with SLNs, and fluorescence quenching did not occur for P4 probes loaded in SLNs during storage.

### 3.2. ACQ Property Verification of P4

The photophysical properties and ACQ properties of the P4 probes were investigated to confirm their feasibility in bioimaging (Figure S1A–C). Figure S1A,B show the contour fluorescence spectra and fluorescence emission spectra of P4 probes, respectively. It demonstrated that the maximum excitation and emission wavelength of P4 probes were 640 nm and 660 nm, respectively, which is similar to the previous study [26]. As shown in

Figure S1C, the fluorescence emission intensities of P4 decreased as the proportion of water content increased. In particular, when the proportion of water reached 90% ($v/v$, turning point) or higher, only the baseline signal was detected in the spectrum. These results indicated that the P4 probes underwent complete quenching in the biological environment (e.g., skin tissue fluid) with nearly 100% water content.

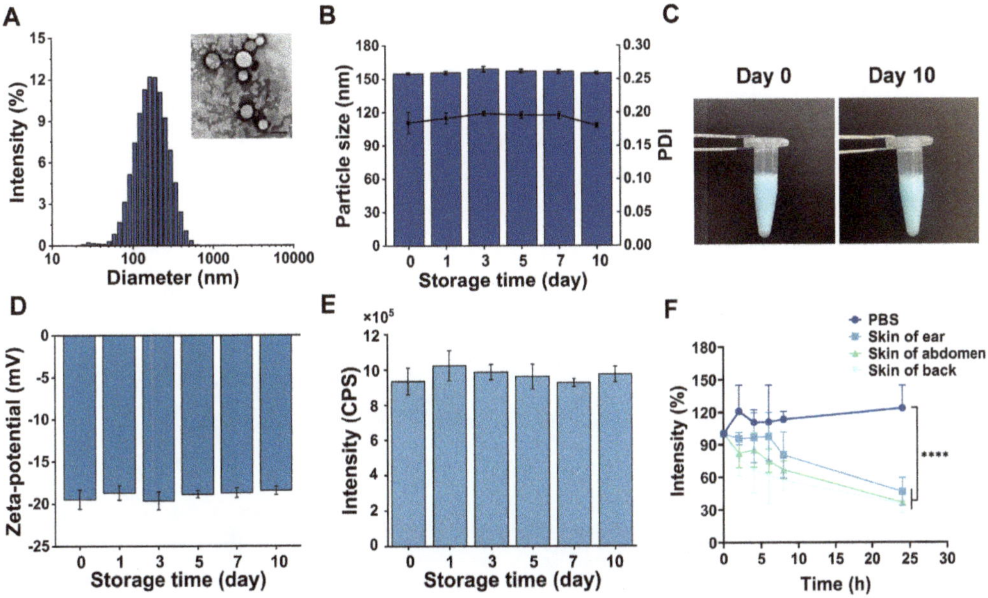


**Figure 2.** Preparation and characterization of P4 SLNs. (**A**) Particle size distribution and TEM image of P4 SLNs (scale bar: 200 nm). (**B**) Stability of the averaged particle size and PDI of P4 SLNs ($n$ = 3). (**C**) The appearance of P4 SLNs before and after ten days. (**D**) Stability of zeta potential of P4 SLNs ($n$ = 3). (**E**) Peak values of emission spectra of P4 SLNs over ten days ($n$ = 3). (**F**) Fluorescence quenching of P4 SLNs in biological matrices ($n$ = 3). Data are expressed as mean ± SD. Note: **** denotes $p < 0.0001$ vs. group of PBS.

To further investigate the quenching behavior of P4 SLNs in skin tissue fluid, P4 SLNs were co-incubated with homogenates from different parts of the rat skin (Figure 2F). The fluorescence intensity of P4 SLNs co-incubated with different skin homogenates significantly reduced compared to PBS. It was possibly due to the degradation of P4 SLNs by enzymes in the skin tissue fluid leading to the subsequent release of P4, which resulted in fluorescence quenching. At 24 h, the fluorescence intensity of the back, abdomen, and ear skin homogenate groups decreased to 35%, 36%, and 45%, respectively. In contrast, the fluorescence intensity of the PBS group showed essentially no decrease. As shown in Figure S2, when the P4 solution was incubated with phosphate-buffered saline solution, the fluorescence signal of the P4 solution group almost completely disappeared at 0.5 h. Hence, the results indicated that SLNs could be degraded by biological matrices such as skin tissue fluids, resulting in the ACQ phenomenon of P4.

### *3.3. Fabrication and Characterization of P4 SLNs@DMNs*

In order to improve the loading rate of P4 SLNs in DMNs, this study used multiple centrifugation steps to enrich P4 SLNs at the tip of the needle, as described in our previous study [34] (Figure 3A). The DMNs patch consisted of 144 needles (12 × 12) with a height of 800 μm in the shape of a quadrilateral cone. The fluorescence images of P4 SLNs@DMNs

(Figure 3B) captured by CLSM depicted that the P4 SLNs were mainly concentrated in the tips of needles.

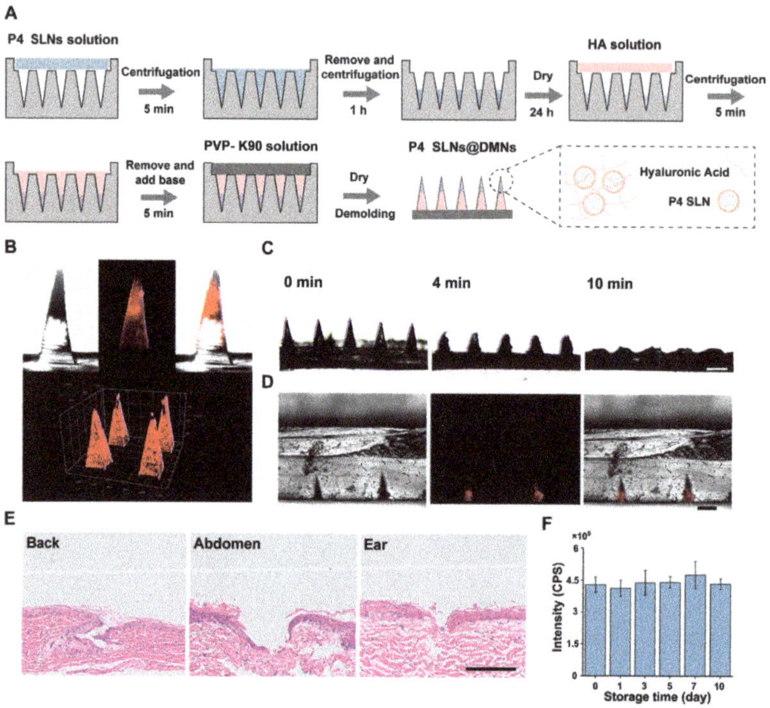


**Figure 3.** Preparation and characterization of P4 SLNs@DMNs. (**A**) Scheme of preparation process of P4 SLNs@DMNs. (**B**) The fluorescence images of P4 SLNs@DMNs (scale bar: 200 μm). (**C**) Optical microscopy images of P4 SLN@DMNs before and after insertion into gelatin (scale bar: 500 μm). (**D**) The fluorescence images of gelatin block after insertion of P4 SLNs@DMNs for 10 min (scale bar: 200 μm). (**E**) The histological section of back, abdomen, and ear skin of rats after P4 SLNs@DMNs application (scale bar: 100 μm) (**F**) Peak values of emission spectra of dissolved P4 SLNs@DMNs dispersions within ten days ($n$ = 3). Data are expressed as mean ± SD.

To assess the dissolution behavior of P4 SLNs@DMNs, a DMNs patch was inserted into a gelatin block with a similar level of hydration to that of the skin stratum corneum [35] and removed at predetermined time points. The side view of the microscope in Figure 3C shows that the P4 SLN@DMNs could dissolve completely within 10 min. Figure 3D shows the fluorescence image of P4 SLNs remaining in the gelatin block after the removal of the base of DMNs. These results demonstrated that the DMNs were able to penetrate the gelatin block and dissolve rapidly and deliver the P4 SLNs inside the gelatin block.

### *3.4. Insertion Ability of P4 SLNs@DMNs*

The photograph after trypan blue staining (Figure S3A) and H&E-stained section (Figure 3E) of the skin after insertion with DMNs show that DMNs patch could form microchannels in rat skin. These results demonstrated that DMNs could successfully penetrate the epidermis of different parts of the rat skin, which was the prerequisite to the study of the fate of NC delivered in vivo by DMNs. Taken together, DMNs have been demonstrated to be mechanically strong enough to pierce the skin and subsequently dissolve rapidly through the skin tissue fluid, allowing for effective delivery of P4 SLNs.

### 3.5. Stability of P4 SLNs@DMNs

We investigated the stability of P4 SLNs@DMNs to ensure that the physicochemical properties of P4 SLNs did not change after they were loaded into DMNs. As shown in Figure S3B, no significant change in the morphology of P4 SLNs@DMNs was observed over ten days. TEM image showed a slight increase in particle size after P4 SLNs were loaded into DMNs (Figure S3C), probably due to HA adhesion to its surface, which did not affect the property of P4 SLNs themselves.

Moreover, the fluorescence intensity of dissolved P4 SLNs@DMNs suspension was measured during the 10-day storage period. As indicated in Figure 3F, the fluorescence intensity of P4 within P4 SLNs@DMNs was still maintained unaltered during storage for ten days. In general, the prepared DMNs exhibited superior stability and would not alter the structure and fluorescence properties of the encapsulated P4 SLNs.

### 3.6. In Vivo Live Imaging

The diffusion rate of P4 SLNs delivered via different skin sites by DMNs was monitored by the IVIS system in rats. Figure 4A shows the live images of rats treated with P4 SLNs@DMNs at different skin sites. In the group without any treatment on the skin of the back, abdomen, and ear, no fluorescent signal associated with the P4 probe was detected (Figure S4). Over time, the fluorescence intensity indicated by the retention of P4 SLNs in different parts of the rat skin gradually decreased (Figure 4B–D), associated with particle diffusion. The results of live imaging implied differences in the retention profile of P4 SLNs in the rats.

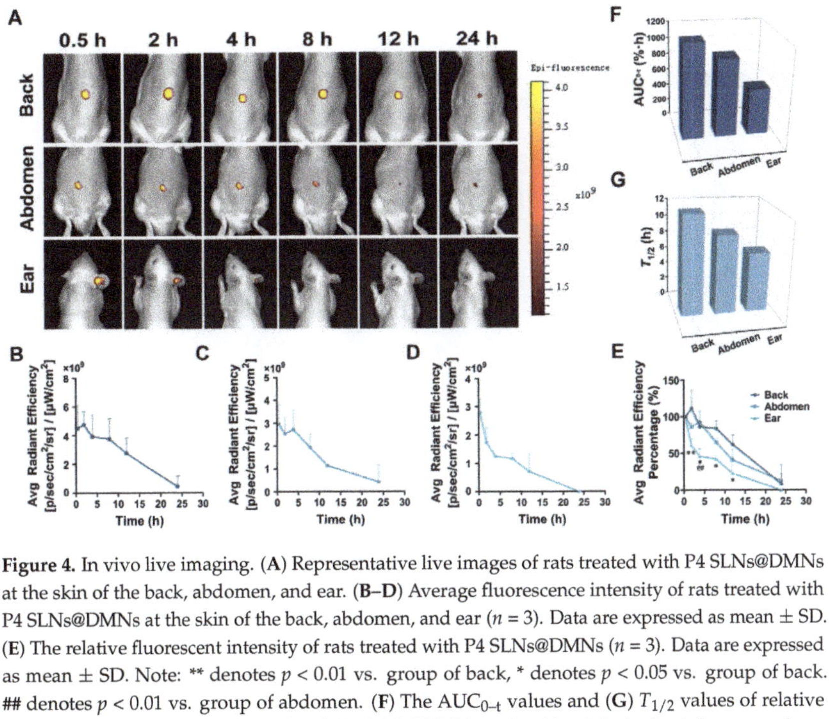

**Figure 4.** In vivo live imaging. (**A**) Representative live images of rats treated with P4 SLNs@DMNs at the skin of the back, abdomen, and ear. (**B–D**) Average fluorescence intensity of rats treated with P4 SLNs@DMNs at the skin of the back, abdomen, and ear ($n$ = 3). Data are expressed as mean ± SD. (**E**) The relative fluorescent intensity of rats treated with P4 SLNs@DMNs ($n$ = 3). Data are expressed as mean ± SD. Note: ** denotes $p < 0.01$ vs. group of back, * denotes $p < 0.05$ vs. group of back. ## denotes $p < 0.01$ vs. group of abdomen. (**F**) The $AUC_{0\text{-}t}$ values and (**G**) $T_{1/2}$ values of relative fluorescent intensity of rats treated with P4 SLNs@DMNs at the skin of the back, abdomen, and ear.

The fluorescence intensity measured at different time points for each group was normalized to the fluorescence intensity of the first time point (0.5 h) and assigned an intensity value of 100%. Plotting the fluorescence intensity over time showed a significant decreasing trend for all groups (Figure 4E). After 8 h of administration, the percentage of fluorescence intensity decreased to 83.72 ± 0.10%, 65.07 ± 0.06%, and 41.92 ± 0.04% for back, abdomen, and ear skin, respectively. The rate of decrease in relative fluorescence intensity was in the order of ear > abdomen > back. Furthermore, within 24 h, the $AUC_{0-t}$ values of the back, abdomen, and ear were 1146.40%·h, 952.16%·h, and 560.99%·h, respectively (Figure 4F). The $T_{1/2}$ values of the back, abdomen and ear were calculated to be 11.85 h, 9.39 h, and 7.08 h, respectively (Figure 4G).

### 3.7. Ex Vivo Imaging

To visualize the diffusion rate of P4 SLNs, CLSM was used to observe the diffusion of P4 SLNs after treatment at different sites in rats. As shown in Figure 5A, the group of back remained high fluorescence after 4 h of administration, implying that P4 SLNs maintained a certain degree of integrity. In contrast, the group of ear exhibited weaker fluorescence, indicating that most of the P4 SLNs were degraded after 4 h of administration, resulting in P4 leakage and quenching of fluorescence. Moreover, compared to the group of abdomen and ear, the group of the back could observe the fluorescent signal deepening in the skin after 4 h of administration by DMNs. The retention of fluorescence signal was in the order of back > abdomen > ear. Furthermore, the fluorescent signal of the back could be detected at a deeper level of the skin. The maximum skin depth of fluorescent signals detected in the back, abdomen, and ear were 140 μm, 120 μm, and 100 μm, respectively. In addition, almost no fluorescence signal was detected in major organs such as the heart, liver, spleen, lung, and kidney after 4, 12, and 24 h of administration with P4 SLNs@DMNs (Figure 5B). Moreover, there was still no fluorescent signal of skin and organs observed in the group without any treatment (Figure S5A,B).

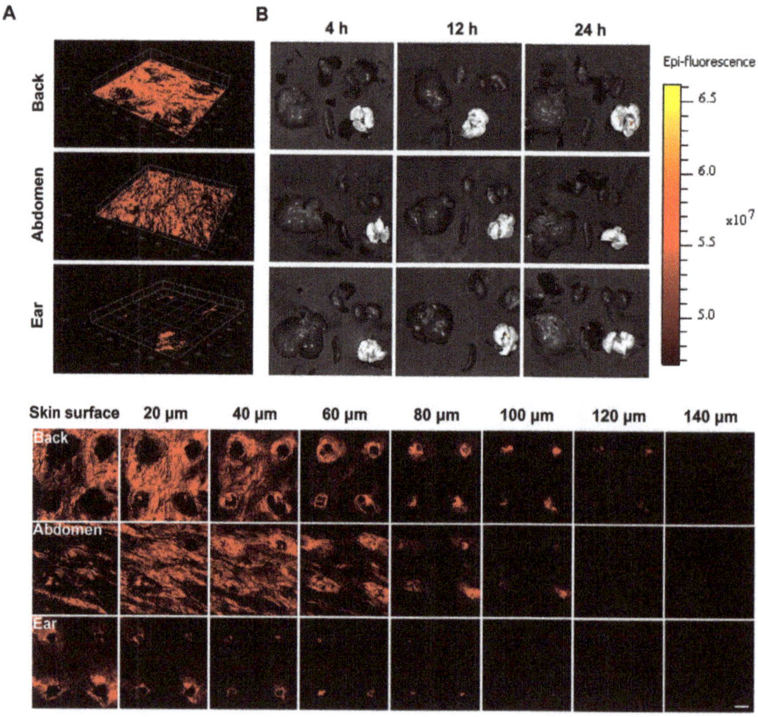


**Figure 5.** Ex vivo imaging. (**A**) Representative CLSM 3D reconstruction images (up) and 2D fluorescent images (down) of the skin of the back, abdomen, and ear of rats after being treated with P4 SLNs@DMNs at 4 h (scale bar: 100 μm). (**B**) Representative fluorescent images of major organs after being treated with P4 SLNs@DMNs at 4, 12, and 24 h.

## 4. Discussion

In the past few decades, the rapid development of pharmaceutical and material technology has made it possible to combine DMNs with novel NC, and the combination of the two has significantly broadened the application of TDD and demonstrated significant efficacy in various disease models [36–38]. However, there are few products of NC-loaded DMNs currently on the market, and they still face many challenges in practical application. First, there are a limited number of studies concerning in vivo fate of NC-loaded DMNs. Moreover, in previous studies [39,40], the fluorescent signals detected were a mixture of NC and free probes, which could not represent intact NC and did not accurately elucidate the in vivo fate of NC. Thus, there is an urgent need for a reliable bioimaging tool for holistic identification and accurate detection of NC to facilitate the clinical translation of NC-loaded DMNs. Second, current studies [26,28,41] on the in vivo fate of NC have focused more on the delivery system itself, ignoring the influence of the complex biological environment. The skin is the largest organ of the body, and the sites of DMNs application may affect the in vivo fate of NC-loaded DMNs, mainly because at different skin sites: (1) Different thicknesses of the epidermis and dermis meant that the area where the needle tips enter the dermis after insertion of DMNs was different; (2) Different classes of cells and matrices in the dermal region implied different interactions with NC; (3) Different mechanical strength meant different shear forces on the DMNs [23]. The above factors might mutually affect the transdermal absorption rate of NC-loaded DMNs, and it was necessary to investigate the role of the site of administration on the fate of NC in vivo. Based on this rationale, we chose P4 probes with ACQ effect as a bioimaging tool for in vivo fate of intact NC. Moreover, we constructed P4 SLNs@DMNs that were applied to the back, abdomen, and ear skin of rats, respectively, to investigate the effects of different skin sites on the in vivo fate of P4 SLNs@DMNs (Figure 1).

Based on the previous study of our group [34], we have prepared SLNs@DMNs systems with excellent biocompatibility and safety. Furthermore, we have demonstrated the storage stability of P4 SLNs through experiments (Figure 2B–E). During the storage period, the particle size, PDI, and fluorescence intensity of P4 SLNs did not change significantly. In addition, the fluorescence quenching occurred when P4 probes loaded into SLNs were exposed to biological matrices (Figure 2F), which not only validated the ACQ properties of P4 probes but also demonstrated the feasibility of P4 probes in bioimaging. Furthermore, we also investigated the physicochemical properties of P4 SLNs@DMNs. The results showed that the morphology of the microneedles was intact, P4 SLN was mainly distributed at the needle tip (Figure 3B,C), and the microneedles had good puncture ability and stability (Figure 3D–F), which ensured the effective transdermal delivery of P4 SLN.

In the in vivo live imaging study (Figure 4A), we found significant differences in the diffusion rates of SLNs loaded in DMNs applied at different sites, and the order of the rate of diffusion was as follows: ear > abdomen > back. The application of P4 SLNs@DMNs to the back resulted in higher $AUC_{0\text{–}t}$ and $T_{1/2}$, while the application to the ear resulted in the lowest $AUC_{0\text{–}t}$ and $T_{1/2}$ (Figure 4F,G), which is consistent with the previous findings [42]. A reasonable explanation is that ear has the thinnest thickness of the stratum corneum, the least number of cell layers, and the lowest elastic properties compared to the back and abdomen [43,44], and thus SLNs are more likely to enter the dermal region of the ear. Moreover, the capillaries are most abundant in the dermal region of the ear compared to the back and abdomen [45], and therefore, SLNs are more likely to enter the body's circulation through the capillaries. In the ex vivo imaging study of rat skin (Figure 5A), we found that the most fluorescence remained in the back skin after 4 h of application with P4 SLNs@DMNs, while the fluorescence signal in the ear almost disappeared. This is similar to the trend of fluorescence reduction in the in vivo live imaging study. These results suggest that SLNs are more likely to accumulate in thicker skin areas.

In addition, no strong fluorescent signal was detected in the major organs after applying P4 SLNs@DMNs to different skin sites (Figure 5B), and there was almost no distribution of integrated SLNs in the major organs. It seems to indicate that most NC are degraded after entering the body circulation via DMNs administration, which further suggests that the target-modified ligands may be lost, and perhaps off-target effects may occur after the administration of target-modified NCs-loaded DMNs. Therefore, more attention should be paid when designing NCs-loaded DMNs.

In general, our results have implications for the selection of transdermal delivery sites for the therapy of different diseases (Figure 6). For example, for chronic diseases in which patients require long-term medication, such as hypertension, diabetes, rheumatoid arthritis, etc., perhaps the application of NC-loaded DMNs via the thicker skin areas of the back and forearm is an option to consider. Instead, for acute diseases, in which the drug needs to work quickly, such as motion sickness, coronary heart disease, acute pains, etc., the skin of the posterior auricle and forehead, which are rich in capillaries, is ideal [46,47]. Overall, the difference in NC-loaded DMNs diffusion rates observed at different sites of the skin can provide a theoretical basis for the design of selective therapies. What is more, it indicates the importance of clearly defining the site of administration for different indications during the formulation development process, and relevant standard operating procedures or clinical practices should be put forward, and then the therapeutic effect could be maximized. We also suggest that when the product of NC-loaded DMNs is launched in the future, the site of administration could be specified in the instructions in order to improve the treatment effect of patients.

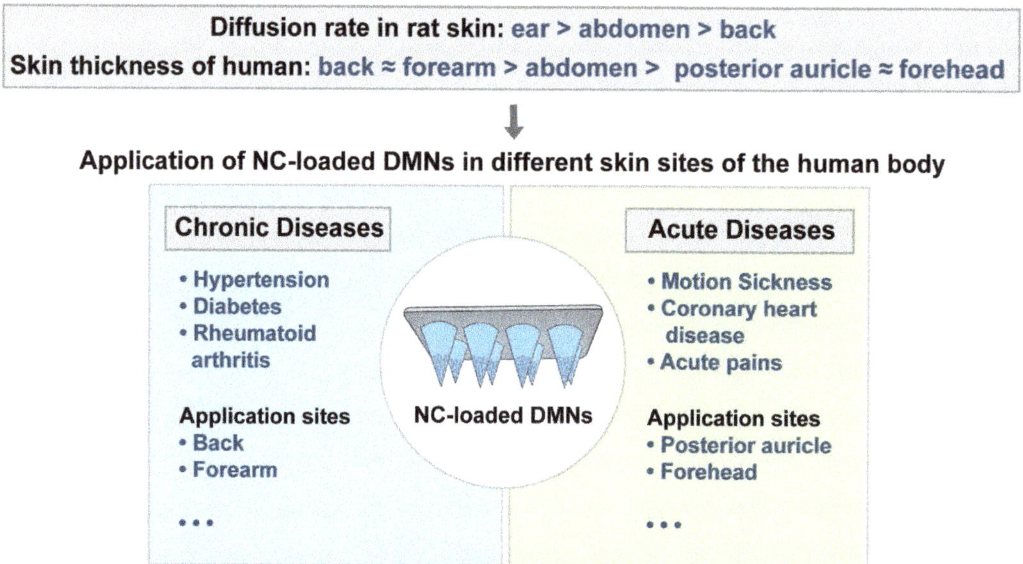


**Figure 6.** Potential application of NC-loaded DMNs at different skin sites.

In conclusion, different skin sites are important factors influencing the fate of transdermal delivery of NC-loaded DMNs. Apart from differences between sites, skin varies in different disease conditions (such as psoriasis, proliferative scarring, and subcutaneous tumors) and even in people of different ages and genders [23,48,49]. Therefore, the in vivo fate of NCs loaded in DMNs needs to be further investigated in such different cases. Furthermore, our study mainly analyzed the transdermal delivery efficiency of NC-loaded DMNs at different skin sites from a macroscopic perspective. We will expand our study to explore the interactions between NC-loaded DMNs and different skin tissue cells from a microscopic perspective in ongoing studies.

## 5. Conclusions

In this study, P4 SLNs@DMNs with good stability was successfully constructed, which exhibited the good compatibility of SLNs with DMNs. Moreover, DMNs could effectively pierce different sites of rat skin, followed by the rapid dissolution and release of the loaded SLNs. The results of in vivo live imaging and ex vivo imaging showed that the order of the rate of diffusion was as follows: ear > abdomen > back, and NCs were more likely to accumulate in the back skin. Therefore, the appropriate site of drug delivery can be selected according to the rate and maintenance time of drug onset required for different diseases. These findings can provide a strong theoretical basis for the clinical application of NC-loaded DMNs. In addition, the effects of skin in different disease states, different ages, and genders on the in vivo fate of NC-loaded DMNs should be further explored to promote clinical translation.

**Supplementary Materials:** The following supporting information can be downloaded at: https://www.mdpi.com/article/10.3390/pharmaceutics15010169/s1, Figure S1: (A) Fluorescence emission contour map of P4 probes. (B) The fluorescence emission spectrum of P4 probes. (C) Fluorescence emission spectra (left) and peak intensity transition (right) of P4 probes in water-acetonitrile co-solvent with 10–100% ($v/v$) water content. Figure S2: Fluorescence intensity of P4 and P4 SLNs incubated with phosphate-buffered saline solution for 0.5 h, respectively ($n = 3$). Data are expressed as mean ± SD. Figure S3: (A) The photographs of the skin by trypan blue staining (up) and the base of DMNs (down) after inserting with P4 SLNs@DMNs. (B) The appearance of P4 SLNs@DMNs before and after ten days. (C) TEM image of dissolved P4 SLNs from P4 SLNs@DMNs (scale bar: 200 nm). Figure S4: In vivo live imaging. Representative live images of rats without any treatment. Figure S5: Ex vivo imaging. (A) Representative CLSM 3D reconstruction images of the skin of the back, abdomen, and ear without any treatment at 4 h. (B) Representative fluorescent images of major organs without any treatment at 4 h.

**Author Contributions:** Conceptualization, Y.F., Q.W., Z.H. and G.Q.; Data curation, Y.F. and C.S.; Formal analysis, Y.F., C.S., X.L. and T.W.; Funding acquisition, Q.W., Z.H. and G.Q.; Investigation, Y.F., C.S., X.L. and A.Z.; Methodology, Y.F., C.S., X.L. and T.W.; Project administration, P.H., C.W., X.P., Z.H. and G.Q.; Resources, Q.W., P.H., C.W. and X.P.; Software, Y.F., C.S., X.L. and T.W.; Supervision, C.W., X.P., Z.H. and G.Q.; Validation, C.S., T.W. and A.Z.; Visualization, Y.F., X.L. and A.Z.; Writing—original draft, Y.F.; Writing—review & editing, P.H., Z.H. and G.Q. All authors have read and agreed to the published version of the manuscript.

**Funding:** This work was supported by the National Natural Science Foundation of China [Grant No. 82104070, 82173747], and the Guangzhou Science and Technology Plan Project [Grant No. 202201010589, 202102020635, 202102080535].

**Institutional Review Board Statement:** All the experimental procedures were approved by the Institutional Animal Care and Use Committee of Sun Yat-sen University in accordance with the National Institute of Health and Nutrition Guidelines for the care and use of laboratory animals (Approval No. SYSU-IACUC-2022-001225).

**Informed Consent Statement:** Not applicable.

**Data Availability Statement:** Not applicable.

**Acknowledgments:** The authors would like to thank Wei Wu's group at Fudan University for the donation of P4 probes.

**Conflicts of Interest:** The authors declare no conflict of interest.

## References

1. Ranade, V.V. Drug delivery systems. 6. Transdermal drug delivery. *J. Clin. Pharmacol.* **1991**, *31*, 401–418. [CrossRef] [PubMed]
2. Lee, H.; Song, C.; Baik, S.; Kim, D.; Hyeon, T.; Kim, D.-H. Device-assisted transdermal drug delivery. *Adv. Drug Deliv. Rev.* **2018**, *127*, 35–45. [CrossRef] [PubMed]
3. Prausnitz, M.R.; Langer, R. Transdermal drug delivery. *Nat. Biotechnol.* **2008**, *26*, 1261–1268. [CrossRef] [PubMed]
4. Benson, H.A. Transdermal drug delivery: Penetration enhancement techniques. *Curr. Drug Deliv.* **2005**, *2*, 23–33. [CrossRef]

5. Phatale, V.; Vaiphei, K.K.; Jha, S.; Patil, D.; Agrawal, M.; Alexander, A. Overcoming skin barriers through advanced transdermal drug delivery approaches. *J. Control. Release* **2022**, *351*, 361–380. [CrossRef]
6. Jeong, W.Y.; Kwon, M.; Choi, H.E.; Kim, K.S. Recent advances in transdermal drug delivery systems: A review. *Biomater. Res.* **2021**, *25*, 24. [CrossRef]
7. Indermun, S.; Luttge, R.; Choonara, Y.E.; Kumar, P.; du Toit, L.C.; Modi, G.; Pillay, V. Current advances in the fabrication of microneedles for transdermal delivery. *J. Control. Release* **2014**, *185*, 130–138. [CrossRef]
8. Zhang, L.; Guo, R.; Wang, S.; Yang, X.; Ling, G.; Zhang, P. Fabrication, evaluation and applications of dissolving microneedles. *Int. J. Pharm.* **2021**, *604*, 120749. [CrossRef]
9. Chen, M.; Yang, D.; Sun, Y.; Liu, T.; Wang, W.; Fu, J.; Wang, Q.; Bai, X.; Quan, G.; Pan, X.; et al. In Situ Self-Assembly Nanomicelle Microneedles for Enhanced Photoimmunotherapy via Autophagy Regulation Strategy. *ACS Nano* **2021**, *15*, 3387–3401. [CrossRef]
10. Kim, N.W.; Kim, S.-Y.; Lee, J.E.; Yin, Y.; Lee, J.H.; Lim, S.Y.; Kim, E.S.; Duong, H.T.T.; Kim, H.K.; Kim, S.; et al. Enhanced Cancer Vaccination by In Situ Nanomicelle-Generating Dissolving Microneedles. *ACS Nano* **2018**, *12*, 9702–9713. [CrossRef]
11. Ling, M.-H.; Chen, M.-C. Dissolving polymer microneedle patches for rapid and efficient transdermal delivery of insulin to diabetic rats. *Acta Biomater.* **2013**, *9*, 8952–8961. [CrossRef] [PubMed]
12. Wan, T.; Pan, Q.; Ping, Y. Microneedle-assisted genome editing: A transdermal strategy of targeting NLRP3 by CRISPR-Cas9 for synergistic therapy of inflammatory skin disorders. *Sci. Adv.* **2021**, *7*, eabe2888. [CrossRef]
13. Chen, M.; Quan, G.; Sun, Y.; Yang, D.; Pan, X.; Wu, C. Nanoparticles-encapsulated polymeric microneedles for transdermal drug delivery. *J. Control. Release* **2020**, *325*, 163–175. [CrossRef] [PubMed]
14. Qu, F.; Geng, R.; Liu, Y.; Zhu, J. Advanced nanocarrier- and microneedle-based transdermal drug delivery strategies for skin diseases treatment. *Theranostics* **2022**, *12*, 3372–3406. [CrossRef]
15. Ventola, C.L. The nanomedicine revolution: Part 1: Emerging concepts. *P T Peer-Rev. J. Formul. Manag.* **2012**, *37*, 582–591.
16. Yoon, H.J.; Lee, H.S.; Jung, J.H.; Kim, H.K.; Park, J.H. Photothermally Amplified Therapeutic Liposomes for Effective Combination Treatment of Cancer. *ACS Appl. Mater. Interfaces* **2018**, *10*, 6118–6123. [CrossRef]
17. Fathy Abd-Ellatef, G.-E.; Gazzano, E.; Chirio, D.; Ragab Hamed, A.; Belisario, D.C.; Zuddas, C.; Peira, E.; Rolando, B.; Kopecka, J.; Assem Said Marie, M.; et al. Curcumin-Loaded Solid Lipid Nanoparticles Bypass P-Glycoprotein Mediated Doxorubicin Resistance in Triple Negative Breast Cancer Cells. *Pharmaceutics* **2020**, *12*, 96. [CrossRef]
18. Wen, T.; Lin, Z.; Zhao, Y.; Zhou, Y.; Niu, B.; Shi, C.; Lu, C.; Wen, X.; Zhang, M.; Quan, G.; et al. Bioresponsive Nanoarchitectonics-Integrated Microneedles for Amplified Chemo-Photodynamic Therapy against Acne Vulgaris. *ACS Appl. Mater. Interfaces* **2021**, *13*, 48433–48448. [CrossRef]
19. Espinosa, A.; Reguera, J.; Curcio, A.; Muñoz-Noval, Á.; Kuttner, C.; Van de Walle, A.; Liz-Marzán, L.M.; Wilhelm, C. Janus Magnetic-Plasmonic Nanoparticles for Magnetically Guided and Thermally Activated Cancer Therapy. *Small* **2020**, *16*, 1904960. [CrossRef]
20. Faridi Esfanjani, A.; Assadpour, E.; Jafari, S.M. Improving the bioavailability of phenolic compounds by loading them within lipid-based nanocarriers. *Trends Food Sci. Technol.* **2018**, *76*, 56–66. [CrossRef]
21. Lee, J.H.; Yeo, Y. Controlled drug release from pharmaceutical nanocarriers. *Chem. Eng. Sci.* **2015**, *125*, 75–84. [CrossRef] [PubMed]
22. Shi, C.; Yang, D.; Zhao, Y.; Wen, T.; Zhao, W.; Hu, P.; Huang, Z.; Quan, G.; Wu, C.; Pan, X. The spatial-dimensional and temporal-dimensional fate of nanocarrier-loaded dissolving microneedles with different lengths of needles. *Med. Drug Discov.* **2022**, *14*, 100124. [CrossRef]
23. Darlenski, R.; Fluhr, J.W. Influence of skin type, race, sex, and anatomic location on epidermal barrier function. *Clin. Dermatol.* **2012**, *30*, 269–273. [CrossRef] [PubMed]
24. Yaghmur, A.; Mu, H. Recent advances in drug delivery applications of cubosomes, hexosomes, and solid lipid nanoparticles. *Acta Pharm. Sin. B* **2021**, *11*, 871–885. [CrossRef] [PubMed]
25. Bouchaala, R.; Mercier, L.; Andreiuk, B.; Mély, Y.; Vandamme, T.; Anton, N.; Goetz, J.G.; Klymchenko, A.S. Integrity of lipid nanocarriers in bloodstream and tumor quantified by near-infrared ratiometric FRET imaging in living mice. *J. Control. Release* **2016**, *236*, 57–67. [CrossRef]
26. Xia, F.; Fan, W.F.; Jiang, S.F.; Ma, Y.H.; Lu, Y.; Qi, J.P.; Ahmad, E.; Dong, X.C.; Zhao, W.L.; Wu, W. Size-Dependent Translocation of Nanoemulsions via Oral Delivery. *ACS Appl. Mater. Interfaces* **2017**, *9*, 21660–21672. [CrossRef]
27. Wang, Y.; Zhang, Y.; Wang, J.; Liang, X.J. Aggregation-induced emission (AIE) fluorophores as imaging tools to trace the biological fate of nano-based drug delivery systems. *Adv. Drug Deliv. Rev.* **2019**, *143*, 161–176. [CrossRef]
28. Huang, Z.; Huang, Y.; Wang, W.; Fu, F.; Wang, W.; Dang, S.; Li, C.; Ma, C.; Zhang, X.; Zhao, Z.; et al. Relationship between particle size and lung retention time of intact solid lipid nanoparticle suspensions after pulmonary delivery. *J. Control. Release* **2020**, *325*, 206–222. [CrossRef]
29. Cai, Y.; Ji, X.; Zhang, Y.; Liu, C.; Zhang, Z.; Lv, Y.; Dong, X.; He, H.; Qi, J.; Lu, Y.; et al. Near-infrared fluorophores with absolute aggregation-caused quenching and negligible fluorescence re-illumination for in vivo bioimaging of nanocarriers. *Aggregate* **2022**, *3*, e277. [CrossRef]
30. Fan, W.; Peng, H.; Yu, Z.; Wang, L.; He, H.; Ma, Y.; Qi, J.; Lu, Y.; Wu, W. The long-circulating effect of pegylated nanoparticles revisited via simultaneous monitoring of both the drug payloads and nanocarriers. *Acta Pharm. Sin. B* **2022**, *12*, 2479–2493. [CrossRef]

31. Qi, J.; Hu, X.; Dong, X.; Lu, Y.; Lu, H.; Zhao, W.; Wu, W. Towards more accurate bioimaging of drug nanocarriers: Turning aggregation-caused quenching into a useful tool. *Adv. Drug Deliv. Rev.* **2019**, *143*, 206–225. [CrossRef] [PubMed]
32. He, H.; Liu, C.; Ming, J.; Lv, Y.; Qi, J.; Lu, Y.; Dong, X.; Zhao, W.; Wu, W. Accurate and sensitive probing of onset of micellization based on absolute aggregation-caused quenching effect. *Aggregate* **2022**, *3*, e163. [CrossRef]
33. Satapathy, M.K.; Yen, T.-L.; Jan, J.-S.; Tang, R.-D.; Wang, J.-Y.; Taliyan, R.; Yang, C.-H. Solid Lipid Nanoparticles (SLNs): An Advanced Drug Delivery System Targeting Brain through BBB. *Pharmaceutics* **2021**, *13*, 1183. [CrossRef] [PubMed]
34. Qin, W.; Quan, G.; Sun, Y.; Chen, M.; Yang, P.; Feng, D.; Wen, T.; Hu, X.; Pan, X.; Wu, C. Dissolving Microneedles with Spatiotemporally controlled pulsatile release Nanosystem for Synergistic Chemo-photothermal Therapy of Melanoma. *Theranostics* **2020**, *10*, 8179–8196. [CrossRef] [PubMed]
35. Amodwala, S.; Kumar, P.; Thakkar, H.P. Statistically optimized fast dissolving microneedle transdermal patch of meloxicam: A patient friendly approach to manage arthritis. *Eur. J. Pharm. Sci.* **2017**, *104*, 114–123. [CrossRef] [PubMed]
36. Zhang, Y.; Feng, P.; Yu, J.; Yang, J.; Zhao, J.; Wang, J.; Shen, Q.; Gu, Z. ROS-Responsive Microneedle Patch for Acne Vulgaris Treatment. *Adv. Ther.* **2018**, *1*, 1800035. [CrossRef]
37. Yang, P.; Lu, C.; Qin, W.; Chen, M.; Quan, G.; Liu, H.; Wang, L.; Bai, X.; Pan, X.; Wu, C. Construction of a core-shell microneedle system to achieve targeted co-delivery of checkpoint inhibitors for melanoma immunotherapy. *Acta Biomater.* **2020**, *104*, 147–157. [CrossRef]
38. Yang, G.; Chen, Q.; Wen, D.; Chen, Z.; Wang, J.; Chen, G.; Wang, Z.; Zhang, X.; Zhang, Y.; Hu, Q.; et al. A Therapeutic Microneedle Patch Made from Hair-Derived Keratin for Promoting Hair Regrowth. *ACS Nano* **2019**, *13*, 4354–4360. [CrossRef]
39. Kennedy, J.; Larrañeta, E.; McCrudden, M.T.C.; McCrudden, C.M.; Brady, A.J.; Fallows, S.J.; McCarthy, H.O.; Kissenpfennig, A.; Donnelly, R.F. In vivo studies investigating biodistribution of nanoparticle-encapsulated rhodamine B delivered via dissolving microneedles. *J. Control. Release* **2017**, *265*, 57–65. [CrossRef]
40. Hollis, C.P.; Weiss, H.L.; Leggas, M.; Evers, B.M.; Gemeinhart, R.A.; Li, T. Biodistribution and bioimaging studies of hybrid paclitaxel nanocrystals: Lessons learned of the EPR effect and image-guided drug delivery. *J. Control. Release* **2013**, *172*, 12–21. [CrossRef]
41. Cai, Y.; Qi, J.; Lu, Y.; He, H.; Wu, W. The in vivo fate of polymeric micelles. *Adv. Drug Deliv. Rev.* **2022**, *188*, 114463. [CrossRef]
42. Zhang, Y.T.; Han, M.Q.; Shen, L.N.; Zhao, J.H.; Feng, N.P. Solid lipid nanoparticles formulated for transdermal aconitine administration and evaluated in vitro and in vivo. *J. Biomed. Nanotechnol.* **2015**, *11*, 351–361. [CrossRef] [PubMed]
43. Holbrook, K.A.; Odland, G.F. Regional Differences in the Thickness (Cell Layers) of the Human Stratum Corneum: An Ultrastructural Analysis. *J. Investig. Dermatol.* **1974**, *62*, 415–422. [CrossRef] [PubMed]
44. Wei, J.C.J.; Edwards, G.A.; Martin, D.J.; Huang, H.; Crichton, M.L.; Kendall, M.A.F. Allometric scaling of skin thickness, elasticity, viscoelasticity to mass for micro-medical device translation: From mice, rats, rabbits, pigs to humans. *Sci. Rep.* **2017**, *7*, 15885. [CrossRef] [PubMed]
45. Landis, E.M. The Capillaries of the Skin: A Review. *J. Investig. Dermatol.* **1938**, *1*, 295–311. [CrossRef]
46. Bormann, J.L.; Maibach, H.I. Effects of anatomical location on in vivo percutaneous penetration in man. *Cutan. Ocul. Toxicol.* **2020**, *39*, 213–222. [CrossRef] [PubMed]
47. Maibach, H.I.; Feldmann, R.J.; Milby, T.H.; Serat, W.F. Regional Variation in Percutaneous Penetration in Man. *Arch. Environ. Health Int. J.* **1971**, *23*, 208–211. [CrossRef] [PubMed]
48. Man, M.Q.; Xin, S.J.; Song, S.P.; Cho, S.Y.; Zhang, X.J.; Tu, C.X.; Feingold, K.R.; Elias, P.M. Variation of Skin Surface pH, Sebum Content and Stratum Corneum Hydration with Age and Gender in a Large Chinese Population. *Ski. Pharmacol. Physiol.* **2009**, *22*, 190–199. [CrossRef]
49. Reed, J.T.; Ghadially, R.; Elias, P.M. Skin type, but neither race nor gender, influence epidermal permeability barrier function. *Arch. Dermatol.* **1995**, *131*, 1134–1138. [CrossRef]

pharmaceutics

MDPI

*Article*

# An Adjuvanted Inactivated SARS-CoV-2 Microparticulate Vaccine Delivered Using Microneedles Induces a Robust Immune Response in Vaccinated Mice

**Sharon Vijayanand [1], Smital Patil [1], Ipshita Menon [1], Keegan Braz Gomes [1], Akanksha Kale [1], Priyal Bagwe [1], Mohammad N. Uddin [1], Susu M. Zughaier [2,*] and Martin J. D'Souza [1]**

[1] Vaccine Nanotechnology Laboratory, Center for Drug Delivery and Research, College of Pharmacy, Mercer University, Atlanta, GA 30341, USA

[2] College of Medicine, QU Health, Qatar University, Doha P.O. Box 2713, Qatar

* Correspondence: szughaier@qu.edu.qa

**Abstract:** SARS-CoV-2, the causal agent of COVID-19, is a contagious respiratory virus that frequently mutates, giving rise to variant strains and leading to reduced vaccine efficacy against the variants. Frequent vaccination against the emerging variants may be necessary; thus, an efficient vaccination system is needed. A microneedle (MN) vaccine delivery system is non-invasive, patient-friendly, and can be self-administered. Here, we tested the immune response produced by an adjuvanted inactivated SARS-CoV-2 microparticulate vaccine administered via the transdermal route using a dissolving MN. The inactivated SARS-CoV-2 vaccine antigen and adjuvants (Alhydrogel® and AddaVax™) were encapsulated in poly(lactic-co-glycolic acid) (PLGA) polymer matrices. The resulting MP were approximately 910 nm in size, with a high percentage yield and percent encapsulation efficiency of 90.4%. In vitro, the vaccine MP was non-cytotoxic and increased the immunostimulatory activity measured as nitric oxide release from dendritic cells. The adjuvant MP potentiated the immune response of the vaccine MP in vitro. In vivo, the adjuvanted SARS-CoV-2 MP vaccine induced high levels of IgM, IgG, IgA, IgG1, and IgG2a antibodies and $CD4^+$ and $CD8^+$ T-cell responses in immunized mice. In conclusion, the adjuvanted inactivated SARS-CoV-2 MP vaccine delivered using MN induced a robust immune response in vaccinated mice.

**Keywords:** microneedles; microparticles; SARS-CoV-2; immunogenicity; cytotoxicity; antibody response; T-cell response

## 1. Introduction

Severe acute respiratory syndrome coronavirus-2 (SARS-CoV-2) infection causes COVID-19 in humans and has globally affected the health of individuals with over 1,083,2791 deaths in the United States alone (as of 20 December 2022) [1]. Vaccination against SARS-CoV-2 is the most effective tool used to protect against lower respiratory tract infection or severe disease caused by the virus [2]. Currently, several vaccines for COVID-19 have been approved for use in humans [3]. However, through mutations and immune evasion, SARS-CoV-2 and its variants remain a significant global threat [4]. Therefore, much like the flu shot, frequent vaccination against SARS-CoV-2 may be necessary. With routine immunizations, there is a lack of efficiency during mass vaccination, not to mention the burden on healthcare professionals to administer the vaccines. From a patient's perspective, individuals face several challenges while vaccinating. Individuals suffering from needle phobia refuse to vaccinate; needle injections are often painful and are not desired by older patients, young children, and toddlers. Therefore, an improvised and patient-friendly vaccination system that can maintain vaccine efficacy while being pain-free and efficient for mass vaccination and frequent immunization is highly desirable.

Recently, the microneedle (MN) system for vaccine delivery has gained much attention, as it is a non-invasive approach with the possibility of self-administration [5–7]. Such a versatile system for vaccine delivery is suitable for mass vaccination and frequent immunization and will positively influence the global vaccination rate. From an immunological standpoint, MN administration is advantageous, as the epidermal and dermal layers of the skin are enriched with Langerhans's cells and circulating dendritic cells that can readily recognize the vaccine antigen, thus activating an immune response [8–10]. Here, we explore the use of dissolving MN for administering an inactivated microparticulate SARS-CoV-2 vaccine. These dissolving MN are composed of biodegradable polymers, which are very safe for human use and dissolve within 5 min upon application to deliver the vaccine antigen.

When an inactivated virus vaccine is administered to an individual, the virus is presented as a whole to the immune system, resulting in a broader immune response [11]. SARS-CoV-2 consists of several structural proteins, including the spike (S) protein, membrane (M) protein, nucleoprotein (N), and envelope (E) protein [12,13]. Heat inactivation of the virus destroys the viral RNA, thus preventing the virus from replicating in the host cell while conserving the other structural proteins [14,15]. With relevance to SARS-CoV-2, when an inactivated vaccine is administered, the immune system may generate antibodies and cellular responses against the N protein, M protein, and E protein, in addition to the S protein [11,15,16]. Recent studies have shown that the SARS-CoV-2 variants predominantly harbor spike RBD mutations, resulting in reduced vaccine efficacy against the variants [17–19]. Therefore, a vaccine targeting different structural proteins may be more efficacious against the emerging variants [20–23]. However, to generate responses against the other structural proteins, all the proteins must be presented to the immune system without being degraded or destroyed by the tissue fluids upon vaccine administration [24]. Here, we propose a microparticulate vaccine delivery system encapsulating the inactivated SARS-CoV-2 virus in a polymer matrix.

Encapsulating the vaccine antigen in a biodegradable polymer matrix protects it by providing sustained release, thereby preventing antigen degradation by enzymes in the tissue fluids [25–27]. Microparticulate vaccines have also been reported to be better taken up by the circulating dendritic cells (DCs), resulting in more significant translocation to immune organs (draining lymph nodes and spleen) and allowing for increased antigen presentation to the T-cells [28–31]. In contrast to microparticulate antigens, antigens in the suspension form are smaller in size and are less immunogenic. Therefore, they are poorly recognized and are rapidly cleared by the host' immune system [32]. In the past, we have demonstrated that encapsulating the vaccine antigen in a polymer matrix can enhance the immunostimulatory activity of the antigen [26,33–35]. In the present study, the vaccine antigen and adjuvants are encapsulated in polymer matrices using poly(lactic-co-glycolic acid) (PLGA) to form an effective carrier system. Microparticulate vaccines have previously been reported to be stable at room temperature and thus may be favorable during vaccine storage and distribution for mass vaccinations and global immunization [36–40].

Adjuvants have long been used in vaccines to boost the immune response produced by the vaccine antigen [41]. The adjuvants Alhydrogel® and AddaVax™ are approved for use in licensed vaccines and have been documented to enhance the vaccine response [42]. Alhydrogel® forms a depot when injected and recruits APCs to the site of administration, increasing cellular uptake and antigen presentation to T-cells [43–45]. AddaVax™ (MF59-like) is a squalene-based nano-emulsion that induces cytokines and chemokines involved in the recruitment, activation, and maturation of APCs [46–48]. Previously, we have tested the adjuvants Alhydrogel® and AddaVax™, encapsulated in polymer matrices in a model microparticulate vaccine formulation [35]. We observed that adjuvants and an inactivated model antigen yielded increased antibody levels in vaccinated mice [35]. Therefore, Alhydrogel® and AddaVax™ were used in this study as adjuvants to enhance the immunogenicity of the inactivated SARS-CoV-2 antigen.

Previously, as a proof of concept, we demonstrated that MN administration of an inactivated microparticulate vaccine utilizing canine coronavirus (CCoV) as a model antigen increased antibody levels in vaccinated mice [35]. In this current follow-up study, we have summarized the results of testing an adjuvanted inactivated SARS-CoV-2 MP vaccine administered to mice using quick-dissolving MNs. First, the vaccine and adjuvant MP were formulated, characterized, and assessed in vitro for immunogenicity and cytotoxicity. The vaccine-loaded MN was then prepared and administered to mice via the skin. The MN quickly dissolves to release the vaccine MP, which may then be taken up by the dendritic cells or macrophages in the skin, subsequently activating the host immune responses against the vaccine antigen. The SARS-CoV-2 specific antibody levels and T-cell responses following MN vaccination were evaluated and are reported in this article.

## 2. Materials and Methods

### 2.1. Materials

Sodium hyaluronate (100 kDa) was obtained from Lifecore Biomedical (Chaska, MN, USA). Poly(lactic-co-glycolic acid) (75:25) was procured from Evonik Industries (Essen, Germany). Polyvinyl alcohol (PVA) (Avg Mol Wt. 30,000–70,000), dichloromethane (DCM), trehalose dihydrate, and lipopolysaccharides (LPSs) from Escherichia coli O111:B4 were purchased from Sigma-Aldrich (St. Louis, MO, USA). The heat-inactivated SARS-CoV-2 antigen was obtained from BEI Resources (NIAID, NIH: Heat Inactivated, SARS-Related Coronavirus 2, Isolate USA-WA1/2020, NR-52286). Alhydrogel® and AddaVax™ were purchased from InvivoGen (San Diego, CA, USA). Pierce Micro BCA™ Assay Kit was obtained from Thermo Fisher Scientific (Waltham, MA, USA). The 8 × 8 array poly dimethyl siloxane (PDMS) MN templates were obtained from Micropoint Technologies (Singapore). Fetal bovine serum (FBS), Dulbecco's Modified Eagle's Medium (DMEM), non-essential amino acids, and penicillin/streptomycin were procured from American Type Culture Collection (ATCC) (Manassas, VA, USA). Murine dendritic cells (DCs) were a gift from Kenneth L. Rock at the Dana-Farber Cancer Institute, Inc. (Boston, MA, USA). Six- to eight-week-old Swiss Webster mice were procured from Charles River Laboratories (Wilmington, MA, USA). HRP-tagged secondary goat anti-mouse antibodies IgG, IgM, IgA, IgG1, and IgG2a, were procured from Invitrogen (Rockford, IL, USA). Allophycocyanin (APC)-labeled anti-mouse CD4 and fluorescein isothiocyanate (FITC)-labeled anti-mouse CD8 antibodies were obtained from Invitrogen™, Thermofisher Scientific (Waltham, MA, USA).

### 2.2. Methods

#### 2.2.1. Preparation and Characterization of Microparticles (MP)

The heat-inactivated SARS-CoV-2 (iSARS-CoV-2) vaccine MP and adjuvant MP (Alhydrogel® and AddaVax™) were prepared using a double emulsion method with solvent evaporation as described previously [9,33–35]. First, the inactivated SARS-CoV-2 antigen (1% loading) in a pH 7.4 phosphate buffer was added to PLGA in DCM solution (2% $w/v$) and probe-homogenized at 17,000 RPM using a 30 s on/30 s off cycle for 2 min (primary emulsion). Next, the primary emulsion was probe-homogenized with the PVA solution in deionized water (0.1% $w/v$) for 2 min at 17,000 RPM (double emulsion). The final emulsion was stirred at 500 RPM for 5 h to remove the residual DCM via solvent evaporation. The excess PVA was removed by washing with deionized water followed by centrifugation at 17,000 RPM for 10 min. The MP was resuspended with 1 mL of trehalose solution (2% $w/v$) to serve as a cryoprotectant. The Alhydrogel® MP (10% loading) and AddaVax™ (5% loading) MP were prepared similarly by substituting the antigen with the adjuvant in the primary emulsion. The final vaccine MP and adjuvant MP formulations were freeze-dried to obtain the dry product. The percent recovery yield of the lyophilized product was calculated using the following formula as described previously [35,49,50].

$$\text{Percent Recovery yield} = \frac{\text{Weight of lyophilized MP} * 100}{\text{Weight of all ingredients in the formulation}} \quad (1)$$

The MP were observed under the scanning electron microscope and characterized for size and shape. The MP size and the surface charge were measured using a Malvern Zetasizer Nano ZS (Malvern Panalytical Ltd., Worcestershire, UK), as described previously [35]. The encapsulation efficiency (EE) of the inactivated SARS-CoV-2 antigen in the MP was assessed as described previously [33–35,51]. Briefly, DCM was added to 5 mg of the vaccine MP to dissolve the PLGA matrix. The solution was centrifuged to concentrate the antigen into a pellet. The supernatant was discarded, and the concentrated antigen pellet was placed in a vacuum chamber for 30 min to remove the residual DCM by evaporation. The antigen was resuspended using 1 mL PBS and analyzed using a micro-Bicinchoninic acid (BCA) assay per the manufacturer's instructions. The concentration per ml (conc/mL) was determined by plotting a standard curve. The percentage encapsulation efficiency (% EE) was calculated using the following formula, as described previously [34,35,51].

$$\%\text{EE} = \frac{\text{Practical concentration of antigen in 5mg of MP} \times 100}{\text{Theoretical concentration of antigen in 5mg of MP}} \quad (2)$$

2.2.2. Evaluating the In Vitro Immunostimulatory Activity of the Vaccine MP

The in vitro immunogenicity of the MP was assessed by measuring the nitrite released by the DCs exposed to the different MP groups. As described previously, the nitrite accumulated consequent to nitric oxide production by the DCs was quantified using Griess' nitrite assay [26,33–35]. Briefly, in a 96-well plate, murine DCs were plated at a density of $1 \times 10^4$ cells/well. The cells were then pulsed with a calculated amount of antigen MP and adjuvant MP and were incubated for 24 h at 37 °C. The groups tested and their corresponding dose/wells are listed as follows: lipopolysaccharide (LPS) from *Escherichia coli* (positive control) (2 µg), no treatment (negative control), blank MP, Alhydrogel® MP (3 µg), AddaVax™ MP (0.5 µg), inactivated SARS-CoV-2 (iSARS-CoV-2) suspension (2 µg), iSARS-CoV-2 MP vaccine (2 µg), adjuvanted iSARS-CoV-2 MP vaccine (iSARS-CoV-2 (2 µg) + Alhydrogel® (3 µg) + AddaVax™ (0.5 µg)). After the 24 h incubation, the supernatants (50 µL/well) were transferred to a fresh 96-well plate. To each well, 50 µL of sulfanilamide (1%) in phosphoric acid (5%) was added and incubated for 5–10 min, protected from light at room temperature. Next, 50 µL of NED (0.1%) (*N*-1-naphthyl ethylenediamine dihydrochloride) solution in deionized water was added and kept at room temperature for 5–10 min, protected from light. The appearance of a purple/magenta color indicated nitrite release. The absorbance (540 nm) was read using a plate reader (Bio Tek Synergy, BIO-TEK Instruments, Winooski, VT, USA). A sodium nitrite standard curve was plotted from which the nitrite content was quantified.

2.2.3. Determining the In Vitro Cytotoxicity of the Vaccine MP

The cytotoxicity of the inactivated SARS-CoV-2 MP to DCs was assessed in vitro using an MTT assay (3-(4,5-Dimethylthiazol-2-yl)-2,5-diphenyltetrazolium bromide) described previously [33–35]. The cytotoxicity of the adjuvant MP (Alhydrogel® MP and AddaVax™ MP) has been previously tested and was found to be non-cytotoxic in varying concentrations [35]. To assess the cytotoxicity of the inactivated SARS-CoV-2 MP, DCs were plated at a cell density of $1 \times 10^4$ cells/well in a 96-well plate. Then, two-fold serial dilutions of the inactivated SARS-CoV-2 MP (31.25 ug/mL to 500 µg/mL) were prepared in cDMEM (DMEM high glucose medium with 2 mM L-glut, 1% penicillin–streptomycin, sodium pyruvate, 10% FBS). The diluted MP suspensions were added in triplicate to each well and incubated for 24 h at 37 °C. Cells that received no treatment were used as the positive control, and cells treated with 50 µL of DMSO were used as the negative control. After the incubation period, the media containing the suspended MP were removed gently using a pipette. Next, 10 µL MTT reagent (5 mg/mL) was added to every well, and the volume was made up to 100 µL/well with cDMEM. The plate was kept for incubation at 37 °C for 4 h, protected from light. Following incubation, 100 µL/well of DMSO was added, and the absorbance (570 nm) was measured using a plate reader.

2.2.4. Preparation of Vaccine-Loaded MNs

As described previously, a spin casting method was used to prepare the vaccine-loaded quick-dissolving MN [9,35]. Then, 10% *w/v* sodium hyaluronate and 5% *w/v* trehalose in deionized water constituted the MN gel base. Then, the vaccine MP and the adjuvants MP required for each patch were weighed and dispersed into the MN gel base. Then, 25 mg of gel was added to each pre-weighed PDMS MN mold and centrifuged at 4000 rpm for 15 min at 15 °C to form the MN. The MN molds were kept overnight for drying, and 10% HA gel was added as backing the following day. The dried MN were removed from the molds and observed under the scanning electron microscope for its physical appearance.

2.2.5. In Vivo Immunization Procedure and Dosing Regimen

The vaccine efficacy of the adjuvanted inactivated SARS-CoV-2 MP vaccine administered using dissolving MN was tested in vivo in 6–8-week-old male Swiss Webster (CFW) mice, $n = 4$. The mice were immunized via the skin with the vaccine-loaded MN patches. The testing was performed as per the approved Mercer University IACUC protocol (animal protocol #A2004006). The antigen dose was 20 µg/mouse of inactivated SARS-CoV-2, the Alhydrogel® dose was 30 µg/mouse, and the AddaVax™ dose was 5 µg/mouse. The animals were divided into two groups: a no treatment control group and the adjuvanted inactivated SARS-CoV-2 vaccine MP group. The vaccine group received the adjuvanted MP vaccine using the dissolving MNs via the transdermal route. Before immunization, a 2 × 2 cm patch of the fur was removed from the back of the anesthetized mice (inhalational Isoflurane) using a depilatory cream for ease of MN application. The animals received three doses of the vaccine at weeks 0, 3, and 5. The mice were bled bi-weekly, and the serum was collected for determining the antibody levels. The animals were sacrificed at week 10, and their immune organs, including the spleen and lymph node, were isolated and processed into single-cell suspensions to analyze T-cell responses (Figure 1).

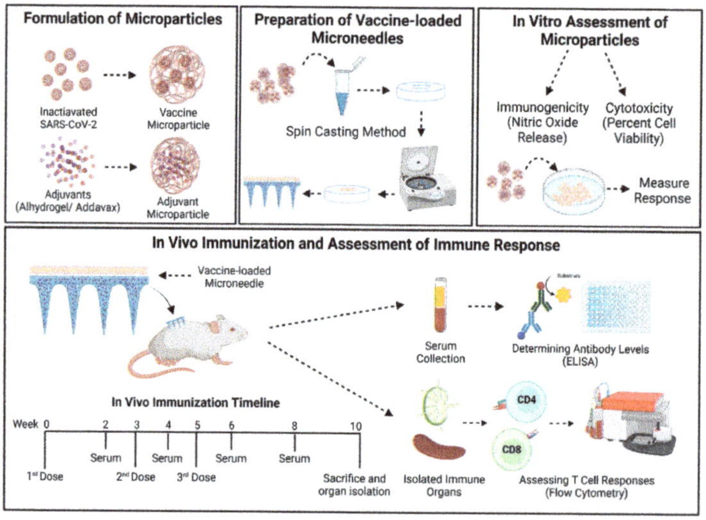


**Figure 1.** Schematics of methodology used in this study. The vaccine MP and adjuvant MP were formulated and characterized. The vaccine-loaded quick-dissolving MN were prepared using a spin casting method. The MP were assessed in vitro for their immunogenicity and cytotoxicity. The vaccine-loaded MN were administered to mice following which both antibody levels and cellular responses were assessed and reported. The mice received three doses of the adjuvanted inactivated SARS-CoV-2 MP MN vaccine at weeks 0, 3, and 5. The mice were sacrificed at week 10, and the immune organs (spleen and lymph node) were isolated and processed into single-cell suspensions to analyze T-cell responses. The image was created using BioRender.com (accessed on 7 March 2023).

2.2.6. Determining the Serum Antibody Levels in Immunized Mice

The mice were bled bi-weekly, and the serum was isolated to evaluate the SARS-CoV-2-specific antibody responses. An enzyme-linked immunosorbent assay was used to determine the serum IgM, IgG, IgA, IgG1, and IgG2a levels described previously [35]. For this purpose, high-binding 96-well plates (MICROLON®, 96-well plate, High binding, Greiner bio one) were coated with 50 µL/well of the inactivated SARS-CoV-2 antigen (0.2 µg/well) in a pH 9.6 carbonate buffer solution. The coated plates were kept overnight at 4 °C to facilitate attachment of the antigen. Following incubation, plates were washed with 200 µL of 0.01% Tween-20 PBS (T-PBS) solution and blocked with 50 µL/well of 3% Bovine Serum Albumin (BSA) in T-PBS (blocking solution) for 3 h at 37 °C. The plates were rewashed, and the diluted serum sample (50 µL/well) was added to the wells and incubated overnight at 4 °C. The plates were washed again, and 50 µL/well of the HRP-tagged secondary goat anti-mouse IgM, IgG, IgA, IgG1, and IgG2a antibodies (1:2000 to 1:4000) were added and incubated at 37 °C for 90 min. Next, the plates were washed, and 50 µL/well of the TMB (3,3′,5,5′′-tetramethyl benzidine) substrate reagent (BD OptEIA™, BD Biosciences, San Jose, CA, USA) was added to each well and kept at room temperature for 10 min. The reaction was stopped by adding 50 µL of 0.3 M $H_2SO_4$ to each well. The absorbance was read at 450 nm using a plate reader.

2.2.7. Evaluating the T-Cell Responses in Immunized Mice

The mice were sacrificed during week 10, and spleen and lymph nodes (inguinal and brachial) were isolated and processed into single-cell suspensions as described previously [26,52]. The red blood cells (RBCs) in the spleen were lysed by adding ammonium chloride potassium (ACK) lysis buffer. The cells were centrifuged to remove the lysed RBCs at 1200 rpm for 10 min, and the splenocytes were resuspended in DMEM containing 70% fetal bovine serum (FBS). Then, 5% $v/v$ DMSO was added to the cells as a cryoprotectant, frozen at −80 °C. The percentage (%) expression of $CD4^+$ and $CD8^+$ T-cells in the lymph nodes and spleen cells was evaluated using a flow cytometer. First, the cell suspensions were quickly thawed and centrifuged at 1200 rpm to remove the media and DMSO. The cells were resuspended using fresh DMEM and stimulated with 5 ng/mL IL-2 overnight. The following day, the cells were centrifuged at 1200 rpm to remove the IL-2, and the cells were resuspended using fresh DMEM. The cells were then stimulated with 5 µg/mL of the inactivated SARS-CoV-2 antigen overnight. As the mice were not challenged with the live SARS-CoV-2 virus, the splenocytes and lymphocytes were stimulated in vitro with the vaccine antigen to test the specificity of the CD4+ and CD8+ T-cells toward SARS-CoV-2. Following incubation with the antigen, the cells were centrifuged at 1200 rpm to form a pellet. The cells were resuspended in 100 µL of the marker solution containing APC-labeled anti-mouse CD4 and FITC-labeled anti-mouse CD8 antibodies in PBS. The cells were incubated for 1 h on ice, protected from light, and gently vortexed every 15 min. Following incubation, the cells were washed 3 times and analyzed using flow cytometry.

2.2.8. Statistical Analysis

Statistical analysis was performed using GraphPad Prism 9.2.0 software (GraphPad Software, San Diego, CA, USA). One-way ANOVA was used for normally distributed data with independent groups. Two-way ANOVA was used for dependent groups. A post hoc Sidak's test was used for multiple comparisons between the two groups. For multiple comparisons between three or more groups, a post hoc Tukey test (to compare between means) or post hoc Dunnett test (to compare means to control) was used. The following $p$ values were used, $p > 0.05$ (ns—non-significant), $p \leq 0.05$ (*), $p \leq 0.01$ (**), $p \leq 0.001$ (***), and $p \leq 0.001$ (****). A $p$ value < 0.05 is considered statistically significant. Data are expressed as mean ± standard error mean (SEM).

## 3. Results

### *3.1. Characterization of Vaccine MP and MN*

The percentage yield of the inactivated SARS-CoV-2 MP was 83%, with an encapsulation efficiency of 90.4%, size of approximately 910 nm, and surface charge of −23.11 mV. The percentage yield of the Alhydrogel® MP was 93%, with a size of roughly 1.3 µm and a surface charge of 12 mV. The percentage yield of the AddaVax™ MP was 90.5%, with an approximate size of 1.2 µm and a surface charge of −12.5 mV. Scanning electron microscope images show that the inactivated SARS-CoV-2 MP were spherical with smooth surfaces (Figure 2A). The dissolving MNs were also observed under the scanning electron microscope. The images show the formation of sharp needles with a length of approximately 482 µm (Figure 2B). A detailed characterization analysis of dissolving MNs was previously published by our group [9].

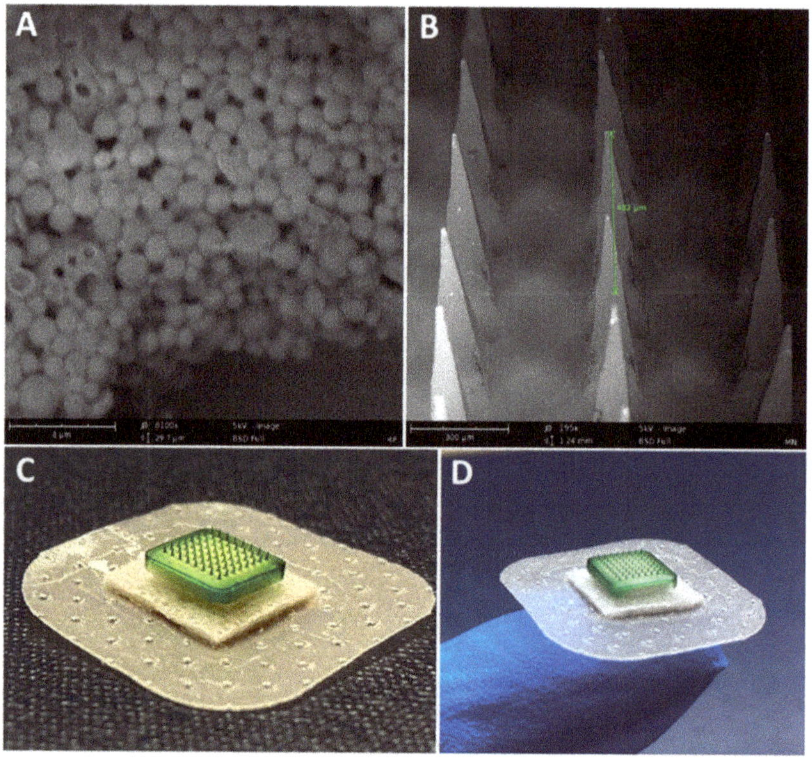


**Figure 2.** Characterization of vaccine MP and vaccine-loaded MN. (**A**) Scanning electron microscope image of the vaccine MP (magnification—8100×). The vaccine MP was spherical with smooth surfaces. (**B**) Scanning electron microscope image of an MN patch (magnification—195×). The MN was approximately 482 µm in length. (**C**,**D**) Indocyanine green (ICG)-loaded MN band-aid patch. ICG was used for better visualization of MN.

### *3.2. Vaccine MP Show Enhanced Immunostimulatory Activity In Vitro*

The immune recognition or biologic activity of the formulated iSARS-CoV2 MP by DC was assessed using an in vitro assay. The nitric oxide (NO) released by the DCs pulsed with vaccine MP was measured and quantified. The blank MP and the AddaVax™ MP did not release significant levels of NO compared to the cells that received no treatment or LPS-treated DC (Figure 3). Alhydrogel® MP produced significant levels of NO compared to the no treatment group. The cells that received the inactivated SARS-CoV-2 antigen suspension had negligible NO. However, the cells that received the inactivated SARS-CoV-2 MP vaccine produced significantly high levels of NO compared to the antigen in the suspension form. Further, adding adjuvants Alhydrogel® and AddaVax™ significantly increased the NO release and resulted in a significant difference compared to the unadjuvanted MP group (Figure 3).

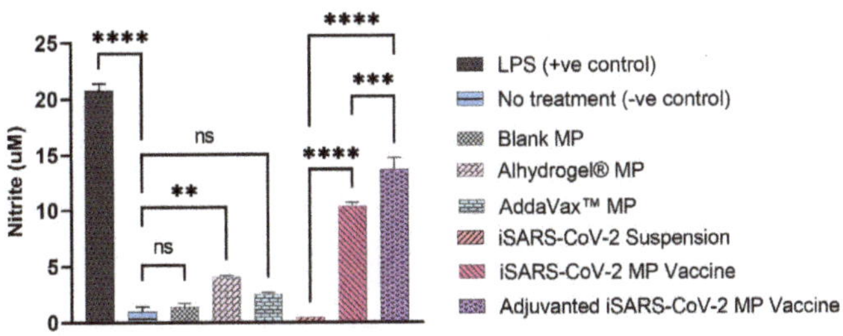


**Figure 3.** Nitric oxide (NO) released by the DCs upon exposure to the different treatment groups. The cell density was adjusted to $1 \times 10^4$ cells/well and treated with the following groups for 24 h: lipopolysaccharide (LPS) (2 µg) (+ve control), no treatment (−ve control), blank MP, Alhydrogel® MP (3 µg), AddaVax™ (0.5 µg), iSARS-CoV-2 suspension (2 µg), iSARS-CoV-2 MP vaccine (2 µg), adjuvanted iSARS-CoV-2 MP vaccine (iSARS-CoV-2 (2 µg) + Alhydrogel® (3 µg) + AddaVax™ (0.5 µg)). The nitrite released in the supernatant was assessed using the Griess' nitrite assay method. Data expressed as mean ± SEM, $n = 3$, one-way ANOVA test, post hoc Dunnett's multiple comparisons test, ns: non-significant, ** $p \leq 0.01$, *** $p \leq 0.001$, and **** $p \leq 0.0001$.

### 3.3. Vaccine MP Are Non-Cytotoxic to DCs

The cytotoxicity of the inactivated SARS-CoV-2 MP was tested in vitro using the MTT assay. The cytotoxicity of the adjuvant MP was previously assessed and reported to be non-toxic to cells in specific concentrations [35]. Consistent with our previously published data, the inactivated SARS-CoV-2 MP vaccine was also found to be non-cytotoxic and resulted in no significant cell death up to a concentration of 500 µg/mL. Dimethyl sulfoxide (DMSO) was used as a positive control and resulted in a significant decrease in the percent cell viability compared to the cells only control (Figure 4).

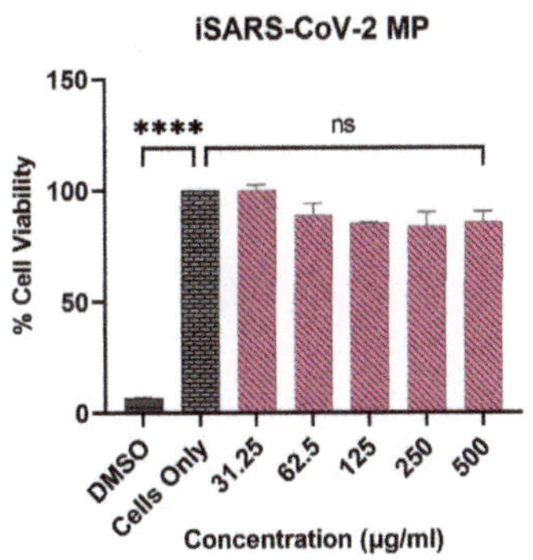


**Figure 4.** Percent cell viability of DCs pulsed with iSARS-CoV-2 MP. The cell density was adjusted to $1 \times 10^4$ cells/well. Two-fold serial dilutions of the iSARS-CoV-2 MP in cDMEM (concentration range: 31.25 to 500 ug/mL) were added to every well at a volume of 100 µL/well and incubated for 24 h. Cell only and cells treated with DMSO (50 µL) were used as positive and negative controls, respectively. Data expressed as mean ± SEM, $n = 3$, one-way ANOVA test, post hoc Dunnett's multiple comparison test, ns: non-significant, **** $p \leq 0.0001$.

*3.4. Adjuvanted Vaccine Increased Antibody Levels in Immunized Mice*

Following immunization of mice with the vaccine MN, the antibody levels in the mice sera were assessed using ELISA. The SARS-CoV-2-specific IgM, IgG, IgA, IgG1, and IgG2a antibody levels were detected and quantified. The serum IgM levels peaked during week 2 following the prime dose and subsequently decreased during the later weeks (Figure 5).

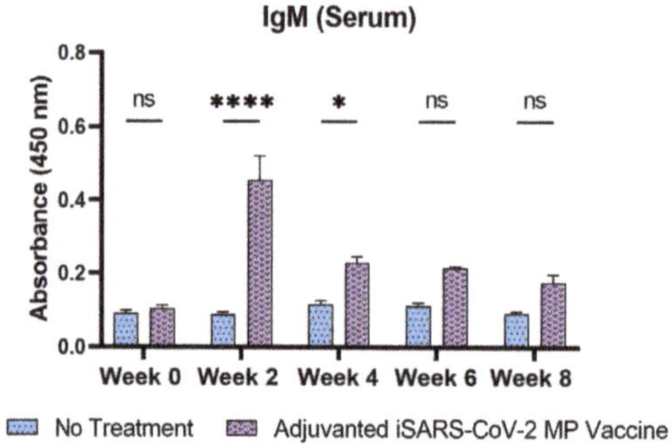


**Figure 5.** Serum IgM antibody levels in vaccinated mice. Responses obtained are compared to the no treatment (control). Data expressed as mean ± SEM, $n = 4$, two-way ANOVA, post hoc Sidak's multiple comparisons test. ns: non-significant, * $p \leq 0.05$, **** $p \leq 0.0001$.

The serum IgG levels increased following the prime dose and remained significantly high until week 8 (Figure 6A). The serum IgA levels increased considerably following the prime dose and remained high until week 8 (Figure 6B).

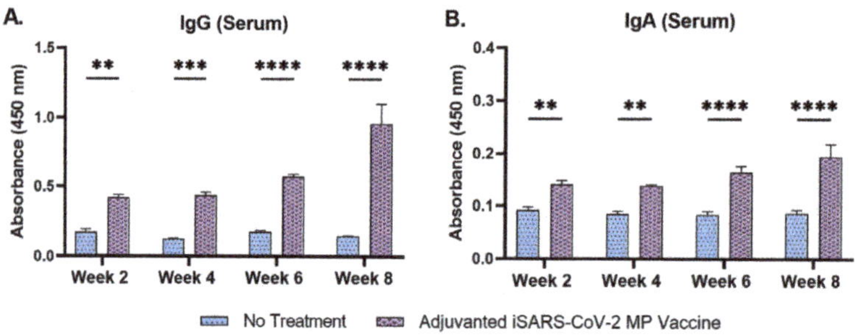


**Figure 6.** Serum IgG and serum IgA antibody levels in vaccinated mice. (**A**) Total IgG in vaccinated mice. (**B**) Total IgA in vaccinated mice. Responses obtained are compared to the no treatment (control). Data expressed as mean ± SEM, $n = 4$, two-way ANOVA, post hoc Sidak's multiple comparisons test. ** $p \leq 0.01$, *** $p \leq 0.001$, **** $p \leq 0.0001$.

IgG subtyping revealed that the serum IgG1 levels increased significantly during weeks 6 and 8 following the second booster dose, administered at week 5 (Figure 7A). Serum IgG2a levels increased significantly at week 8 (Figure 7B). The data show that the adjuvanted iSARS-CoV2 MP delivered by microneedles induced a robust antibody response against the vaccine antigen.

*3.5. Adjuvanted Vaccine Produced T-Cell Responses in Immunized Mice*

The expression of CD4 and CD8 molecules on the surface of the activated T-cells in the splenocytes and lymphocytes of the vaccinated mice was assessed using flow cytometry analysis. The percentages of $CD4^+$ (30.09%) and $CD8^+$ (9.3%) T-cells in the splenocytes of the vaccinated mice were higher compared to the percentage of $CD4^+$ (13.92%) and $CD8^+$ (9.3%) T-cells of the no treatment control group (Figure 8A,C). The percentage of

T-cells expressing CD4 molecules (30.09%) was higher than that of T-cells expressing CD8 molecules (9.3%) in the splenocytes of the vaccinated mice (Figure 8A). The percentage of CD4$^+$ (54%) and CD8$^+$ (18.3%) T-cells in the lymph nodes of the vaccinated mice were higher compared to the percentage of CD4$^+$ (39.5%) and CD8$^+$ (10.4%) T-cells of the no treatment control group (Figure 8B,D). Similar to the results obtained from the splenocytes, the percentage of T-cells expressing CD4 molecules (54%) was higher than that of T-cells expressing CD8 molecules (18.3%) (Figure 8B).

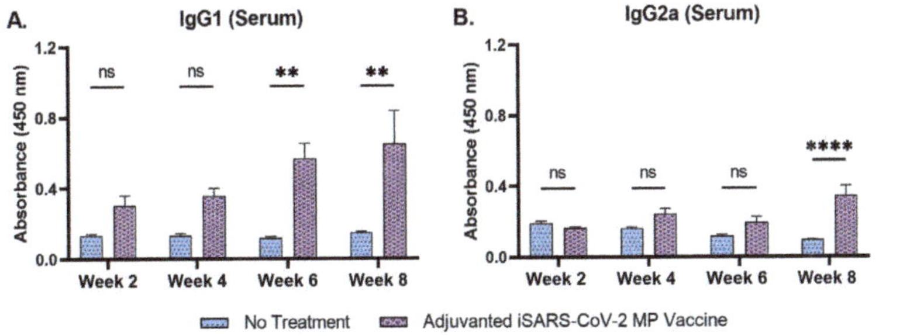


**Figure 7.** Serum IgG1 and serum IgG2a antibody levels in vaccinated mice. (**A**) Serum IgG1 levels in vaccinated mice. (**B**) Serum IgG2a levels in vaccinated mice. Responses obtained are compared to no treatment (control). Data expressed as mean ± SEM, $n = 4$, two-way ANOVA, post hoc Sidak's multiple comparisons test. ns: non-significant, ** $p \leq 0.01$, **** $p \leq 0.0001$.

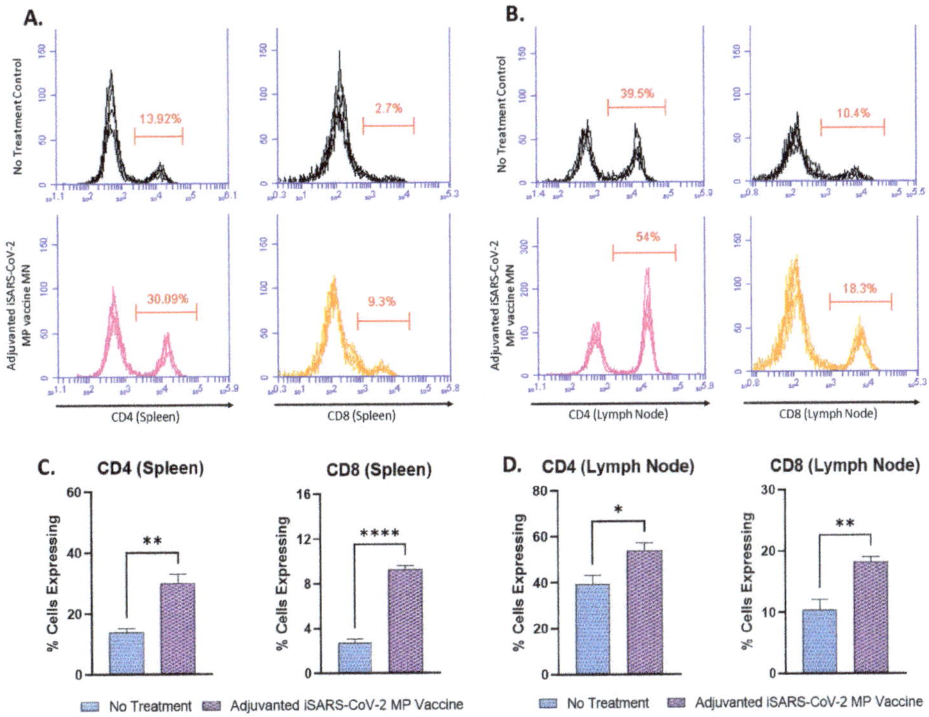


**Figure 8.** CD4$^+$ and CD8$^+$ T-cells in the splenocytes and lymphocytes of immunized mice. Responses obtained are compared to no treatment (control). Data expressed as mean ± SEM, $n = 4$, Student's $t$ test. * $p \leq 0.05$, ** $p \leq 0.01$, **** $p \leq 0.0001$. (**A**,**C**) Percentage of CD+ and CD8+ T-cells in the splenocytes of the vaccinated mice. (**B**,**D**) Percentage of CD+ and CD8+ T-cells in the lymphocytes of the vaccinated mice.

## 4. Discussion

Here, we formulated and characterized an adjuvanted inactivated SARS-CoV-2 microparticulate vaccine and evaluated the immune response generated when administered to mice using MNs. The vaccine was evaluated in vitro for its immunogenicity and cytotoxicity to DC. It was tested in vivo for its ability to induce SARS-CoV-2-specific antibodies and T-cell responses in vaccinated mice.

The inactivated SARS-CoV-2 MP vaccine, Alhydrogel® MP, and AddaVax™ MP were formulated using PLGA as the polymer matrix for encapsulating the antigen or adjuvant. Encapsulating the antigen in a polymer matrix protects the antigen [24]. It has been previously shown to reduce antigen degradation by enzymes present in the tissue fluids while also increasing cellular uptake of the antigen due to its increased size [28,31,40]. The MP product yield using the double emulsion method was greater than 80% with minimal loss during processing. The particles were spherical, with an optimum size ranging from 900 to 1300 nm. MP of 1 to 3 μm size are reported to be efficiently recognized and engulfed by circulating APCs [27]. The charges of the vaccine and adjuvant MP were positive or negative depending on the encapsulated material and were consistent with previously published results [35]. Typically, colloidal suspensions are stable when MP have a high positive or negative charge that prevent agglomeration when the particles are suspended [53]. The %EE of the inactivated SARS-CoV-2 antigen in the PLGA MP was 90.4%, indicating that the double emulsion method's formulation process results in an effectively loaded carrier system.

Particulate vaccines are more immunogenic than antigens in suspension and are thus capable of producing a more robust immune response [32]. Previously, we have shown that the double emulsion method of encapsulating vaccine antigens in a polymer matrix increases the immunogenicity, cellular uptake, and antigen presentation compared to the antigen suspension [26,33–35]. We tested the in vitro immunogenicity of the MP using a Griess' nitrite assay. APCs such as DCs and macrophages release NO, a non-specific innate immune marker when encountered with an invading pathogen [54,55]. NO is crucial in recruiting APCs and releasing cytokines upon infection, triggering the host cells to produce a robust immune response against the invading pathogen [56,57]. Consistent with our previously published results, we observed that the particulate vaccine was better able to stimulate DCs than the inactivated SARS-CoV-2 antigen suspension [35].

The adjuvant MP was evaluated individually to assess for NO release in pulsed DCs. Alhydrogel® MP (3 μg) induced higher NO levels than the AddaVax™ MP (0.5 μg) due to the differences in the adjuvant concentrations tested. Previously, we tested the in vitro cytotoxicity of varying concentrations of the adjuvant MP (Alhydrogel® and AddaVax™) in DCs [35]. The metabolically active cells (live cells) can reduce MTT salts to purple formazan crystals, which were used to assess the cytotoxicity of the vaccine MP. We observed that increased concentrations of AddaVax™ MP (>0.625 μg) resulted in significant cytotoxicity, whereas Alhydrogel® MP was non-cytotoxic even at higher concentrations [35]. Since it is essential for the vaccine MP and adjuvant MP to be non-cytotoxic to the target cells, we evaluated a lower dose of the AddaVax™ MP for its in vitro immunogenicity, which explains the negligible NO release from the DCs pulsed with just the AddaVax™ MP. However, the Alhydrogel® MP and AddaVax™ MP, when combined with the SARS-CoV-2 vaccine MP, significantly increased the immunogenicity of the vaccine MP. We further tested the percent viability of the cells exposed to the SARS-CoV-2 vaccine MP. The cytotoxicity study suggested that the vaccine MP was non-cytotoxic at a wide range of concentrations (31.25 to 500 μg/mL). The in vitro studies indicated that the MP vaccine was immunogenic and non-cytotoxic at various doses.

We then evaluated the in vivo immune response produced by the adjuvanted inactivated SARS-CoV-2 MP vaccine administered to mice using quick-dissolving MN. Vaccine administration via the skin is promising, as the immune-rich layers of the skin contain several APCs, such as Langerhans cells and DCs, that can promptly recognize and engulf the microparticulate vaccine, thereby triggering robust immune response activation [5,6,58]. After vaccine administration, the mice were bled biweekly, and the serum was evaluated for antigen-specific antibody levels. A functional vaccine needs to generate antibodies specific to the vaccine antigen, as it can recognize and bind to the invading pathogen, thereby preventing it from infecting the host.

It has been reported that IgM appears during the early weeks of vaccination and undergoes isotype class switching to IgG and IgA antibodies [59]. Consistent with the published literature, our vaccine produced high IgM levels during week 2, which decreased significantly in the following weeks. The serum IgG and the serum IgA antibody levels increased following the prime dose and remained significantly high up to week 10. Serum IgA and IgG have been reported to play a critical role in SARS-CoV-2 binding and neutralization [60,61]. MN administration of the adjuvanted iSARS-CoV-2 MP vaccine increased IgG and IgA antibody levels. Here, the antibodies were evaluated in terms of their capacity to bind to the inactivated virus efficiently, as IgG and IgA are the primary humoral antibodies conferencing protection in tissues and at mucosal surfaces. The vaccine's efficacy will be established by assessing the neutralization capacity of the IgG and IgA antibodies as a follow-up in our future studies. IgG subtyping was performed to characterize and understand the type of Th-mediated (Th1 and Th2) responses produced upon vaccination. Typically, a Th2-type response is associated with increased IgG1 levels [62,63]. Th2-type responses signal the helper T-cells, which play a vital role in activating host immune responses against the invading pathogen [62]. The IgG2a levels are often associated with Th-1 type response [64]. Such a response will trigger cellular responses, predominantly signaling the cytotoxic T-cells and APCs, causing their migration to the invading pathogen [65]. We observed that MN vaccination increased serum IgG1 levels during weeks 6 and 8 following the second booster dose administration at week 5. The serum IgG2a levels increased only during week 8. The IgG1 antibody levels were higher than the IgG2a antibody levels, suggesting that the immune responses produced by the vaccine may be predominantly of Th-2 type.

To further corroborate the results obtained from the antibody assessment, we characterized the cell-mediated immune responses produced upon vaccination. The percentage of CD4+ and CD8+ T-cells in the splenocytes and lymphocytes was assessed using flow cytometry analysis. The Results section shows that the vaccine induced significant levels of SARS-CoV-2-specific CD4+ and CD8+ T-cells. Similar to the results obtained from the antibody analysis, the percentage of CD4+ T-cells was higher than that of CD8+ T-cells. The increased percentage of CD4+ T-cells confirms that the Th-2 type responses are higher than the Th-1 type responses.

Further, CD4+ helper T-cells play a crucial role in the activation and maturation of plasma B-cells responsible for antibody production [63]. Our results suggest that the increased antibody levels may be attributed to the increased CD4+ T-cells. Although the CD4+ T-cells are higher in number, the vaccine is not devoid of CD8+ T-cells. MN vaccine administration produced significant CD4+ and CD8+ T-cells, and both responses are necessary for an efficacious vaccine.

In future work and follow-up studies, we will evaluate the vaccine's efficacy by assessing the neutralizing antibody titers using a pseudovirus neutralization assay (PVNA). We will further test the durability of the antibody responses generated by the microparticulate method of vaccine formulation. The microparticulate vaccine will also be evaluated for memory responses by assessing the memory markers in the isolated B-cells and T-cells.

## 5. Conclusions

In summary, the adjuvanted inactivated SARS-CoV-2 MP vaccine was formulated and characterized. The microparticulate vaccine was non-cytotoxic and more immunogenic than the soluble antigen suspension in vitro. The vaccine MP delivered via microneedles effectively induced humoral and cell-mediated immune responses in vaccinated mice. When combined with MN administration, the microparticulate method for vaccine delivery can be an effective tool for frequent immunization and mass vaccination. However, like every vaccine, these novel strategies require significant groundwork and validation to be utilized in the marketed formulations.

**Author Contributions:** Conceptualization, S.V. and M.J.D.; methodology, S.V., S.P., I.M., K.B.G., A.K., P.B., M.J.D. and S.M.Z.; validation, S.V. and M.J.D.; formal analysis, S.V.; investigation, S.V. and S.P.; resources, M.J.D.; data curation, S.V.; writing—original draft preparation, S.V.; writing—review and editing, M.N.U., S.V., S.P., I.M., K.B.G., A.K., P.B., M.J.D. and S.M.Z.; visualization, S.V.; supervision, M.J.D.; project administration, M.J.D.; funding acquisition, M.J.D. All authors have read and agreed to the published version of the manuscript.

**Funding:** This research received no external funding.

**Institutional Review Board Statement:** This study was conducted in accordance with the Declaration of Helsinki and was approved by the IACUC Review Board of Mercer University (animal protocol #A2004006, date of approval—23 April 2020).

**Informed Consent Statement:** Not applicable.

**Data Availability Statement:** Data will be made available on reasonable request.

**Acknowledgments:** The following reagent was deposited by the Centers for Disease Control and Prevention and was obtained through BEI Resources, NIAID, NIH: SARS-Related Coronavirus 2, Isolate USA-WA1/2020, Heat Inactivated, NR-52286. Graphics were created using Bio Render, https://biorender.com (accessed on 7 March 2023).

**Conflicts of Interest:** The authors declare no conflict of interest. The authors are responsible for the contents and writing of this article.

## References

1. CDC. COVID Data Tracker. Centers for Disease Control and Prevention 2020. Available online: https://covid.cdc.gov/covid-data-tracker (accessed on 22 February 2021).
2. CDC. COVID-19 Vaccination. Centers for Disease Control and Prevention 2020. Available online: https://www.cdc.gov/coronavirus/2019-ncov/vaccines/effectiveness/why-measure-effectiveness/breakthrough-cases.html (accessed on 6 January 2022).
3. COVID-19 Vaccines | FDA, n.d. Available online: https://www.fda.gov/emergency-preparedness-and-response/coronavirus-disease-2019-covid-19/covid-19-vaccines (accessed on 19 December 2022).
4. Science Brief: Emerging SARS-CoV-2 Variants | CDC n.d. Available online: https://www.cdc.gov/coronavirus/2019-ncov/science/science-briefs/scientific-brief-emerging-variants.html (accessed on 2 November 2021).
5. Menon, I.; Bagwe, P.; Gomes, K.B.; Bajaj, L.; Gala, R.; Uddin, M.N.; D'souza, M.J.; Zughaier, S.M. Microneedles: A New Generation Vaccine Delivery System. *Micromachines* **2021**, *12*, 435. [CrossRef] [PubMed]
6. Prausnitz, M.R.; Mikszta, J.A.; Cormier, M.; Andrianov, A.K. Microneedle-based vaccines. *Curr. Top. Microbiol. Immunol.* **2009**, *333*, 369–393. [CrossRef] [PubMed]
7. Prausnitz, M. A Phase I Study of the Safety, Reactogenicity, Acceptability and Immunogenicity of Inactivated Influenza Vaccine Delivered by Microneedle Patch or by Hypodermic Needle. 2019. Available online: clinicaltrials.gov (accessed on 7 March 2023).
8. Kim, Y.-C.; Prausnitz, M.R. Enabling skin vaccination using new delivery technologies. *Drug Deliv. Transl. Res.* **2011**, *1*, 7–12. [CrossRef] [PubMed]
9. Braz Gomes, K.; D'Souza, B.; Vijayanand, S.; Menon, I.; D'Souza, M.J. A dual-delivery platform for vaccination using antigen-loaded nanoparticles in dissolving microneedles. *Int. J. Pharm.* **2022**, *613*, 121393. [CrossRef] [PubMed]
10. Aldawood, F.K.; Andar, A.; Desai, S. A Comprehensive Review of Microneedles: Types, Materials, Processes, Characterizations and Applications. *Polymers* **2021**, *13*, 2815. [CrossRef]
11. Li, Z.; Xiang, T.; Liang, B.; Deng, H.; Wang, H.; Feng, X.; Quan, X.; Wang, X.; Li, S.; Lu, S.; et al. Characterization of SARS-CoV-2-Specific Humoral and Cellular Immune Responses Induced by Inactivated COVID-19 Vaccines in a Real-World Setting. *Front. Immunol.* **2021**, *12*, 802858. [CrossRef]
12. Satarker, S.; Nampoothiri, M. Structural Proteins in Severe Acute Respiratory Syndrome Coronavirus-2. *Arch. Med. Res.* **2020**, *51*, 482–491. [CrossRef]
13. Yadav, R.; Chaudhary, J.K.; Jain, N.; Chaudhary, P.K.; Khanra, S.; Dhamija, P.; Sharma, A.; Kumar, A.; Handu, S. Role of Structural and Non-Structural Proteins and Therapeutic Targets of SARS-CoV-2 for COVID-19. *Cells* **2021**, *10*, 821. [CrossRef]
14. Batéjat, C.; Grassin, Q.; Manuguerra, J.-C.; Leclercq, I. Heat inactivation of the severe acute respiratory syndrome coronavirus 2. *J. Biosaf. Biosecur.* **2021**, *3*, 1–3. [CrossRef]
15. Li, X.N.; Huang, Y.; Wang, W.; Jing, Q.L.; Zhang, C.H.; Qin, P.Z.; Guan, W.J.; Gan, L.; Li, Y.L.; Liu, W.H.; et al. Effectiveness of inactivated SARS-CoV-2 vaccines against the Delta variant infection in Guangzhou: A test-negative case-control real-world study. *Emerg. Microbes Infect.* **2021**, *10*, 1751–1759. [CrossRef]
16. Gao, Q.; Bao, L.; Mao, H.; Wang, L.; Xu, K.; Yang, M.; Li, Y.; Zhu, L.; Wang, N.; Lv, Z.; et al. Development of an inactivated vaccine candidate for SARS-CoV-2. *Science* **2020**, *369*, 77–81. [CrossRef]

17. Ding, C.; He, J.; Zhang, X.; Jiang, C.; Sun, Y.; Zhang, Y.; Chen, Q.; He, H.; Li, W.; Xie, J.; et al. Crucial Mutations of Spike Protein on SARS-CoV-2 Evolved to Variant Strains Escaping Neutralization of Convalescent Plasmas and RBD-Specific Monoclonal Antibodies. *Front. Immunol.* **2021**, *12*, 693775. [CrossRef] [PubMed]
18. Harvey, W.T.; Carabelli, A.M.; Jackson, B.; Gupta, R.K.; Thomson, E.C.; Harrison, E.M.; Ludden, C.; Reeve, R.; Rambaut, A.; COVID-19 Genomics UK (COG-UK) Consortium; et al. SARS-CoV-2 variants, spike mutations and immune escape. *Nat. Rev. Microbiol.* **2021**, *19*, 409–424. [CrossRef] [PubMed]
19. Magazine, N.; Zhang, T.; Wu, Y.; McGee, M.C.; Veggiani, G.; Huang, W. Mutations and Evolution of the SARS-CoV-2 Spike Protein. *Viruses* **2022**, *14*, 640. [CrossRef] [PubMed]
20. Viral Targets for Vaccines against COVID-19 | Nature Reviews Immunology n.d. Available online: https://www.nature.com/articles/s41577-020-00480-0 (accessed on 19 December 2022).
21. Fan, S.; Sun, W.; Fan, L.; Wu, N.; Sun, W.; Ma, H.; Chen, S.; Li, Z.; Li, Y.; Zhang, J.; et al. The highly conserved RNA-binding specificity of nucleocapsid protein facilitates the identification of drugs with broad anti-coronavirus activity. *Comput. Struct. Biotechnol. J.* **2022**, *20*, 5040–5044. [CrossRef] [PubMed]
22. Ye, Q.; Lu, S.; Corbett, K.D. Structural Basis for SARS-CoV-2 Nucleocapsid Protein Recognition by Single-Domain Antibodies. *Front. Immunol.* **2021**, *12*, 719037. [CrossRef]
23. Lopandić, Z.; Protić-Rosić, I.; Todorović, A.; Glamočlija, S.; Gnjatović, M.; Ćujic, D.; Gavrović-Jankulović, M. IgM and IgG Immunoreactivity of SARS-CoV-2 Recombinant M Protein. *Int. J. Mol. Sci.* **2021**, *22*, 4951. [CrossRef]
24. Waeckerle-Men, Y.; Uetz-von Allmen, E.; Gander, B.; Scandella, E.; Schlosser, E.; Schmidtke, G.; Merkle, H.P.; Groettrup, M. Encapsulation of proteins and peptides into biodegradable poly(D,L-lactide-co-glycolide) microspheres prolongs and enhances antigen presentation by human dendritic cells. *Vaccine* **2006**, *24*, 1847–1857. [CrossRef]
25. Shastri, P.N.; Kim, M.-C.; Quan, F.-S.; D'Souza, M.J.; Kang, S.-M. Immunogenicity and protection of oral influenza vaccines formulated into microparticles. *J. Pharm. Sci.* **2012**, *101*, 3623–3635. [CrossRef]
26. Gomes, K.B.; Menon, I.; Bagwe, P.; Bajaj, L.; Kang, S.-M.; D'Souza, M.J. Enhanced Immunogenicity of an Influenza Ectodomain Matrix-2 Protein Virus-like Particle (M2e VLP) Using Polymeric Microparticles for Vaccine Delivery. *Viruses* **2022**, *14*, 1920. [CrossRef]
27. Joshi, V.B.; Geary, S.M.; Salem, A.K. Biodegradable Particles as Vaccine Delivery Systems: Size Matters. *AAPS J.* **2012**, *15*, 85–94. [CrossRef] [PubMed]
28. Behzadi, S.; Serpooshan, V.; Tao, W.; Hamaly, M.A.; Alkawareek, M.Y.; Dreaden, E.C.; Brown, D.; Alkilany, A.M.; Farokhzad, O.C.; Mahmoudi, M. Cellular uptake of nanoparticles: Journey inside the cell. *Chem. Soc. Rev.* **2017**, *46*, 4218–4244. [CrossRef] [PubMed]
29. Gregory, A.; Williamson, D.; Titball, R. Vaccine delivery using nanoparticles. *Front. Cell. Infect. Microbiol.* **2013**, *3*, 13. [CrossRef]
30. He, Y.; Park, K. Effects of the Microparticle Shape on Cellular Uptake. *Mol. Pharm.* **2016**, *13*, 2164–2171. [CrossRef] [PubMed]
31. Sun, H.-F.; Pollock, K.; Brewer, J. Effects of PLGA microparticles on antigen presentation of bone marrow-derived dendritic cells in vitro. *Chin. J. Biomed. Eng.* **2005**, *24*, 35–37.
32. Snapper, C.M. Distinct Immunologic Properties of Soluble Versus Particulate Antigens. *Front. Immunol.* **2018**, *9*, 598. [CrossRef]
33. Menon, I.; Moo Kang, S.; D'Souza, M. Nanoparticle formulation of the fusion protein virus like particles of respiratory syncytial virus stimulates enhanced in vitro antigen presentation and autophagy. *Int. J. Pharm.* **2022**, *623*, 121919. [CrossRef]
34. Kale, A.; Joshi, D.; Menon, I.; Bagwe, P.; Patil, S.; Vijayanand, S.; Gomes, K.B.; D'Souza, M. Novel microparticulate Zika vaccine induces a significant immune response in a preclinical murine model after intramuscular administration. *Int. J. Pharm.* **2022**, *624*, 121975. [CrossRef]
35. Vijayanand, S.; Patil, S.; Joshi, D.; Menon, I.; Braz Gomes, K.; Kale, A.; Bagwe, P.; Yacoub, S.; Uddin, M.N.; D'Souza, M.J. Microneedle Delivery of an Adjuvanted Microparticulate Vaccine Induces High Antibody Levels in Mice Vaccinated against Coronavirus. *Vaccines* **2022**, *10*, 1491. [CrossRef]
36. Escobar-García, J.D.; Prieto, C.; Pardo-Figuerez, M.; Lagaron, J.M. Room Temperature Nanoencapsulation of Bioactive Eicosapentaenoic Acid Rich Oil within Whey Protein Microparticles. *Nanomaterials* **2021**, *11*, 575. [CrossRef]
37. Thomas, H.; Fries, F.; Gmelch, M.; Bärschneider, T.; Kroll, M.; Vavaleskou, T.; Reineke, S. Purely Organic Microparticles Showing Ultralong Room Temperature Phosphorescence. *ACS Omega* **2021**, *6*, 13087–13093. [CrossRef]
38. Kaplan, I.; Yüksel, H.; Evliyaoğlu, O.; Basarali, M.K.; Toprak, G.; Çolpan, L.; Şen, V. Effects of Storage Temperature and Time on Stability of Serum Tacrolimus and Cyclosporine A Levels in Whole Blood by LC-MS/MS. *Int. J. Anal. Chem.* **2015**, *2015*, 956389. [CrossRef] [PubMed]
39. Hines, D.J.; Kaplan, D.L. Poly (lactic-co-glycolic acid) controlled release systems: Experimental and modeling insights. *Crit. Rev. Ther. Drug Carrier Syst.* **2013**, *30*, 257–276. [CrossRef] [PubMed]
40. Lengyel, M.; Kállai-Szabó, N.; Antal, V.; Laki, A.J.; Antal, I. Microparticles, Microspheres, and Microcapsules for Advanced Drug Delivery. *Sci. Pharm.* **2019**, *87*, 20. [CrossRef]
41. Liang, Z.; Zhu, H.; Wang, X.; Jing, B.; Li, Z.; Xia, X.; Sun, H.; Yang, Y.; Zhang, W.; Shi, L.; et al. Adjuvants for Coronavirus Vaccines. *Front. Immunol.* **2020**, *11*, 589833. [CrossRef]
42. Adjuvants and Vaccines | Vaccine Safety | CDC 2020. Available online: https://www.cdc.gov/vaccinesafety/concerns/adjuvants.html (accessed on 1 July 2022).
43. Alhydrogel® Adjuvant 2%. InvivoGen 2016. Available online: https://www.invivogen.com/alhydrogel (accessed on 1 July 2022).

44. Brewer, J.M. (How) do Aluminium Adjuvants Work? *Immunol. Lett.* **2006**, *102*, 10–15. [CrossRef]
45. He, P.; Zou, Y.; Hu, Z. Advances in aluminum hydroxide-based adjuvant research and its mechanism. *Hum. Vaccin. Immunother.* **2015**, *11*, 477–488. [CrossRef] [PubMed]
46. Nian, X.; Zhang, J.; Deng, T.; Liu, J.; Gong, Z.; Lv, C.; Yao, L.; Li, J.; Huang, S.; Yang, X. AddaVax Formulated with PolyI:C as a Potential Adjuvant of MDCK-based Influenza Vaccine Enhances Local, Cellular, and Antibody Protective Immune Response in Mice. *AAPS PharmSciTech* **2021**, *22*, 270. [CrossRef]
47. AddaVax$^{TM}$. InvivoGen 2016. Available online: https://www.invivogen.com/addavax (accessed on 1 July 2022).
48. Wilkins, A.L.; Kazmin, D.; Napolitani, G.; Clutterbuck, E.A.; Pulendran, B.; Siegrist, C.A.; Pollard, A.J. AS03- and MF59-Adjuvanted Influenza Vaccines in Children. *Front. Immunol.* **2017**, *8*, 1760. [CrossRef] [PubMed]
49. Joshi, D.; Gala, R.P.; Uddin, M.N.; D'Souza, M.J. Novel ablative laser mediated transdermal immunization for microparticulate measles vaccine. *Int. J. Pharm.* **2021**, *606*, 120882. [CrossRef]
50. Gala, R.P.; Zaman, R.U.; D'Souza, M.J.; Zughaier, S.M. Novel Whole-Cell Inactivated Neisseria Gonorrhoeae Microparticles as Vaccine Formulation in Microneedle-Based Transdermal Immunization. *Vaccines* **2018**, *6*, 60. [CrossRef] [PubMed]
51. Joshi, D.; Chbib, C.; Uddin, M.N.; D'Souza, M.J. Evaluation of Microparticulate (S)-4,5-Dihydroxy-2,3-pentanedione (DPD) as a Potential Vaccine Adjuvant. *AAPS J.* **2021**, *23*, 84. [CrossRef]
52. Braz Gomes, K.; D'Sa, S.; Allotey-Babington, G.L.; Kang, S.-M.; D'Souza, M.J. Transdermal Vaccination with the Matrix-2 Protein Virus-like Particle (M2e VLP) Induces Immunity in Mice against Influenza A Virus. *Vaccines* **2021**, *9*, 1324. [CrossRef]
53. Samimi, S.; Maghsoudnia, N.; Eftekhari, R.B.; Dorkoosh, F. Chapter 3—Lipid-Based Nanoparticles for Drug Delivery Systems. In *Characterization and Biology of Nanomaterials for Drug Delivery*; Mohapatra, S.S., Ranjan, S., Dasgupta, N., Mishra, R.K., Thomas, S., Eds.; Elsevier: Amsterdam, The Netherlands, 2019; pp. 47–76. [CrossRef]
54. Uehara, E.U.; Shida, B.D.; de Brito, C.A. Role of nitric oxide in immune responses against viruses: Beyond microbicidal activity. *Inflamm. Res.* **2015**, *64*, 845–852. [CrossRef]
55. Wink, D.A.; Hines, H.B.; Cheng, R.Y.; Switzer, C.H.; Flores-Santana, W.; Vitek, M.P.; Ridnour, L.A.; Colton, C.A. Nitric oxide and redox mechanisms in the immune response. *J. Leukoc. Biol.* **2011**, *89*, 873–891. [CrossRef] [PubMed]
56. Bogdan, C.; Röllinghoff, M.; Diefenbach, A. The role of nitric oxide in innate immunity. *Immunol. Rev.* **2000**, *173*, 17–26. [CrossRef] [PubMed]
57. Tripathi, P. Nitric oxide and immune response. *Indian J. Biochem. Biophys.* **2007**, *44*, 310–319.
58. Frontiers | Redefining the Role of Langerhans Cells as Immune Regulators within the Skin n.d. Available online: https://www.frontiersin.org/articles/10.3389/fimmu.2017.01941/full (accessed on 4 August 2022).
59. Mazzini, L.; Martinuzzi, D.; Hyseni, I.; Benincasa, L.; Molesti, E.; Casa, E.; Lapini, G.; Piu, P.; Trombetta, C.M.; Marchi, S.; et al. Comparative analyses of SARS-CoV-2 binding (IgG, IgM, IgA) and neutralizing antibodies from human serum samples. *J. Immunol. Methods* **2021**, *489*, 112937. [CrossRef]
60. Nie, J.; Li, Q.; Wu, J.; Zhao, C.; Hao, H.; Liu, H.; Zhang, L.; Nie, L.; Qin, H.; Wang, M.; et al. Quantification of SARS-CoV-2 neutralizing antibody by a pseudotyped virus-based assay. *Nat. Protoc.* **2020**, *15*, 3699–3715. [CrossRef]
61. Sterlin, D.; Mathian, A.; Miyara, M.; Mohr, A.; Anna, F.; Claër, L.; Quentric, P.; Fadlallah, J.; Devilliers, H.; Ghillani, P.; et al. IgA dominates the early neutralizing antibody response to SARS-CoV-2. *Sci. Transl. Med.* **2021**, *13*, eabd2223. [CrossRef]
62. Aleebrahim-Dehkordi, E.; Molavi, B.; Mokhtari, M.; Deravi, N.; Fathi, M.; Fazel, T.; Mohebalizadeh, M.; Koochaki, P.; Shobeiri, P.; Hasanpour-Dehkordi, A. T helper type (Th1/Th2) responses to SARS-CoV-2 and influenza A (H1N1) virus: From cytokines produced to immune responses. *Transpl. Immunol.* **2022**, *70*, 101495. [CrossRef] [PubMed]
63. Carty, S.A.; Riese, M.J.; Koretzky, G.A. Chapter 21—T-Cell Immunity. In *Hematology*, 7th ed.; Hoffman, R., Benz, E.J., Silberstein, L.E., Heslop, H.E., Weitz, J.I., Anastasi, J., Salama, M.E., Abutalib, S.A., Eds.; Elsevier: Amsterdam, The Netherlands, 2018; pp. 221–239. [CrossRef]
64. Ganneru, B.; Jogdand, H.; Daram, V.K.; Das, D.; Molugu, N.R.; Prasad, S.D.; Kannappa, S.V.; Ella, K.M.; Ravikrishnan, R.; Awasthi, A.; et al. Th1 skewed immune response of whole virion inactivated SARS CoV 2 vaccine and its safety evaluation. *IScience* **2021**, *24*, 102298. [CrossRef] [PubMed]
65. Getahun, A.; Dahlström, J.; Wernersson, S.; Heyman, B. IgG2a-Mediated Enhancement of Antibody and T Cell Responses and Its Relation to Inhibitory and Activating Fc$\gamma$ Receptors1. *J. Immunol.* **2004**, *172*, 5269–5276. [CrossRef] [PubMed]

pharmaceutics

Article

# Biocontrol Microneedle Patch: A Promising Agent for Protecting Citrus Fruits from Postharvest Infection

Ling Jiang [1,2], Huan Huang [1], Xingyu Shi [1], Jian Wu [3], Juexian Ye [1], Qian Xu [1,4], Shaobin Fang [5], Chuanbin Wu [2], Rui Luo [2,*], Chao Lu [2,4,*] and Daojun Liu [1,*]

1 Department of Pharmacy, Shantou University Medical College, Shantou 515041, China
2 College of Pharmacy, Jinan University, Guangzhou 511436, China
3 Shantou Central Hospital, Shantou 515041, China
4 Guangdong Provincial Key Laboratory of Infectious Diseases and Molecular Immunopathology, Shantou University Medical College, Shantou 515041, China
5 The Second Affiliated Hospital of Shantou University Medical College, Shantou 515000, China
* Correspondence: luocq1989@163.com (R.L.); chaolu@jnu.edu.cn (C.L.); liudj@stu.edu.cn (D.L.)

**Abstract:** With increasing human awareness of food safety, the replacement of highly toxic pesticides with biocompatible antimicrobials has become a trend. This study proposes a biocontrol microneedle (BMN) to expand the application of the food-grade preservative epsilon-poly-L-lysine (ε-PL) in fruit preservatives by utilizing a dissolving microneedle system. The macromolecular polymer ε-PL not only possesses broad-spectrum antimicrobial activity but also exhibits good mechanical properties. With the addition of a small amount of polyvinyl alcohol, the mechanical strength of the ε-PL-based microneedle patch could be further improved to achieve an enhanced failure force of needles at 1.6 N/needle and induce an approximately 96% insertion rate in citrus fruit pericarps. An ex vivo insertion test revealed that the microneedle tips could be effectively inserted into the citrus fruit pericarp, rapidly dissolve within 3 min, and produce inconspicuous needle holes. Moreover, the high drug loading capacity of BMN was observed to reach approximately 1890 μg/patch, which is essential for enhancing the concentration-dependent antifungal activity of ε-PL. The drug distribution study has confirmed the feasibility of mediating the local diffusion of EPL in the pericarp through BMN. Therefore, BMN has great potential to reduce the incidence of invasive fungal infections in local areas of citrus fruit pericarp.

**Keywords:** biocontrol microneedle patch; antifungal agent; ε-poly-lysine; citrus fruit; postharvest infection

## 1. Introduction

Fruits (e.g., citrus, grapes, and apples) have high economic and nutritional values but high nutrient and water contents, which make them susceptible to postharvest mold infections [1–3]. Numerous types of pathogens exist that induce fruit diseases in nature, including *Penicillium digitatum*, *Penicillium italicum*, *Penicillium expansum*, *Botrytis cinerea*, and *Alternaria alternata* [4–8]. Therefore, the application of broad-spectrum antifungals is important for the postharvest disease control of fruits.

Artificial fungicides, including thiabendazole, sodium ortho-phenylphenol, and imazalil, have been extensively used to inhibit the spread of postharvest fruit diseases. However, residues of these chemical fungicides are usually toxic and carcinogenic and may induce chronic or acute toxicity in humans [9–11]. In contrast, epsilon-poly-L-lysine (ε-PL), which typically consists of 25–40 L-lysine residues, has been approved by the US Food and Drug Administration (FDA) as a food-grade preservative because of its broad-spectrum activity, biodegradability, and biocompatibility [12]. Recently, ε-PL has been widely used in the preservation of instant rice, cooked noodles, cooked vegetables, seafood, sauces, soy sauce, and crackers [13,14]. However, fruit cuticles primarily composed of polymer cutin and cuticular wax provide effective surface barriers, which are not conducive to the penetration of polar macromolecules such as ε-PL [15,16]. The low percutaneous efficiency of ε-PL may severely hinder its inhibition of pathogens colonizing the deep pericarp. Therefore, the application of ε-PL in controlling the postharvest decay of fruits is still limited and remains only in the field of basic research.

The microneedle patch is a novel topical drug delivery system in which the drug is incorporated into tiny needles at the micron level and the needles are attached to a base-supporting patch. Drugs can pass through the tissue barrier via needle tips by pressing the microneedle patch onto the tissue surface with significantly improved transdermal delivery efficiency [17,18]. Owing to the recent increase in the level of mass production, the reduction in production costs, and the advantages of its universality, microneedle patches have been developed for skin disease treatment [19–22], blood alcohol and glucose detection [23–25], and vaccination [26–29].

Considering the above-mentioned advantages of microneedles, this study proposes the construction of a biocontrol microneedle-array patch (BMN) based on the food-grade preservative ε-PL to explore its potential application in controlling the decay of fruits, particularly citrus fruits (Scheme 1). An ex vivo insertion test of various microneedles in pericarp was first carried out to screen the optimal microneedle formulation. Subsequently, the drug loading amount, microneedle mechanics, and insertion ability of the ε-PL-based BMN were characterized. To elucidate the mode of action after microneedle administration, the dissolution and diffusion behavior of BMN have been investigated. Finally, cytotoxicity experiments were conducted to demonstrate the safety of BMN. This ε-PL-based microneedle patch is expected to exhibit the following advantages: (1) In addition to serving as a broad-spectrum antimicrobial, ε-PL with a molecular weight of 3.2~4.4 kDa possesses the mechanical properties of polymeric materials [30], which can improve the drug loading capacity by reducing the amount of microneedle tip excipients. (2) Using the dissolving microneedle patch system, ε-PL can efficiently penetrate into the citrus pericarp to exert better mold prevention and control. (3) ε-PL can be degraded into natural amino acids required by the human body in the gastrointestinal tract after oral administration, and its safety is much higher than that of traditional pesticides [31]. (4) The micron-level pores produced by microneedle piercing will naturally shrink with the evaporation of water on the pericarp surface, which is conducive to reducing the entry of microorganisms into the citrus through the pores, while ensuring the aesthetics of the fruit surfaces. (5) The improvements of large-scale production, the reduction in production costs, and the development of potential advertising uses in recent years are expected to reduce the cost of antimicrobial microneedles in fruit preservation.

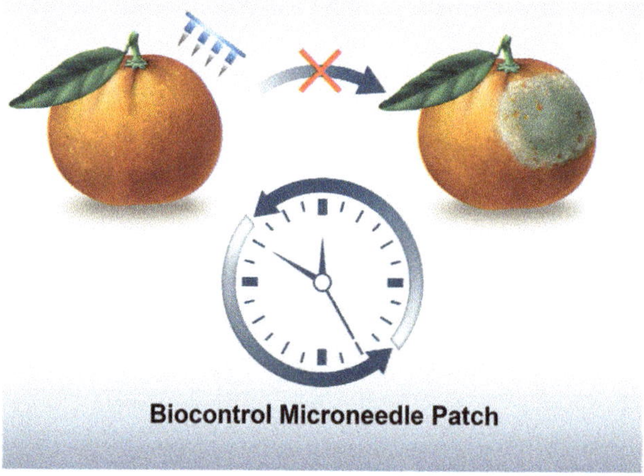


**Scheme 1.** Schematic illustration of using BMN to protect fruits from infection.

## 2. Materials and Methods

### 2.1. Materials

Polyvinyl alcohol (PVA, 103) and trypan blue were obtained from Aladdin (Shanghai, China). Polyvinyl pyrrolidone (PVP K90) were kindly donated by BASF (Ludwigshafen, Germany). ε-PL was purchased from Binafo Biology Co., Ltd. (Zhengzhou, China). L-lysine hydrochloride and 4% paraformaldehyde were purchased from Sigma-Aldrich (Shanghai, China). An adhesive label was purchased from Deli (Ningbo, China). Sulfo-Cyanine-7 NHS ester (Cy7) was purchased from Xi'an Qianghua Biological Technology Co., Ltd. (Xi'an, China). All the other solvents and materials used were of analytical grade.

### 2.2. Fabrication and Imaging Study of Various Microneedles

BMN were prepared by a multi-step centrifugation method using female polydimethylsiloxane (PDMS) molds fabricated by replica molding from a microneedle array template. First, a template of a microneedle patch with a 12 × 12 array of tetragonal pyramidal needles was fabricated using computer-aided design and computer-aided manufacturing cutting operations with brass as the raw material.

The master molds were placed in anhydrous ethanol and cleaned via ultrasonication. Then, a 10:1 mixture of polydimethylsiloxane (PDMS) monomer and curing agent (Dow Corning Slygard 184) was poured into the mold, degassed under vacuum for 30 min, and cured at 80 °C for 2 h. After cooling to room temperature, a PDMS mold with a morphology complementary to that of the master mold was obtained.

Subsequently, ε-PL was mixed with ultrapure water at a ratio of 1:1.8 ($w/v$) and stirred until completely dissolved. PVA solution was obtained by mixing PVA with ultrapure water at a ratio of 1:1.8 ($w/v$) and water bath at 90 °C for 2 h. Needle tip solutions containing different amounts of ε-PL were obtained by mixing ε-PL solution with PVA solution at the mass ratios of 1:9, 3:7, 5:5, 7:3, and 9:1, respectively. After a water bath at 65 °C for 1 h, 250 μL of the needle tip solution was added to the PDMS molds and centrifuged at 3500× $g$ at 20–30 °C for 10 min. After removing excess needle tip solution from the molds, the drug-containing needle tips were centrifuged at 3500× $g$ at 20–30 °C for 10 min to allow the molds to be filled and properly concentrated. Further, 26.2% ethanolic solution of PVP K90 was added to the PDMS molds and centrifuged at 3500× $g$ for 45 min at 0–10 °C. Finally, the BMN were gently separated from the PDMS molds by drying in a desiccator for 72 h at room temperature. To evaluate the distribution of ε-PL in the tip, microneedles with a PVP layer stained with trypan blue were prepared using a method similar to that described above, except that an appropriate amount of trypan blue dye was dissolved in the PVP K90 ethanol solution.

A digital camera and inverted microscope (Eclipse Ts2, Nikon Corporation, Japan) were used to observe the morphology of the different microneedles. In addition, the newly prepared microneedles were sputter-coated and imaged using a SU8010 scanning electron microscope (SEM, Hitachi, Tokyo, Japan).

### 2.3. Fruit Treatment

Organically farmed lemons and Satsuma mandarins were purchased from a local citrus farm in Sichuan and Guangxi provinces in China, respectively. Valencia oranges and green pomelos imported from South Africa and Thailand, respectively, were purchased in a local supermarket. All citrus fruits of the four species without any apparent surface damage and infection were chosen, washed with deionized water, and drained until dryness.

### 2.4. An Ex Vivo Insertion Test of Various Microneedles in Pericarp

To evaluate the insertion ability of the different dissolving microneedles in citrus fruits, different microneedles were inserted into the pericarp of freshly separated citrus fruits for 5 min. After removing the microneedles, a 4% ($w/v$) solution of trypan blue was added dropwise to the pericarp, where the microneedles were inserted for 2 min. The excess dye solution was washed with distilled water. Stained pores on the pericarp surface were observed and photographed using a digital camera. The efficiency of microneedle tip insertion into the pericarp was calculated as follows:

$$\text{Insertion efficacy (\%)} = N_p/N_n \times 100\% \tag{1}$$

where $N_p$ and $N_n$ are the number of stained pores on the pericarp surface and needle tips on the microneedles, respectively.

## 2.5. Determination of the Thickness and Water Content of Various Pericarp

To evaluate the pericarp thickness of the different fruits, pericarp discs with a diameter of 3 cm were cut and separated from the equatorial plane of the different citrus fruits, and the pericarp thickness was measured using Vernier calipers.

To evaluate the moisture content of the different pericarps, freshly obtained pericarps were weighed and dried in an oven (Boxun, Shanghai, China) at 70 °C until they reached a constant weight. The water content of the pericarp was then determined and calculated as follows:

$$\text{Water content (\%)} = (W_0 - W)/W_0 \times 100\% \tag{2}$$

where $W_0$ and W are the pericarp weights before and after drying, respectively.

## 2.6. Drug Loading Amount of BMN

To evaluate the loading amount of ε-PL in BMN, the needle part of the BMN was carefully separated using a scalpel blade and dissolved in $H_2O$. Subsequently, the ε-PL content of the samples was analyzed by high-performance liquid chromatography (HPLC, Agilent technologies, Santa Clara, CA, USA) using a Waters X-Bridge TM C18 analytical column (4.6 mm × 150 mm, 3.5 μm). The samples were eluted with a linear gradient of water-acetonitrile with 0.1% trifluoroacetic acid at a flow rate of 1 mL/min and were detected at 215 nm.

## 2.7. Microneedle Mechanics

The mechanical strength of the various microneedles was measured using a texture analyzer (TA-XT Plus, Stable Micro Systems, Godalming, UK) [32]. Briefly, the microneedle was placed on the surface of the metallic platform of the texture analyzer. The probe was programmed to move down toward the microneedles patches at a rate of 0.1 mm/s until mechanical fracture occurred. In this study, force was applied parallel to the microneedle axis. Stress versus strain curves were obtained by measuring the force and displacement.

## 2.8. Pericarp Morphology after Microneedle Insertion

To further observe the effect of microneedle insertion on pericarp morphology, fresh pericarps of Satsuma mandarins were obtained. The microneedles were inserted into the surface of the pericarp using thumb pressure for 2 min. After removing the microneedle patches, the pericarp was dried naturally in the air for 30 min and then fixed in 4% paraformaldehyde. Subsequently, pericarp sections were prepared and stained with hematoxylin and eosin (H&E, Beyotime, Shanghai, China) for histopathological observation.

## 2.9. Dissolution Rate of Microneedle Tip in Pericarp

Fresh pericarps of Satsuma mandarin were harvested to investigate the dissolution rate of the microneedle tip in the pericarp. Briefly, microneedles were inserted into the pericarp surface using thumb pressure. At pre-set time points (1, 3, 5, 10, 15, and 30 min), the microneedles were removed and the tip of the microneedle was imaged using an inverted microscope system (Eclipse Ts2, Nikon, Tokyo, Japan).

## 2.10. Study of Drug Distribution after Microneedle Administration

To study the distribution of ε-PL in intact citrus and isolated pericarp, Cy7 was immobilized onto ε-PL and then Cy7-labeled BMN was fabricated. Then, the microneedles were, respectively, inserted into the surface of intact citrus and isolated pericarp for 5 min. At predetermined time points, the fluorescence imaging of citrus and isolated pericarp was conducted using an in vivo imaging system (Lumina III, Perkin Elmer, Waltham, MA, USA).

### 2.11. In Vitro Cytotoxicity Assay

The cytotoxicity of needle-tip excipients on human-originated colon epithelial cells (NCM460) was studied using the cell counting kit-8 (CCK-8) method (Dojindo, Kumamoto, Japan) [33,34]. Briefly, cells were inoculated into 96-well plates and incubated overnight at 37 °C in 5% $CO_2$. After 24 h, the medium was removed, and 100 μL of fresh medium containing different concentrations of ε-PL/PVA mixture or L-lysine hydrochloride was added. After another 24 h of incubation, the medium was replaced with 100 μL of fresh DMEM containing 10% fetal bovine serum (Gibco, Grand Island, NY, USA), followed by the addition of 10 μL of CCK-8 solution. After 4 h of incubation, relative cell viability was calculated by measuring the absorbance at 450 nm. The cell viability was calculated as follows:

$$\text{Cell viability (\%)} = (A_{sample} - A_{blank})/(A_{control} - A_{blank}) \times 100\% \quad (3)$$

where $A_{sample}$ is the absorbance of wells containing cells, CCK-8 solution, and sample solution; $A_{blank}$ indicates the absorbance of wells containing medium and CCK-8 solution without cells; and $A_{control}$ indicates the absorbance of wells containing cells and CCK-8 solution but not the sample solution.

### 2.12. Fabrication of Microneedles with an Adhesive Label

An adhesive label was used to wrap the microneedle patch and improve its adherence to the fruit surface. The text and pattern describing the product information were printed on the adhesive label using a printer. The label was then cut into the desired shape. After removing the anti-sticking layer of the adhesive label, microneedle patches were attached to the center of the label.

## 3. Results and Discussion

### 3.1. Preparation of Microneedles Loaded with ε-PL

We designed a brass template of a microneedle patch with a 12 × 12 array of tetragonal pyramidal needles with a base width of 300 μm and a height of 1200 μm (600 μm pyramidal tip; 600 μm base column). Meanwhile, the tip diameter of the needles was controlled to be no greater than 30 μm, ensuring that the microneedle is sharp enough. PDMS molds fabricated by replica molding from the microneedle array template were used for the fabrication of the ε-PL-loaded microneedles (Figure 1A). As shown in Figure 1B, the microneedles fabricated from pure ε-PL had a high needle breakage rate, and the texture of the tip was extremely brittle. Therefore, we chose PVA, which is a tougher polymer, to improve the tip formability of ε-PL microneedles. The introduction of PVA significantly improved the microneedle shape, resulting in microneedle patches with almost no needle breakage (Figure 1C,D).

### 3.2. Pericarp Insertion Performance and Optimization of Various Microneedles

To determine the optimal ratio of ε-PL and PVA, microneedles with different ratios of ε-PL and PVA were prepared. Citrus fruits such as lemon, Satsuma mandarin, Valencia oranges, and green pomelo were selected for this study and characterized for their basic pericarp properties (Figure 2A–C). Because trypan blue can stain broken tissues [35], the pericarp insertion performance of different microneedles was evaluated using trypan blue staining (Figure 2D,E).

As shown in Figure 2D,E, different ratios of ε-PL and PVA had a greater impact on the pericarp insertion performance. At a 9:1 ratio between ε-PL and PVA, the microneedles with lower PVA content may be brittle, resulting in easy breakage of the microneedles during skin puncture. Moreover, owing to the high hygroscopicity of ε-PL, premature dissolution of microneedles during skin puncture may also significantly affect the insertion depth of the microneedles. Conversely, lower skin puncture at high-PVA-specific gravity may be due to the lack of sufficient stiffness of the microneedle to puncture the fruit pericarp.

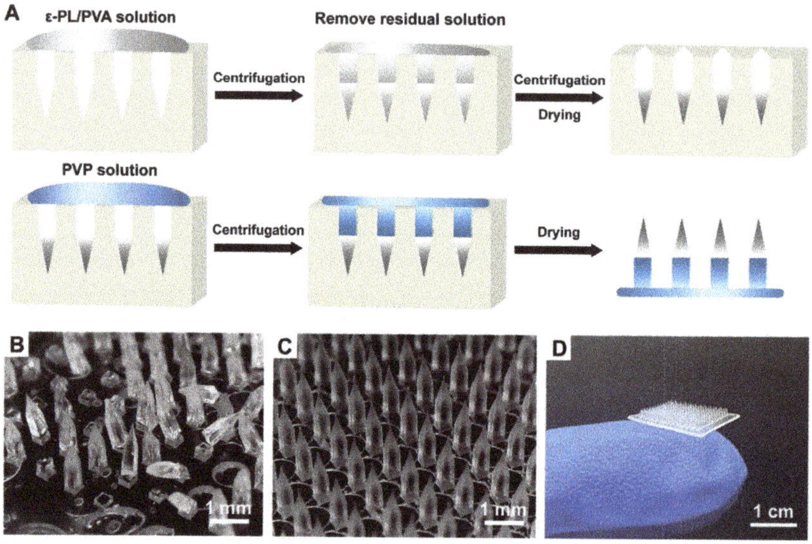


**Figure 1.** Preparation of ε-PL-loaded microneedles. (**A**) Schematic of the preparation process of ε-PL-loaded microneedles; digital microscope photographs of microneedles with ε-PL to PVA ratio of 10:0 (**B**) and 5:5 (**C**). (**D**) Macroscopic morphology of ε-PL/PVA hybridized microneedles.

Because the thickness of the pericarp is related to its mechanical properties, the moisture content of the pericarp also affects the dissolution rate of microneedles [36,37]. We compared the skin thickness and water content of four fruits: lemon, Satsuma mandarin, Valencia oranges, and green pomelo. The fruits with the thinnest and thickest pericarps included Satsuma mandarin and green pomelo, respectively. In addition, the fruits with the smallest and largest water content included Satsuma mandarin and Valencia oranges, respectively. However, the highest insertion rate of approximately 96% was obtained for microneedles with a 7:3 ratio of ε-PL to PVA in all the fruit puncture tests (Figure 2E). This result indicates that microneedles with a 7:3 ratio of ε-PL to PVA possess both good mechanical properties and resistance to moisture. Thus, we selected this formulation as the optimal formulation for the BMN construction and used it in the subsequent evaluation.

### *3.3. Characterization of BMN*

BMN is expected to have a well-defined structure, with ε-PL being enriched at the tip of the needle (Figure 3A). Therefore, we stained the PVP-based substrate layer with trypan blue. As shown in Figure 3B,C, the microneedle tip of ε-PL and PVA hybridization had an intact needle shape, no air bubbles at the tip, and a clear partitioning between the ε-PL-containing layer of the tip and the substrate layer. The ε-PL-containing tip layer was distributed in the region 0~600 μm from the tip. SEM images of this microneedle were obtained to observe the microstructure of the BMNs. Figure 3D shows that the BMN tip was intact with no obvious fine defects, indicating that ε-PL is compatible with PVA.

We quantified the mechanical properties of the needle tip of the BMN using a texture analyzer and measured the force that a microneedle could withstand before failure using the method of Park et al. [36]. Stress versus strain curves of the BMN were thus obtained, and the maximum force applied immediately before dropping was identified as the force of needle failure. As shown in Figure 3E, the prepared BMN microneedles showed a failure force of 1.6 N per needle, indicating that the microneedles should have sufficient strength to penetrate the pericarp without breaking.

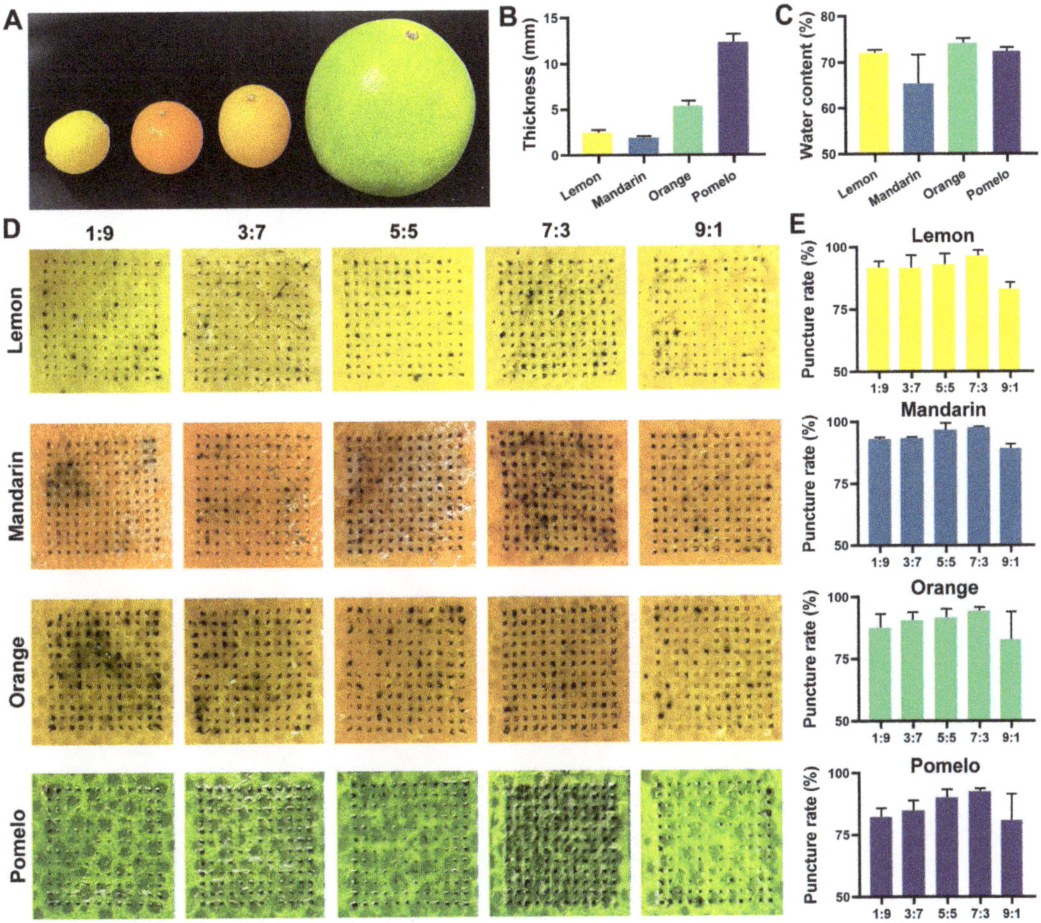


**Figure 2.** Characterization of pericarp insertion performance of different microneedles in citrus fruits. (**A**) Photographs of lemon, Satsuma mandarin, Valencia oranges and green pomelo. Water content (**B**) and pericarp thickness (**C**) of different fruits. (**D**) Photographs of the pericarp after the treatment of different microneedles and stained with Trypan blue. (**E**) Pericarp insertion rates of different microneedles in different fruits.

To further investigate the insertion performance of BMN into the pericarp, we collected Satsuma mandarin pericarps after microneedle administration for H&E staining (Figure 3F,G). Figure 3H,I shows that BMN could form distinct micropore channels in the Satsuma mandarin pericarp after puncture, reaching depths between 660 and 920 μm. Notably, microneedle systems usually penetrate mammalian skin with a penetration depth of merely 50–400 μm, because the skin surface is more deformable than fruit pericarps [17–21]. The deeper micropore channels caused by the microneedle penetration into the pericarp imply that ε-PL could be delivered to deeper tissues via BMN, which also illustrated the great application potential of the microneedle system in protecting fruits from postharvest infection.

Interestingly, we found that these micropore channels would naturally close after BMN administration, probably because of tissue wrinkling caused by water evaporation from the pericarp surface (Figure 3I). The hole on the pericarp surface gradually became less visible within 3 h (Figure 3J,K), which may have resulted in an improved appearance of the fruit and hindered the invasion of external microorganisms.

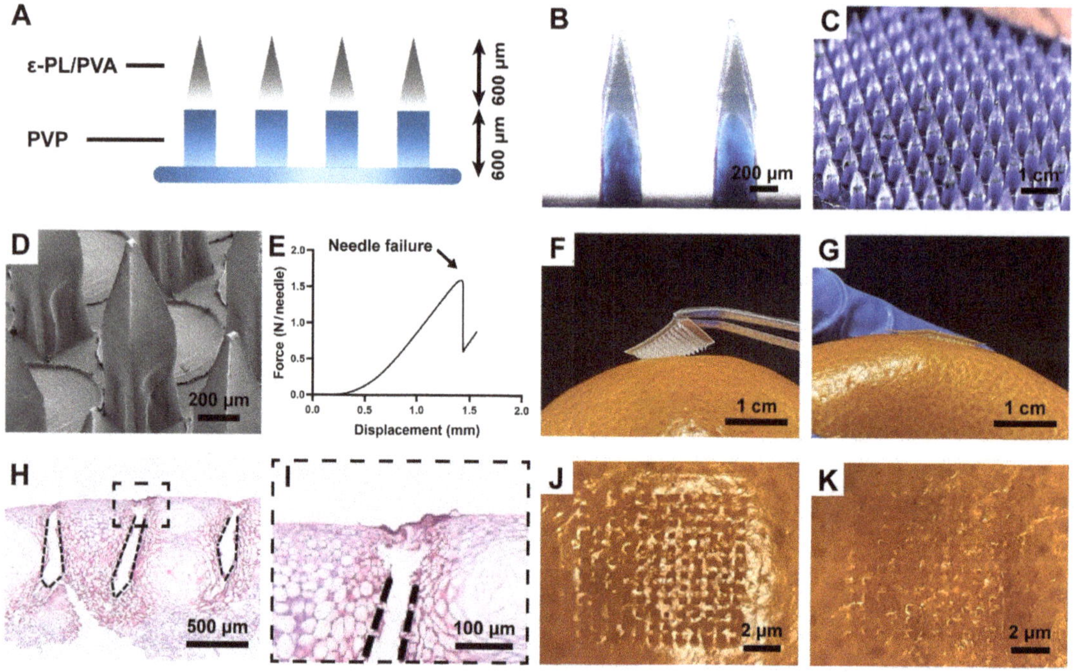


**Figure 3.** Structural characterization and insertion performance of BMN. (**A**) Schematic of the microneedle tip structure. Microscopic (**B**) and camera image (**C**) of BMN with the basal layer stained with trypan blue. (**D**) SEM image of BMN. (**E**) Failure behavior of BMN under axial load. Photograph of Satsuma mandarin before (**F**) and after BMN treatment (**G**). H&E-stained image of BMN after puncture into the pericarp of Satsuma mandarin (**H**) and its local magnification (**I**). Photograph of the pericarp of Satsuma mandarin before (**J**) and after 3 h of BMN insertion (**K**).

### *3.4. Dissolution Properties of BMN in Fruit Pericarp*

To evaluate the dissolution behavior and dissolution rate of BMN after puncturing the pericarp, the microneedle was observed by microscopy after puncturing the citrus skin at different times. As shown in Figure 4, the ε-PL-containing needle tip dissolved completely after 3 min of BMN piercing the pericarp, and the entire microneedle tip disappeared completely within 30 min. This experiment indicated that the needle tips of BMN have good solubility and that BMN could promote the ε-PL efficiently pass through the outer cuticles of fruit pericarp.

### *3.5. Antifungal Potential of BMN*

As a natural antimicrobial peptide, ε-PL usually kills pathogens through a membrane disruption mechanism [38,39]. While the fungal cell membrane is negatively charged, cationic ε-PL can electrostatically bind to cells with little dependence on specific receptors or essential components of the fungal cell membranes [40]. Therefore, various previous studies have indicated that ε-PL displays effective antifungal activity against a range of plant pathogenic fungi, which may result in cell dysfunction and suppression of spore germination or mycelial growth [41–46]. ε-PL can inhibit common postharvest pathogens, including *Alternaria alternata*, *Botrytis cinerea*, *Penicillium expansum*, and *Penicillium digitatum*, with half-maximal inhibitory concentration ($IC_{50}$) values of 30–200 μg/mL [46].

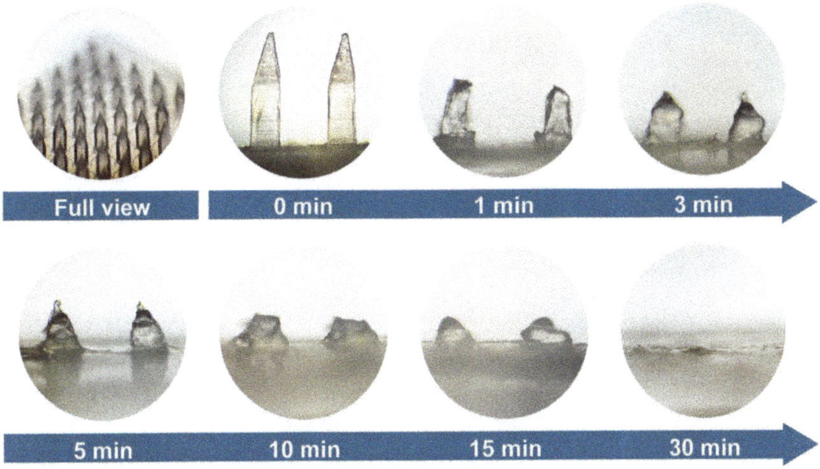


**Figure 4.** Appearance of BMN and its needle tip length after insertion into citrus pericarp for different times.

To investigate the antifungal potential of BMN, we separated the needle tips of BMN and measured the ε-PL content using HPLC. We found that the drug-loading capacity of BMN was very high, and the microneedle patch contained up to 1890 μg of ε-PL per patch. As ε-PL could suppress fungal cell viability in a concentration-dependent manner, a higher ε-PL loading capacity implies that BMN may be more effective in protecting fruits from postharvest infection.

### 3.6. Drug Distribution Study

Microneedle patches have been widely applied in the treatment of animal diseases, and drugs can be rapidly and systematically distributed through the blood circulation. When microneedles are used to fruit preservatives, drug distribution may be achieved mainly through concentration gradient-mediated drug diffusion. Therefore, to evaluate the unique mode of action of microneedles for topical application in fruits, we constructed a BMN using Cy7-labeled ε-PL, and administered them to the surface of intact citrus and isolated pericarp, respectively. Interestingly, we found that the diffusion of ε-PL was rapid within 6 h of microneedle administration, and the distribution area of ε-PL remained increased over a period of 72 h (Figure 5A). To quantify the distribution of ε-PL on the pericarp, we further isolated the pericarp of citrus, administered microneedles in the center of the pericarp, and measured the diameter of fluorescent area. As shown in Figure 5B,C, a large concentration difference facilitated the rapid diffusion of ε-PL from BMN to the pericarp forming a fluorescent area with a diameter of 51.1 $\pm$ 3.3 mm at 6 h post-BMN administration, and this area could was continuously enlarged to 58 $\pm$ 12.8 mm in diameter after 72 h. These results indicated that although distributed primarily by diffusion, BMN can deliver ε-PL to the pericarp and create a large drug distribution area, and BMN has great potential to reduce the incidence of invasive fungal infections in local areas of citrus fruit pericarp (e.g., areas with localized damage).

### 3.7. Cytocompatibility Study

To investigate whether the tip material of the BMN could induce potential toxicity to cells in the gastrointestinal tract, the CCK-8 method was used to explore the cytocompatibility of the mixture of ε-PL and PVA (7:3) [47]. Figure 6 demonstrates that the mixture of ε-PL and PVA showed little cytotoxicity against NCM460 cells.

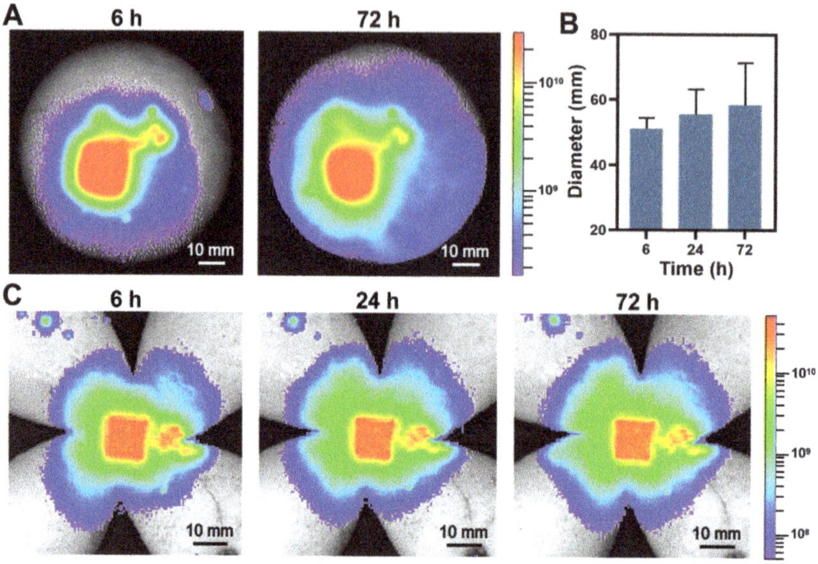


**Figure 5.** Characterization of ε-PL distribution after BMN administration. (**A**) Representative fluorescence images of citrus after Cy7-labeled BMN administration. The diameter changes (**B**) and representative images (**C**) of the fluorescent area on the pericarp of citrus after Cy7-labeled BMN administration.

As lysine-based ε-PL can be degraded by enzymes in the gastrointestinal tract, we further investigated the effect of different concentrations of L-lysine hydrochloride on the viability of NCM460 cells. As shown in Figure 6, the degradation products of ε-PL had little effect on the survival of cells in the gastrointestinal tract, which further suggests that BMN needle-tip excipients may be unlikely to cause significant toxic effects after consumption.

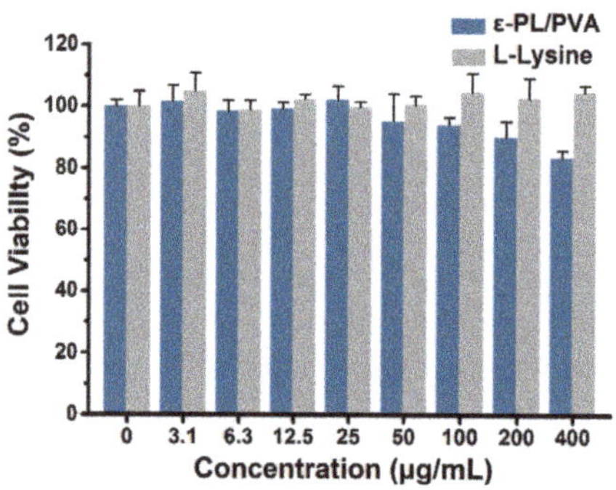


**Figure 6.** Cell viability of NCM460 cells after treatment with different concentrations of ε-PL/PVA mixture or L-lysine hydrochloride.

### 3.8. *Adhesive Outer Layer and Its Potential Applications*

To prevent BMN from falling off during use and to increase the sealing of holes created by the microneedles, an additional layer consisting of an adhesive sticker can be added to the outside of the PVP layer of the BMN. As shown in Figure 7, with the addition of the adhesive outer layer, BMN can be firmly attached to the surface of citrus. By printing text and/or pattern on the surface of the adhesive outer layer, BMN can also be used to provide information on the fruit's production time, preservation conditions, price, and other product information.

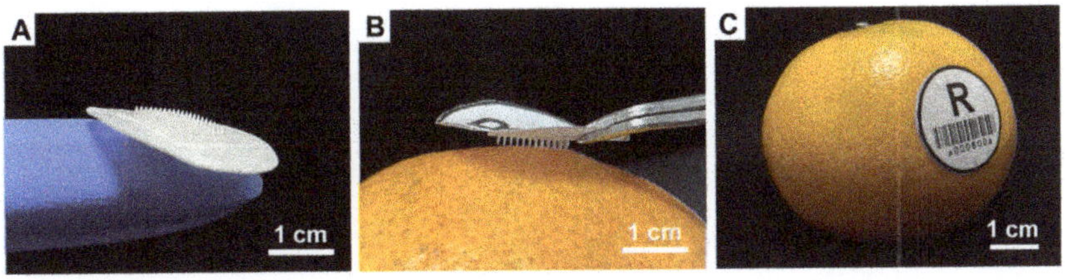


**Figure 7.** Appearance of the adhesive outer layer of BMN (**A**) and the photograph of Satsuma mandarin before (**B**) and after the microneedle patches treatment (**C**).

## 4. Conclusions

In this study, the concept of biocontrol microneedles was proposed to develop a novel biocontrol agent for eliminating postharvest fungal pathogens by exploiting the high drug transdermal delivery properties of the dissolving microneedle system. We successfully optimized the feeding ratio of ε-PL to PVA for the construction of a biocontrol microneedle at 7:3 through an ex vivo insertion test of various microneedles in citrus fruit pericarps. Moreover, BMN was confirmed to have excellent mechanical properties and could be inserted into the pericarp of different citrus fruits with an approximately 96% insertion rate. After insertion into the pericarp, ε-PL located at the tip of the microneedle can be rapidly dissolved and released into the pericarp within 3 min. This microneedle has a high ε-PL loading capacity, which allows a concentration-dependent antimicrobial agent such as ε-PL to exert greater antimicrobial efficacy. The drug distribution study showed that ε-PL could be diffused from the local area after microneedle administration. Moreover, CCK-8 experiments verified the low cytotoxicity of ε-PL and PVA mixtures and the degradation products of ε-PL. Therefore, this study preliminarily confirmed the feasibility and application potential of BMN, and it is believed that it can be applied to protect more types of fruits or vegetables from postharvest infection through further optimization. Notably, we calculated that the raw material cost to produce a BMN is no more than USD 0.005, but the main and high cost of fabricating BMN may be attributed to the manufacturing process. Given that the cost of manufacturing remains a significant uncertainty, robust and cost-effective manufacturing of the BMN may be another important issue needing further study and development.

**Author Contributions:** Conceptualization, C.W., R.L., C.L. and D.L.; methodology, L.J., H.H., S.F., C.W. and C.L.; formal analysis, L.J. and X.S.; investigation, L.J., J.W. and J.Y.; writing—original draft preparation, L.J. and H.H.; writing—review and editing, L.J., S.F., C.L. and D.L.; visualization, L.J. and C.L.; supervision, R.L., C.L. and D.L.; validation, Q.X. and R.L.; project administration, R.L., C.L. and D.L.; funding acquisition, Q.X., C.L. and D.L. All authors have read and agreed to the published version of the manuscript.

**Funding:** This research was funded by the Open Fund of Guangdong Provincial Key Laboratory of Infectious Diseases and Molecular Immunopathology (Grant No. GDKL202207), the Science and Technology Program of Guangzhou (Grant No. 202102020887), and the 2020 Li Ka Shing Foundation Cross-Disciplinary Research Grant, Hong Kong, China (Grant No. 2020LKSFG18B).

**Data Availability Statement:** Data are available on request.

**Acknowledgments:** The authors would like to thank Tingting Peng for her help in writing process.

**Conflicts of Interest:** The authors declare no conflict of interest.

## References


1. Salem, M.F.; Abd-Elraoof, W.A.; Tayel, A.A.; Alzuaibr, F.M.; Abonama, O.M. Antifungal Application of Biosynthesized Selenium Nanoparticles with Pomegranate Peels and Nanochitosan as Edible Coatings for Citrus Green Mold Protection. *J. Nanobiotechnol.* **2022**, *20*, 182. [CrossRef] [PubMed]
2. Tripathi, P.; Dubey, N.K.; Shukla, A.K. Use of some Essential Oils as Post-Harvest Botanical Fungicides in the Management of Grey Mould of Grapes Caused by *Botrytis cinerea*. *World J. Microbiol. Biotechnol.* **2008**, *24*, 39–46. [CrossRef]
3. Wang, K.L.; Ngea, G.L.N.; Godana, E.A.; Shi, Y.; Lanhuang, B.; Zhang, X.Y.; Zhao, L.N.; Yang, Q.Y.; Wang, S.Y.; Zhang, H.Y. Recent Advances in *Penicillium expansum* Infection Mechanisms and Current Methods in Controlling *P. expansum* in Postharvest Apples. *Crit. Rev. Food Sci. Nutr.* **2021**, 1–14. [CrossRef] [PubMed]
4. Zhang, J.; Zhang, B.; Zhu, F.X.; Fu, Y.P. Baseline Sensitivity and Fungicidal Action of Propiconazole against *Penicillium digitatum*. *Pestic. Biochem. Physiol.* **2021**, *172*, 104752. [CrossRef] [PubMed]
5. Guo, J.; Qin, D.K.; Li, W.T.; Wu, F.H.; Li, L.; Liu, X.Q. Inactivation of *Penicillium italicum* on Kumquat via Plasma-Activated Water and Its Effects on Quality Attributes. *Int. J. Food Microbiol.* **2021**, *343*, 109090. [CrossRef]
6. Luciano-Rosario, D.; Keller, N.P.; Jurick, W.M. *Penicillium expansum*: Biology, Omics, and Management Tools for a Global Postharvest Pathogen Causing Blue Mould of Pome Fruit. *Mol. Plant Pathol.* **2020**, *21*, 1391–1404. [CrossRef]
7. Bi, K.; Liang, Y.; Mengiste, T.; Sharon, A. Killing Softly: A Roadmap of *Botrytis cinerea* Pathogenicity. *Trends Plant Sci.* **2022**, *28*, 211–222. [CrossRef]
8. Wang, F.; Saito, S.; Michailides, T.J.; Xiao, C.L. Postharvest Use of Natamycin to Control Alternaria Rot on Blueberry Fruit Caused by *Alternaria alternata* and *A. arborescens*. *Postharvest Biol. Technol.* **2021**, *172*, 111383. [CrossRef]
9. Deng, B.; Wang, W.J.; Ruan, C.Q.; Deng, L.L.; Yao, S.X.; Zeng, K.F. Involvement of CsWRKY70 in Salicylic Acid-Induced Citrus Fruit Resistance against *Penicillium digitatum*. *Hortic. Res.* **2020**, *7*, 157. [CrossRef]
10. Liu, X.; Jiao, W.X.; Du, Y.M.; Chen, Q.M.; Su, Z.B.; Fu, M.R. Chlorine Dioxide Controls Green Mold Caused by *Penicillium digitatum* in Citrus Fruits and the Mechanism Involved. *J. Agric. Food Chem.* **2020**, *68*, 13897–13905. [CrossRef]
11. Bhatta, U.K. Alternative Management Approaches of Citrus Diseases Caused by *Penicillium digitatum* (Green Mold) and *Penicillium italicum* (Blue Mold). *Front. Plant Sci.* **2022**, *12*, 833328. [CrossRef]
12. You, X.M.; Einson, J.E.; Lopez-Pena, C.L.; Song, M.Y.; Xiao, H.; McClements, D.J.; Sela, D.A. Food-Grade Cationic Antimicrobial ε-polylysine Transiently Alters the Gut Microbial Community and Predicted Metagenome Function in CD-1 Mice. *NPJ Sci. Food* **2017**, *1*, 8. [CrossRef]
13. Chang, S.S.; Lu, W.Y.W.; Park, S.H.; Kang, D.H. Control of Foodborne Pathogens on Ready-To-Eat Roast Beef Slurry by Epsilon-polylysine. *Int. J. Food Microbiol.* **2010**, *141*, 236–241. [CrossRef] [PubMed]
14. Wang, L.; Zhang, C.Y.; Zhang, J.H.; Rao, Z.M.; Xu, X.M.; Mao, Z.G.; Chen, X.S. Epsilon-poly-L-lysine: Recent Advances in Biomanufacturing and Applications. *Front. Bioeng. Biotechnol.* **2021**, *9*, 748976. [CrossRef]
15. Li, R.; Sun, S.; Wang, H.J.; Wang, K.T.; Yu, H.; Zhou, Z.; Xin, P.Y.; Chu, J.F.; Zhao, T.M.; Wang, H.Z.; et al. FIS1 Encodes a GA2-oxidase that Regulates Fruit Firmness in Tomato. *Nat. Commun.* **2020**, *11*, 5844. [CrossRef]
16. Ogawa, Y.; Tokunaga, E.; Kobayashi, O.; Hirai, K.; Shibata, N. Current Contributions of Organofluorine Compounds to the Agrochemical Industry. *iScience* **2020**, *23*, 101467. [CrossRef] [PubMed]
17. Liu, T.; Chen, M.L.; Fu, J.T.; Sun, Y.; Lu, C.; Quan, G.L.; Pan, X.; Wu, C.B. Recent Advances in Microneedles-Mediated Transdermal Delivery of Protein and Peptide Drugs. *Acta Pharm. Sin. B* **2021**, *11*, 2326–2343. [CrossRef] [PubMed]
18. Jiang, X.; Zeng, Y.N.; Zhang, W.; Wang, C.Y.; Li, W. Advances in Microneedle Patches for Long-Acting Contraception. *Acta Mater. Med.* **2023**, *2*, 1–8. [CrossRef]
19. Feng, X.Q.; Xian, D.Y.; Fu, J.T.; Luo, R.; Wang, W.H.; Zheng, Y.W.; He, Q.; Ouyang, Z.; Fang, S.B.; Zhang, W.C.; et al. Four-Armed Host-Defense Peptidomimetics-Augmented Vanadium Carbide MXene-Based Microneedle Array for Efficient Photo-Excited Bacteria-Killing. *Chem. Eng. J.* **2023**, *456*, 141121. [CrossRef]
20. Du, H.Y.; Liu, P.; Zhu, J.J.; Lan, J.J.; Li, Y.; Zhang, L.B.; Zhu, J.T.; Tao, J. Hyaluronic Acid-Based Dissolving Microneedle Patch Loaded with Methotrexate for Improved Treatment of Psoriasis. *ACS Appl. Mater. Interfaces* **2019**, *11*, 43588–43598. [CrossRef]
21. Qu, F.; Geng, R.; Liu, Y.J.; Zhu, J.T. Advanced Nanocarrier- and Microneedle-Based Transdermal Drug Delivery Strategies for Skin Diseases Treatment. *Theranostics* **2022**, *12*, 3372–3406. [CrossRef]
22. Jamaledin, R.; Yiu, C.K.Y.; Zare, E.N.; Niu, L.N.; Vecchione, R.; Chen, G.J.; Gu, Z.; Tay, F.R.; Makvandi, P. Advances in Antimicrobial Microneedle Patches for Combating Infections. *Adv. Mater.* **2020**, *32*, 2002129. [CrossRef] [PubMed]
23. Zheng, M.J.; Zhang, Y.Y.; Hu, T.L.; Xu, C.J. A Skin Patch Integrating Swellable Microneedles and Electrochemical Test Strips for Glucose and Alcohol Measurement in Skin Interstitial Fluid. *Bioeng. Transl. Med.* **2022**, 10413. [CrossRef]
24. He, R.Y.; Liu, H.; Fang, T.S.; Niu, Y.; Zhang, H.Q.; Han, F.; Gao, B.; Li, F.; Xu, F. A Colorimetric Dermal Tattoo Biosensor Fabricated by Microneedle Patch for Multiplexed Detection of Health-Related Biomarkers. *Adv. Sci.* **2021**, *8*, 2103030. [CrossRef] [PubMed]
25. Xu, N.; Zhang, M.Y.; Xu, W.X.; Ling, G.X.; Yu, J.; Zhang, P. Swellable PVA/PVP Hydrogel Microneedle Patches for the Extraction of Interstitial Skin Fluid toward Minimally Invasive Monitoring of Blood Glucose Level. *Analyst* **2022**, *147*, 1478–1491. [CrossRef]
26. Creighton, R.L.; Woodrow, K.A. Microneedle-Mediated Vaccine Delivery to the Oral Mucosa. *Adv. Healthcare Mater.* **2019**, *8*, 1801180. [CrossRef]
27. Kolluru, C.; Gomaa, Y.; Prausnitz, M.R. Development of a Thermostable Microneedle Patch for Polio Vaccination. *Drug Deliv. Transl. Res.* **2019**, *9*, 192–203. [CrossRef]

28. Arya, J.M.; Dewitt, K.; Scott-Garrard, M.; Chiang, Y.W.; Prausnitz, M.R. Rabies Vaccination in Dogs Using a Dissolving Microneedle Patch. *J. Control. Release* **2016**, *239*, 19–26. [CrossRef]
29. Kim, K.S.; Kim, H.; Park, Y.; Kong, W.H.; Lee, S.W.; Kwok, S.J.J.; Hahn, S.K.; Yun, S.H. Noninvasive Transdermal Vaccination Using Hyaluronan Nanocarriers and Laser Adjuvant. *Adv. Funct. Mater.* **2016**, *26*, 2512–2522. [CrossRef]
30. Nishikawa, M. Molecular Mass Control Using Polyanionic Cyclodextrin Derivatives for the Epsilon-poly-L-lysine Biosynthesis by Streptomyces. *Enzyme Microb. Technol.* **2009**, *45*, 295–298. [CrossRef]
31. Li, Y.Q.; Han, Q.; Feng, J.L.; Tian, W.L.; Mo, H.Z. Antibacterial Characteristics and Mechanisms of ϵ-psilon-poly-lysine against *Escherichia coli* and *Staphylococcus aureus*. *Food Control* **2014**, *43*, 22–27. [CrossRef]
32. Panda, A.; Shettar, A.; Sharma, P.K.; Repka, M.A.; Murthy, S.N. Development of Lysozyme Loaded Microneedles for Dermal Applications. *Int. J. Pharm.* **2021**, *593*, 120104. [CrossRef] [PubMed]
33. Zheng, Y.W.; Yan, Y.L.; Lin, L.M.; He, Q.; Hu, H.H.; Luo, R.; Xian, D.Y.; Wu, J.Y.; Shi, Y.; Zeng, F.P.; et al. Titanium Carbide MXene-based Hybrid Hydrogel for Chemo-Photothermal Combinational Treatment of Localized Bacterial Infection. *Acta Biomater.* **2022**, *142*, 113–123. [CrossRef] [PubMed]
34. Sun, M.H.; Zhu, C.N.; Long, J.Y.; Lu, C.; Pan, X.; Wu, C.B. PLGA Microsphere-Based Composite Hydrogel for Dual Delivery of Ciprofloxacin and Ginsenoside Rh2 to Treat *Staphylococcus aureus*-Induced Skin Infections. *Drug Deliv.* **2020**, *27*, 632–641. [CrossRef] [PubMed]
35. Wei, S.H.; Quan, G.L.; Lu, C.; Pan, X.; Wu, C.B. Dissolving Microneedles Integrated with pH-Responsive Micelles Containing AIEgen with Ultra-Photostability for Enhancing Melanoma Photothermal Therapy. *Biomater. Sci.* **2020**, *8*, 5739–5750. [CrossRef] [PubMed]
36. Park, J.H.; Allen, M.G.; Prausnitz, M.R. Biodegradable polymer microneedles: Fabrication, Mechanics and Transdermal Drug Delivery. *J. Control. Release* **2005**, *104*, 51–66. [CrossRef] [PubMed]
37. Dillon, C.; Hughes, H.; O'Reilly, N.J.; McLoughlin, P. Formulation and Characterisation of Dissolving Microneedles for the Transdermal Delivery of Therapeutic Peptides. *Int. J. Pharm.* **2017**, *526*, 125–136. [CrossRef]
38. Lin, L.M.; Chi, J.Y.; Yan, Y.L.; Luo, R.; Feng, X.Q.; Zheng, Y.W.; Xian, D.Y.; Li, X.; Quan, G.L.; Liu, D.J.; et al. Membrane-Disruptive Peptides/Peptidomimetics-Based Therapeutics: Promising Systems to Combat Bacteria and Cancer in the Drug-Resistant Era. *Acta Pharm. Sin. B* **2021**, *11*, 2609–2644. [CrossRef]
39. Shi, Y.; Feng, X.Q.; Lin, L.M.; Wang, J.; Chi, J.Y.; Wu, B.Y.; Zhou, G.L.; Yu, F.Y.; Xu, Q.; Liu, D.J.; et al. Virus-Inspired Surface-Nanoengineered Antimicrobial Liposome: A Potential System to Simultaneously Achieve High Activity and Selectivity. *Bioact. Mater.* **2021**, *6*, 3207–3217. [CrossRef]
40. Zhang, D.H.; Shi, C.; Cong, Z.H.; Chen, Q.; Bi, Y.F.; Zhang, J.Y.; Ma, K.Q.; Liu, S.Q.; Gu, J.W.; Chen, M.Z.; et al. Microbial Metabolite Inspired β-Peptide Polymers Displaying Potent and Selective Antifungal Activity. *Adv. Sci.* **2022**, *9*, 2104871. [CrossRef]
41. Liu, K.W.; Zhou, X.J.; Fu, M.R. Inhibiting Effects of Epsilon-poly-lysine (ε-PL) on *Pencillium digitatum* and Its Involved Mechanism. *Postharvest Biol. Technol.* **2017**, *123*, 94–101. [CrossRef]
42. Li, H.; He, C.; Li, G.J.; Zhang, Z.Q.; Li, B.Q.; Tian, S.P. The modes of action of epsilon-polylysine (ε-PL) against *Botrytis cinerea* in jujube fruit. *Postharvest Biol. Technol.* **2019**, *147*, 1–9. [CrossRef]
43. Li, S.F.; Zhang, L.H.; Liu, M.P.; Wang, X.Y.; Zhao, G.Y.; Zong, W. Effect of Poly-ε-lysine Incorporated into Alginate-Based Edible Coatings on Microbial and Physicochemical Properties of Fresh-Cut Kiwifruit. *Postharvest Biol. Technol.* **2017**, *134*, 114–121. [CrossRef]
44. Dou, Y.; Routledge, M.N.; Gong, Y.Y.; Godana, E.A.; Dhanasekaran, S.; Yang, Q.Y.; Zhang, X.Y.; Zhang, H.Y. Efficacy of epsilon-poly-L-lysine inhibition of postharvest blue mold in apples and potential mechanisms. *Postharvest Biol. Technol.* **2021**, *171*, 111346. [CrossRef]
45. Sun, G.Z.; Yang, Q.C.; Zhang, A.C.; Guo, J.; Liu, X.J.; Wang, Y.; Ma, Q. Synergistic Effect of the Combined Bio-Fungicides ε-poly-L-lysine and Chitooligosaccharide in Controlling Grey Mould (*Botrytis cinerea*) in Tomatoes. *Int. J. Food Microbiol.* **2018**, *276*, 46–53. [CrossRef]
46. Shu, C.; Cui, K.B.; Li, Q.Q.; Cao, J.K.; Jiang, W.B. Epsilon-poly-L-lysine (ε-PL) Exhibits Multifaceted Antifungal Mechanisms of Action that Control Postharvest Alternaria Rot. *Int. J. Food Microbiol.* **2021**, *348*, 109224. [CrossRef]
47. Guo, W.T.; Wang, X.C.; Yang, C.Y.; Huang, R.K.; Wang, H.; Zhao, Y.J. Microfluidic 3D Printing Polyhydroxyalkanoates-Based Bionicskin for Wound Healing. *Mater. Futures* **2022**, *1*, 015401. [CrossRef]

MDPI AG
Grosspeteranlage 5
4052 Basel
Switzerland
Tel.: +41 61 683 77 34

*Pharmaceutics* Editorial Office
E-mail: pharmaceutics@mdpi.com
www.mdpi.com/journal/pharmaceutics

www.ingramcontent.com/pod-product-compliance
Lightning Source LLC
Chambersburg PA
CBHW061627210926
51850CB00009B/2462